Practice Development in Nursing

Practice Development in Nursing

Edited by

Brendan McCormack, DPhil (Oxon.),
BSc (Hons.) Nursing, PGCEA, RGN, RMN

Professor of Nursing Research, University of Ulster and
Director of Nursing Research and Practice Development,
Royal Hospitals Trust,
Belfast

Kim Manley, PhD, MN, BA, RGN,
Dip N (Lond.), RCNT, PGCEA, CBE

Head of Practice Development,
RCN Institute London & Visiting Professor,
Bournemouth University

Robert Garbett, RN, BN, MSc

Research Fellow,
University of Ulster and Royal Hospitals Trust,
Belfast

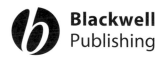
Blackwell
Publishing

© 2004 by Blackwell Publishing Ltd

Editorial offices:
Blackwell Publishing Ltd, 9600 Garsington Road, Oxford OX4 2DQ, UK
  Tel: +44 (0)1865 776868
Blackwell Publishing Inc., 350 Main Street, Malden, MA 02148-5020, USA
  Tel: +1 781 388 8250
Blackwell Publishing Asia Pty Ltd, 550 Swanston Street, Carlton, Victoria 3053,
  Australia
  Tel: +61 (0)3 8359 1011

The right of the Authors to be identified as the Authors of this Work has been asserted
in accordance with the Copyright, Designs and Patents Act 1988.

All rights reserved. No part of this publication may be reproduced, stored in a
retrieval system, or transmitted, in any form or by any means, electronic, mechanical,
photocopying, recording or otherwise, except as permitted by the UK Copyright,
Designs and Patents Act 1988, without the prior permission of the publisher.

First published 2004 by Blackwell Publishing Ltd

Library of Congress Cataloging-in-Publication Data
Practice development in nursing / edited by Brendan McCormack, Kim Manley, and
Robert Garbett. – 1st ed.
      p. ; cm.
Includes bibliographical references and index.
  ISBN 1-4051-1038-4 (pbk : alk. paper)
  1. Nursing.   2. Nurse practitioners.
  [DNLM: 1. Nursing–methods. WY 100 P8945 2004]   I. McCormack, Brendan.
  II. Manley, Kim, RCNT.   III. Garbett, Robert.

    RT82.8.P73   2004
    610.73–dc22
                                                                              2003022155

ISBN 1-4051-1038-4

A catalogue record for this title is available from the British Library

Set in 10.5 on 12.5 pt Palatino
by SNP Best-set Typesetter Ltd., Hong Kong
Printed and bound in India
by Replika Press Pvt. Ltd, Kundli 131028

The publisher's policy is to use permanent paper from mills that operate a sustainable
forestry policy, and which has been manufactured from pulp processed using acid-free
and elementary chlorine-free practices. Furthermore, the publisher ensures that the
text paper and cover board used have met acceptable environmental accreditation
standards.

For further information on Blackwell Publishing, visit our website:
www.blackwellpublishing.com

Contents

Contents

Foreword

I must begin by congratulating all those involved in bringing to health care practice this excellent and long overdue book. The value of its contents is so wide ranging, I could never do it justice in such few words, but hope to highlight why it is a key text for all those engaged in practice development activities.

The nature of practice development is becoming clearer. Indeed, there are now a growing number of texts that focus on change and development for health care practice. However, I believe this book offers something more. It provides an opportunity for individuals to really examine how practice development is approached and the impact it has on individuals, teams and organisations.

The need for the expertise and experience that is found in this book has never been greater. No one could fail to miss the tremendous drive for change led by nurses and other health professionals or the vast investment in leadership development, as part of a commitment to improve and transform the health care services. But, I hesitate to say everything in the garden is rosy! This is not to suggest that the commitment to development and improvement is wrong. Rather, I suggest there are two key inter-linked problems. First, too much responsibility for achieving improvement is placed on individuals changing, rather than organisations. Second, some of the approaches adopted to achieve improvement are ineffective and may have unintended negative consequences for practitioners.

As clearly expounded throughout this book, change and development is complex and workplace culture and context is messy. Change and development challenges us, not simply because we are being asked to change but because it questions fundamentally 'how am I working?' and 'am I providing the best care?'. However open to scrutiny we consider ourselves, challenge can be hard and, without support, can be damaging and demoralising. This is why understanding and using a systematic approach to practice development is more desirable and appropriate than some of the traditional approaches to change still adopted in practice. Furthermore, whilst McCormack, Manley and Garbett emphasise that there is no 'one' right way to develop practice, it is clear that using emancipatory processes within practice development offer greater opportunity for enabling practitioners towards action, transformation and achieving significant cultural change; as well as nurturing and supporting practitioners currently struggling to cope with the demands to improve practice.

The core value within the book towards 'increasing effectiveness in patient-centred care' is particularly evident in the chapters contained in Part 2. These provide detailed, 'warts and all' accounts of practice development. Within each chapter there will be something with which everyone can relate, with activities ranging from strategic trust-wide developments to those addressing to specific clinical needs.

In the 21st Century it is paramount that we:

- examine and understand how we work towards development and improvement of our health care services,
- enable and support practitioners involved in development and change,
- make evaluation integral to our work,
- ensure that the care we provide for patients and service users really is as effective as they tell us they want it to be.

It has been a real privilege to have first sight of this readable book. Over several years I have become familiar with the work of the editors and some of the contributors and this has been a wonderful opportunity to take a fresh look at the work. Whilst each chapter can stand alone, it is fantastic to see them together, intertwined and making this a 'must have' for everyone involved in practice development.

Finally, I note the editors hope to expand, challenge or adjust your understanding of practice development and I am certain it will do at least two if not all three.

Theresa Shaw
Chief Executive
Foundation of Nursing Studies
www.fons.org

February 2004

Contributors

Paddie Blaney (RGN, BSc (Hons) LLM) is Chief Executive of the Northern Ireland Practice and Education Council (NIPEC) for Nursing and Midwifery which was established in April 2002. NIPEC's aim is to improve the quality of health and care by supporting the practice, education and performance of nurses and midwives. NIPEC are particularly keen to support a variety of learning activities. It aims to support all development of practice activities undertaken with the aim of improving patient/client care including audit, benchmarking, care pathways, quality improvement initiatives, practice development and so on. NIPEC appreciates the psychological aspects of undertaking such activities, and seeks to formalise them by building ownership and commitment in order to achieve sustained and meaningful improvements.

Christine Caldwell (MSc, BSc (Hons) PGDip Ed, RSCN, RGN, Senior Nurse/Modern Matron, Great Ormond Street Hospital for Children NHS Trust, Great Ormond Street) works in specialist acute paediatric medicine (immunology/infectious diseases). She is interested in the modern matron role and how it can be implemented to ensure design/redesign, delivery and evaluation of quality patient- and family-centred services and the essentials of care through empowering and transformational leadership approaches. She has a particular interest in practice development in child health through facilitated work-based learning, postgraduate education for children's nurses within a multi-professional context and enabling children and their families to be involved in service/practice development.

Charlotte L. Clarke (PhD, MSc, PGCE, BA, RN, Professor of Nursing Practice Development Research and Head of Nursing, Midwifery and Allied Health Professions Research & Development Unit, School of Health, Community & Education Studies, University of Northumbria, Newcastle) has a clinical and research background working with older people and people with dementia. More recently, her work has embraced a wide range of research projects concerning: people with enduring and chronic health needs; professional and organisational learning. She uses a wide range of socio-critical research methodologies to develop mechanisms for research to be a means of advancing healthcare practices and services based on (re) conceptualisations of the healthcare needs of a service user group.

Patric Devitt (RSCN, BA (Hons), MSc, Senior Lecturer, Salford Centre for Nursing, Midwifery & Collaborative Research, Child Health Directorate, School of Nursing, University of Salford, Manchester) undertook a degree in politics and philosophy before becoming a nurse; this earlier work still influences his practice. He trained originally as an RGN, before undertaking an educational programme to become a nurse of sick children. His clinical experience has primarily been in the field of paediatric oncology, and in particular, bone marrow transplantation. Since moving into Higher Education, he has developed an interest in clinical supervision and translating education into practice. He is an active member of the North West Developing Practice Network and the Research in Child Health (RiCH) Network.

Jan Dewing (RGN, BSc, MN, Dip Nurse Ed, RNT, Dip Nurse, PhD candidate, Consultant Nurse, Milton Keynes PCT and General NHS Trust, Associate Fellow Practice Development Royal College of Nursing) has worked in a range of practice education and research posts all around practice development. Her interests lie in working with others to transform the culture of care and experience of care for older people and practitioners. She has a specialist interest in understanding how older people can live with and through a dementia.

Jill Down (BA (Hons), RN, Lead Practice Development Nurse, Associate Fellow Practice Development Royal College of Nursing Institute) is an experienced practice developer with a background in critical care. Her work focused on facilitating staff to develop person-centred care using guided reflection in a technically dominated speciality. Currently she leads a team of practice developers in a Medical unit. She works with staff in clinical areas to improve care in a practical way based in the realities of everyday practice using evidence generated from their patients and staff. Her particular interests are in developing the skills of staff to influence change using critical companionship and action learning.

Contributors

Rob Garbett (MSc, BN, RN, Research Fellow, Royal Hospitals Trust, and University of Ulster) has been involved with practice development since the early 1990s when he was involved with the King's Fund Nursing Development Unit programme. Since then, he has worked in publishing, research, education and as a facilitator of practice development. His current role involves working with clinical teams in an older people's rehabilitation unit through which he is developing work on models of gathering feedback from patients and on the nurse's role in rehabilitation.

Kate Gerrish (PhD, MSc, BNurs, RGN, RM, NDN Cert, Professor of Nursing Practice Development, School of Nursing & Midwifery, University of Sheffield/Northern General Hospital) holds a joint post as Professor of Nursing Practice Development at the School of Nursing and Midwifery, University of Sheffield and Sheffield Teaching Hospitals NHS Trust. She is actively involved in the strategic development of nursing research and practice development with the Trust and has undertaken research on the process of facilitating practice development and evidence-based practice. Her other main research interests concern the interface of ethnicity and culture with nursing, with a particular focus on the interplay of policy and practice, and the organisation and delivery of community nursing services. Kate has published widely and is co-editor of the journal *Ethnicity and Health*.

Mary Golden (RGN, Cert Behavioural Psychotherapy, Cert Further & Higher Education, MSc Sociology and Social Policy, PG Dip in Cognitive Therapy, Nurse Consultant, Adult Mental Health (Cognitive Behaviour Therapy) and Honorary Visiting Lecturer, School of Nursing & Midwifery, Southampton University) became interested in Cognitive Behaviour Therapy in the early 1980s, shortly after qualifying as a nurse, and has continued to develop this throughout her career. Having worked in a variety of posts across service and education, her current Nurse Consultant role provides an opportunity to work across clinical practice, education and service/organisational development. She is particularly interested in issues relating to service user involvement in setting up, delivering and evaluating services and is actively involved in the development of the local Acute Care Forum to achieve full participation from service users and carers. Other current interests relate to the integration of mental health services within a Primary Care Trust, establishing Clinical Supervision as a key professional development activity and the establishment of new roles in mental health.

Ann Jackson (RMN BA (Hons) MA, Senior Fellow Practice Development, Mental Health Programme, Royal College of Nursing Institute, Radcliffe Infirmary, Oxford) clinical background is in acute in-patient care in Leicester. After several years of clinical nursing, she pursued other roles in nursing research and practice development. She has worked with the RCN Institute Mental Health Programme since 1995, and on a permanent basis since 1998 as Senior Practice Development Fellow. Ann's main role is as external facilitator of a range of project-based practice development initiatives within NHS Trusts and the independent sector. These projects provide the opportunity for teams of clinically-based nurses to systematically and reflectively examine their practice, implement research and a range of evidence in their practice and formally evaluate the impact of the change. The primary aim is to enable mental health nurses to achieve their individual and team aspirations of improving practice within a complex, and often compromised, nursing context. Academic interests include feminist and anti-oppressive research methodologies/practice and women's mental health and will be reflected in future PhD work.

Brendan McCormack (DPhil (Oxon.), BSc (Hons), PGCEA, RMN, RGN, Professor/Director of Nursing Research & Practice Development, University of Ulster/Royal Group of Hospitals) current role gives him responsibility for research, practice development and clinical education in the Royal Hospitals, Belfast. In addition, Brendan leads the co-ordination of many research and practice development projects nationally and internationally. He is National Co-ordinator of the UK Developing Practice Network and co-leader of an International Practice Development Collaborative with the Royal College of Nursing and Monash University, Australia. He has written extensively on the subject of practice development and practitioner research.

Kim Manley (PhD, MN, BA, RGN, Dip N (London) RCNT, PGCEA, CBE, Head of Practice Development and Visiting Professor, Bournemouth University) interests are in the processes of cultural change and the attributes of an effective culture, one that is person-centred, evidence-based and realises shared governance principles, now termed a 'transformational culture'. Additionally, her interests lie with emancipatory action research, Fourth Generation Evaluation, practitioner-researcher approaches and practice expertise. Kim's research on the consultant nurse was influential in guiding government policy. In 2000, she was awarded the CBE for quality patient services. Kim is editor of *Nursing in Critical Care* and is in demand internationally as a consultant in practice development.

Emma Pritchard (RMN, BSc (Hons), Consultant Nurse, Admiral Nursing Central and North West London Mental Health NHS Trust for Dementia, Associate Fellow Practice Development RCN) has worked with older persons with mental health needs, particularly those with a dementia, and their supporters and carers, throughout her nursing career. This has been in both practice and service development roles. Her interests include working with multidisciplinary teams to develop person-centred care, and finding credible and genuine ways to work inclusively with service users. She has published articles and reviews and enjoys facilitating and presenting.

Jo Rycroft-Malone (RGN BSc (Hons) MSc, PhD, Senior Research & Development Fellow, Royal College of Nursing Institute, Radcliffe Infirmary, Oxford) has, over the last eight years worked on a number of different research projects which have explored nursing practice and patient care issues. Her main research interests include getting evidence and knowledge into practice, clinical effectiveness, facilitating change and patient participation. Most recently Jo has been working with RCN colleagues on a research project known as the PARIHS project (Promoting Action on Research Implementation in Health Services). PARIHS is developing and testing a framework for implementing evidence-based practice and forms the basis of her contribution to this book.

Kate Sanders (BSc (Hons) Nursing Studies, RGN, HV Cert, Nurse Advisor (Practice Development), The Foundation of Nursing Studies, London). Prior to joining the Foundation, Kate worked in a variety of acute settings before completing her health visitor training in 1990. Over the last ten years, Kate has been actively involved in practice development initiatives in the field of health visiting and community nursing and most recently worked as a nurse prescribing facilitator. In her current post, Kate has a key role in supporting nurses, health visitors and midwives to develop practice and improve care by implementing and disseminating evidence.

Jane Stokes (RN, MA, Cert Ed DPSN, Senior Nurse Practice Development, Associate Fellow Practice Development, Royal College of Nursing Institute) works as the senior nurse practice development at Barts and the London NHS Trust. She is on secondment for three years from City University where she holds the post of Lecturer in Adult Nursing with a speciality in Sexual Health. Jane is committed to the principles of shared governance, effective interdisciplinary team working and ensuring the highest standards of patient-centred care, across all services. Passionate about all the fundamental aspects of patient care, Jane is the Trust co-facilitator for Essence of Care and a member of the Clinical Governance Committee.

Steve Tee (RMN Dip Professional Studies in Nursing – Community Mental Health BA (Hons) MA, PGCE, Head of Mental Health Care Division, School of Nursing & Midwifery, University of Southampton) is currently working within a university academic department and has an honorary appointment with West Hampshire Mental Health and Learning Disability (NHS) Trust. As head of the mental health care division he has operational responsibility for the design, delivery and evaluation of a range of pre-registration, undergraduate and postgraduate education programmes in mental healthcare. He is the programme leader for Cognitive Behavioural Approaches in Mental Health, Psychosocial Interventions and Clinical Leadership and also leads a number of practice development initiatives that include the assessment and management of risk, developing new roles in mental health and service user and carer involvement. These projects reflect his research interests which are primarily concerned with the development of partnerships in mental health and extending knowledge of the involvement of service users in clinical decision-making.

Angie Titchen (DPhil (Oxon.), MSc, MCSP, Senior Research & Practice Development Fellow, Royal College of Nursing Institute, London, Joint Clinical Chair, Knowledge Centre for Evidence-based Practice, Fontys University of Professional Education, Eindhoven, The Netherlands) work is rooted in clinical experience as a physiotherapist and in her high challenge/high support facilitation of healthcare professionals who are developing evidence-based, person-centred care. Her research interests focus around the facilitation of transformational, learning cultures, experiential learning and the use of creative arts in research, practice development and education. She has published widely in these areas. She loves to walk, dance, paint and practise Tai Chi.

Val Wilson (RN, RSCN, BAEdSt, MN (Research), Lecturer & PhD candidate, School of Nursing, Faculty of Medicine, Nursing &

Health Science, Monash University, Australia) is currently studying for her PhD full-time. She is researching in the area of implementation and evaluation of Practice Development strategies. She is a paediatric nurse and continues to practice clinically.

Acknowledgements

Our thanks must go to all the contributors to this book who have shared their practice development knowledge and expertise in a generous way. Their collective experiences provide inspiration to others to take on what might seem to be insurmountable challenges.

We would also like to thank the many inspirational and transformational leaders we have worked with over the years who have mentored, coached and supported us in developing our understandings of practice development.

We would like to acknowledge the participants and facilitators in practice development programmes across the UK and Ireland who have bravely worked and persevered with implementing the evidence base of practice development within individual teams and across whole organisations seeking to improve patients' experiences and outcomes. A particular mention should be made of the staff of Chelsea & Westminster intensive care and nursing development unit who contributed as co-researchers to our understanding of the attributes of an effective culture and the processes of cultural change towards a person-centred, evidence-based and effective culture.

We would like to thank our employing organisations (The Royal College of Nursing Institute; The School of Nursing, University of Ulster and the Royal Hospitals Trust, Belfast) for their commitment to creating and supporting innovative ways of working that are amenable to sustaining a vision of critical inquiry in practice.

A special thanks must go to Gillian Graham, Royal Hospitals, Belfast, for the management of the writing team, ensuring deadlines were met and for formatting the many drafts of the manuscript. Her patience, expertise and collaborative working is greatly appreciated and the book could not have happened without her support.

Finally, thank you to our families and friends who supported us in this project and endured our 'burning of the midnight oil' in order to complete the work. Thank you.

Part 1

1. *Introduction*

Brendan McCormack, Kim Manley and
Rob Garbett

This book is concerned with the development of practice. In particular, it strives to develop our understanding of that commonly used term – 'practice development'. To contemplate the idea of clarifying a concept such as practice development when it is inherently nebulous and complex may appear to be a somewhat naïve project. However, we hope that by the time you have read this book, you will at least have had your understanding of practice development expanded, challenged or adjusted.

The intention of this book is to provide a resource that locates practice development in an integrated theoretical and practice context. We specifically set out to provide a resource that has an explicit theoretical foundation, as currently such a resource does not exist. However, we have endeavoured to apply this theory to practice throughout. Whilst the second part of the book is explicitly practice focused, wherever appropriate, we offer examples of the theory being used in practice. It is also important to state what this book is *not* concerned with, i.e. practice development roles. In the United Kingdom, a lot of practice development literature in nursing has been concerned with the roles of 'practice development nurses' as a defined role in organisations. Whilst some of the chapters in this book are written by people who undertake such roles, we do not intend to debate the merits or otherwise of these roles. Developing practice (with its explicit focus on improving patients' experiences of healthcare) is everyone's responsibility. Whilst many nurses occupy formal practice development roles, we believe that all nurses need to be aware of the processes of practice development and to embrace a commitment to continuous improvement.

The book is presented in two parts. Part 1 focuses on making explicit key concepts of practice development. In addition we hope that the book provides a resource that helps make sense of practice development in all its guises and this is the focus of Part 2 of the book. In these chapters, practice developers describe their experiences of developing practice from a variety of perspectives. We do not intend to provide the definitive guide to practice development, but in being consistent with the idea of critical social science (a philosophy that guides the theoretical framework of this book) we hope to add to the increasing body of knowledge that is contributing to greater clarity about practice development. But why bother?

Besides the fact that the term 'practice development' is so poorly understood, there is a constant emphasis on the development of practice in contemporary healthcare. This is not surprising given the language of modernisation, effectiveness, collaboration, accountability and user involvement that underpins healthcare policy. Developing practice is one component of organisational change, clinical governance, clinical effectiveness and patient-centredness that are currently widespread. This movement is not accidental. Instead, it represents a concerted effort by government to personalise healthcare services whilst simultaneously ensuring efficiency and effectiveness.

Over the last 25 years the formation of caring helping relationships has increasingly become central to the practice of healthcare. Growing dissatisfaction with the limitations of task focused approaches to care underlay the upsurge in interests in approaches to organising practices oriented to the needs of the individual patient. In the United Kingdom, reforms within the National Health Service (NHS), for example the emphasis placed on professional accountability, have provided a more favourable environment for 'person-centred' care characterised by a carer–patient relationship built on continuity of, and accountability for, care. This environment has resulted in greater emphasis on accountability for care through clinical effectiveness and evidence-based approaches to practice. In the next chapter, we explore the concept of practice development in the context of these changes. The chapter reports the findings of an empirical research study with practice developers and practitioners from across the United Kingdom that set out to analyse the concept of practice development. We believe that this chapter begins a process of concept clarification and a foundation from which practice development programmes can be established as well as a basis for ongoing research and development work.

From the concept analysis of practice development, we will argue that in a modernised healthcare environment with an emphasis on consistent and continuous development, staff involved with developing practice need to operate within a framework that recognises the complexity of bringing about change successfully within large organisations. For the most part it could be argued that practice development in healthcare falls short of such an ideal. In Chapter 3 we challenge the dominant focus on what we have called 'technical practice development' in healthcare. This approach is task based and project specific with little chance of achieving sustainable change in the culture of practice. An alternative approach will be proposed – 'emancipatory practice development' seeks to foster increased effectiveness in patient-centred care through the development of the context and cultures of practice.

A major focus of development in emancipatory practice development is on the transformation of healthcare environments to ensure that they cater for the needs of individual patients. This entails an environment in which practitioners can make and act on decisions about the care given to individuals without being stifled by hierarchical models of reporting and approval. This in turn entails the development of knowledge, skills and decision-making and a context that allows such attributes to be applied with regard to the safety and dignity of individuals. Given the radical nature of the transformation being tackled, the methods employed to bring about such a change need to be carefully chosen. The dominant theme in the literature is for a model of change that develops the attitudes and skills necessary for a more person-centred form of care through the process of change itself. However, changing attitudes and developing skills are not activities that should exist in isolation of carefully planned and systematically evaluated cultural change. In Chapter 4, an in-depth case study of cultural change is presented. Drawing on her empirical research, Kim Manley articulates the complexity of bringing about such change and the challenges and rewards associated with achieving sustainability. This chapter aims to make explicit the need for a systematic emancipatory approach to practice development that is empowering of individuals. Demonstrating the processes and outcomes of this work is complex and challenging. In Chapter 5 we take up this challenge and describe a variety of approaches to evaluating practice developments. A variety of models and frameworks will be presented as well as providing a 'practice development evaluation checklist'.

Part of the process of achieving sustained change is the use of evidence in practice. Emancipatory practice development uses and generates evidence and so Chapter 6 will explore a particular framework (the PARIHS framework) that can be used to explore the use of evidence in practice. The framework is consistent with many of the values of emancipatory practice development and thus is useful for exploring types of evidence, analysing the context of practice and considering the place of facilitation in bringing about sustainable change.

Practice development as a term, has frequently been linked with the notion of professional development and indeed sometimes the terms are used interchangeably. In fact, the concept analysis presented in Chapter 2 argues that professional and practice development is a continuous process, but that the starting point for practice development is the service user and for professional development it is the service provider (i.e. the practitioner). The notion that practice development is concerned with 'increased effectiveness in patient-centred care' is the core value underpinning this book. Nonetheless, the acquisition of skills and knowledge is a central part of practice development, both as a means of moving practice on and as a means of securing support from those who are being expected to change. In Chapter 7, Angie Titchen describes an approach to practice development that fully integrates these two perspectives through the creative process of 'critical companionship'. The processes and outcomes of critical companionship are articulated through exemplars from ongoing research and development work. However, whilst many readers will find the idea of critical companionship an attractive option for continuous development of practice and practitioner expertise, for others, more established education models dominate their work. This is often a reason given by academics with 'heavy' teaching loads for not engaging in practice development work. In Chapter 9, Chris Caldwell demonstrates how an education process itself can be translated into significant development work. Chris shows how *learning about* practice was translated to *learning from* practice and the achievement of sustained developments. This chapter highlights the importance of being open to opportunities to develop practice that may arise surreptitiously.

The increasing emphasis placed on meeting the needs of users is talked about at length in current healthcare agendas, with it increasingly being seen as pivotal to the development of practice within the strategies of organisations. Indeed, the involvement of service users in development work is a key driver in current healthcare policy and practice. Throughout this book there is a focus on involving service users. However, two chapters in particular focus on this issue from differing practice perspectives. In Chapter 8, Jan Dewing and Emma Pritchard explore ways of involving older people with dementia in practice development work. Their approach to this highlights the complexity of such work whilst at the same time emphasising the benefits of using creative approaches to user involvement. Their account is both moving and confirming and challenges all of us to reconsider some of our established assumptions about user involvement. Mary Golden and Steve Tee offer a different perspective, focusing on the involvement of users of mental health services in the planning of practice changes. They outline the steps and stages taken in the involvement of service users and the challenges experienced along the way. Their chapter provides a useful starting point for planning service user involvement and as such should be seen as a 'work in progress'.

Making a difference to the experience of people receiving healthcare is likely to require work at a range of organisational levels involving people working within a number of disciplines. The conceptualisation of practice development occurring at different levels is echoed in many of the chapters in this book, with both explicit and implicit references to the necessity to work at a number of levels to transform the context of care. Defining practice development as being concerned with the development of the care delivered to patients implies that the practice of all those involved with providing that care should be scrutinised. The necessity to think beyond the practice of one group and consider the developmental needs of all those whose work has an impact on patient care was evident in the shift from talk of nursing development units (NDU) to practice development units (PDU) although arguably this shift did not capture popular imagination to the same extent. Practice development that is concerned with the development of one group alone (practising nurses) may be limited in its potential for success. In the concept analysis of practice development we address the contributions of NDUs and PDUs to contemporary understandings of practice development. Whilst recognising that NDUs continue to be formally supported and accredited in the United Kingdom and Australia, we do not intend to critically engage with an analysis of the contributions of NDUs as a defined 'unit'. The conceptualisation of practice development in this book underpinned by critical social science directs us towards a position where *all* clinical settings have the potential to be a development unit (without the formal title) when certain developmental characteristics are in place. The notion of 'transforming the culture and context of care' should be seen as inclusive of all practice that affects patient outcomes. In Chapter 12, Jill Down captures an organisational approach to practice development that is multidisciplinary focused and centred upon the idea of developing organisational characteristics that enable a continuous culture of development to be sustained. Jill and colleagues adopted a strategically focused organisational approach to the organisation of the practice development activities and have been able to demonstrate clear benefits from doing so. The chapter should be a useful resource to all organisations considering the development of strategic frameworks for practice development.

Being strategic is essential to the sustaining of developments in practice. However, being strategic also affords opportunities to proactively adopt developmental approaches to policy drivers. In Chapter 11, Jane Stokes demonstrates how important it is to do this and the impact that this has on both the overall quality of care and the culture of the organisation. Important lessons were learned along the way and these should serve as lessons to us all in planning organisation-wide development initiatives. Jane's chapter complements Jill Down's work as they are both examples of practice development at an organisational level. However, they complement each other because one is focused on a generic organisational framework (Jill Down), whilst the other (Jane Stokes) utilises a specific policy driver (essence of care standards) to create an organisation-wide practice development strategy.

Practice development is associated with questioning the way in which practice takes place in order to attempt some change or improvement. Although the notion of practice development is often only associated with 'innovation', it is also as concerned with ensuring that everyday practice is effective and addressing shortfalls where they occur. It's about working with people to develop their ideas, creating cultures for change and enabling and empowering people to help them develop what they think is important. In Chapter 13, Kate Sanders provides a clear example of how 'ordinary practice' becomes the focus for systematic practice development. Kate utilises a number of conceptual frameworks to shape the questioning of practice and to systematically plan and co-ordinate the development work. This chapter further illustrates an emancipatory approach being taken to a project that set out as a 'technical change' and thus demonstrates the importance of being systematic and rigorous in practice development.

Practice development is often conceptualised as a continuous 'journey' that is complex and multifaceted. This book, too, represents a journey from concept clarification to operational utilisation and further refinement. Part of this process of refinement is the contributions of 'commentators'. Each chapter in Part 2 of this book comes with a commentary from an expert in the particular field of practice. Each of the commentaries provides a critique of the focus of the chapter in the context of wider health and social care policy.

In doing this, we hope to engage in ongoing debate, development and further refinement of issues raised. The commentaries are not a critique of the specifics of the chapter, as (consistent with practice development) each of these chapters represents a unique journey of discovery. Instead the critique helps to locate the chapter in a wider context and expand the depth of understanding of key drivers for change in healthcare.

This refinement is consolidated in the final chapter of the book, where we bring together all the key concepts addressed in previous chapters. In doing this we aim to challenge the conceptual basis of practice development and its stated characteristics and attributes. In light of the journeys presented in individual chapters, the characteristics and attributes of practice development and practice developers will be further explored and brought to a 'holding place' in this journey. The journey is never ending, however, and we hope that overall, this book adds to the body of existing knowledge, is a useful resource for practice developers and provides a basis for ongoing development and discovery.

2. *A Concept Analysis of Practice Development*

Robert Garbett and Brendan McCormack

Introduction

The term 'practice development' is widely, if inconsistently, used in British nursing. It has been used to address a broad range of educational (McKenna, 1995), research (Rolfe, 1996) and audit (NHSE, 1996) activity. The literature emphasises the use of research evidence in practice (for example, Kitson *et al.*, 1996; Jackson *et al.*, 1999a; McCormack *et al.*, 1999). Nonetheless, there appears to be little consensus as to what practice development involves. This lack of clarity means that the increasing numbers of nurses whose work involves practice development have difficulty in focusing their efforts. At a strategic level it can be difficult to differentiate practice development work from other initiatives intended to promote change within healthcare organisations, for example, those associated with quality initiatives and the implementation of evidence-based practice. As part of its contribution to British nursing, midwifery and health visiting the RCN Institute (RCNI) identified the need to develop greater conceptual clarity in this area to inform and develop theoretical frameworks for practice development to assist the RCNI with its work with care providers and to influence practice development within healthcare organisations. The work reported here, carried out between mid 1999 and early 2000 (work that has appeared subsequently has not therefore been included in this discussion, see also Garbett and McCormack, 2002), was designed and conducted with this purpose in mind. It built on previous work carried out within the RCNI (Kitson *et al.*, 1996; Jackson *et al.*, 1999 a & b; McCormack *et al.*, 1999). The aims of the study were to:

10

- Clarify the concept of practice development
- Describe the foci of practice development work and the approaches used
- Develop a framework to help clarify and focus the work for those who engage in practice development work

This chapter will briefly outline the study's methodology and the major findings.

Study design

Concept analysis is now a widely used approach to research and theory building in nursing. Two main schools of thought around concept analysis have been described: the entity and dispositional views (Rodgers, 1994). In entity views (of which Walker & Avant's (1995) work is an example) the emphasis is on developing an abstract meaning of a concept such as practice development, independent of its context. It is an approach that has been used in the measurement of nursing workloads and practices with the result that nursing practice is reduced to a list of measurable and observable tasks. The staged approach that they advocate has been described as static and objective, and inadequate in representing the dynamic and evolving nature of concepts (Morse, 1995). By contrast, the dispositional view is concerned with how concepts are used in the 'real world' rather than with their objective reality. The aim of analysis in this approach is to capture the meanings of the concepts as articulated by those who use them. To this end, Morse (1995) argues for an approach that uses qualitative research methods to analyse both primary and secondary sources of data about the concept. The concept may be present in different forms within such data according to the context in which the concept is used. To help identify these features Morse draws on Bolton's (1977) 'rules of relation':

- Concepts are expressions of the organisation of a person's experience.
- All concepts are the results of particular experiences becoming general.
- Concepts are the results of the co-ordination of their key elements.
- A concept is used to organise events and therefore must be capable of being applied to fresh instances.
- Concepts are formed by the application of a rule to a particular situation and the results of that application.

(Bolton, 1977)

Box 2.1   Approaches to concept analysis (Morse, 1995).

Concept development

Where a concept is considered to be nebulous and ill-defined after a review of the literature.

Concept delineation

Where two concepts are merged and used interchangeably so that the concepts can be differentiated.

Concept comparison

Where an area is not well understood and various approaches have been proposed to fill the gap, for example competing concepts of inference, intuition and insight.

Concept clarification

Where there appears to be a large amount of rich data but where the concept is nevertheless confused and murky and requires careful unpicking. Morse gives the example of caring as a concept requiring clarification.

Concept correction

Where a concept that is well described does not fit with clinical experience or observation and needs to be adjusted.

Concept identification

Where, after qualitative investigation, a category of data remains that is not described or accounted for in the literature. This data may then need to be developed as a new concept.

Analysing the ways in which the term practice development is used helped us to understand the extent to which it can be considered a concept. The rules also helped us to clarify which of Morse's six approaches (see Box 2.1) should be adopted as a framework for concept analysis.

First, the term practice development can be seen as an expression of an individual's experience, it is used as a job title and as a descriptor of activities within the workplace. However, it has been noted that the application of the term as a job descriptor is diverse and context specific with practice development staff working at a range of organisational levels (Mallett *et al.*, 1997). The increasingly common use of the term over a period of nearly 20 years suggests that practice development is an example of a particular experience becoming general. Although once again, on preliminary examination the applications made of the term seem diverse. The growing number of publications on the subject suggests attempts at co-ordinating key elements of the concept, although, as will be discussed, different emphases are present within the literature. For example, both in the literature and in practice there are those who consider practice development as being concerned primarily with the continuing education of practitioners (for example, Hanily, 1995). While another school of thought is that practice development is concerned primarily with development of patient care, a project in which education plays a necessary but supportive role (see for example, Binnie & Titchen, 1999). The use of the concept to organise events is apparent in the application of practice development as a related term to new ideas that have emerged since it was first used; for example evidence-based practice and clinical effectiveness. But the final rule arguably presents some difficulty given the fact that, as will be expanded upon below, there seems to be a lack of clear description around practice development that allows its differentiation from related concepts such as quality improvement.

Based on this preliminary analysis we argued that practice development required a concept development approach to its analysis. Concept development involves three stages: identifying attributes, verifying attributes and identifying manifestations of the concept. Morse (1995) describes the initial stage as one of identifying abstract attributes indicative of the concept in question contained within an exemplar of the concept. Previous work summarised conceptual, theoretical and experiential positions on practice development and was used as the basis for initially identifying attributes (McCormack *et al.*, 1999). However, this process was extended by a more deliberate and systematic approach to examination of the literature. The first stage of the study therefore took the form of a literature analysis including 177 items of published material (published between the early 1980s and 1999) (see Table 2.1).

Colleagues critiquing our work have pointed out that some literature that would have been relevant, notably that emerging from the various nursing development unit and practice development programmes of the 1980s and early 1990s were partially absent from the literature identified. After long deliberation we maintained that we wanted to examine the use of the specific term 'practice

Table 2.1 A summary of references found through searching the literature.

Database	References found (duplicated references in brackets)	References duplicated in Cinahl & Medline	References duplicated in Cinahl, Medline & RCN	References rejected from lists generated by databases (duplicated references in brackets)	References retained (duplicated references in brackets)	References incorporated in addition to searches	Total number of references examined
CINAHL	173			79	94		
Medline	46	26		16 (6)	30 (20)		
RCN (journal articles)	137		8	98 (1)	39 (7)		
RCN (books)	56			44	12		
Totals (including duplicates)	412 (34)			238 (7)	175 (27)		
Totals (excluding duplicates)	378			231	148	29	177

Source Data taken from Garbett & McCormack, 2002

development' and since this was not necessarily present in the literature identified in our searches we chose to omit it from this analysis. That is not to ignore the importance of the work. However, our position does reinforce the developmental nature of knowledge in this area.

The second stage, attribute verification, involves looking for the use of concepts identified in the first stage and is seen as a deductive process. In the study described here a selective search of the literature was employed together with focus group interviews involving nursing staff involved with practice development. Twelve focus group interviews were conducted involving 60 participants whose work involved them in practice development activities. This group encompassed people whose work included a range of clinical practice, education, and managerial activities, but all those involved in the study had a practice development remit within their roles.

The final stage, identifying manifestations of the concept, involves refining the components of the concept and describing how they are manifest in different groups and settings. Telephone interviews and focus group interviews were used as a means of exploring the meaning and dimensions of key ideas arising from the study. In addition to the focus groups 25 telephone interviews were carried out with practitioners who had been involved in practice development activity. Fuller details of methodology and method can be found in other publications arising from the project (Garbett & McCormack, 2001; Garbett & McCormack, 2002; McCormack & Garbett, 2003).

The findings

At the time of the study there had been few attempts at defining the purpose of practice development in the literature. From the work that had attempted some form of definition five main themes can be described:

- an emphasis on improving patient care;
- an emphasis on transforming the contexts and cultures in which nursing care takes place;
- the importance of employing a systematic approach to effect changes in practice;
- the continuous nature of practice development activity;
- the nature of the facilitation required for change to take place.

These themes will be used to organise the discussion that follows.

Practice development: the purposes

Increasing effectiveness in patient-centred care

The impetus to improve practice can be attributed to a range of influences:

- Government policy provides context for directions in the development of practice. For example, *Health of the Nation* (Department of Health, 1992) and *Vision for the Future* (Department of Health, 1993) underpinned NDU work in Graham's (1996) report.
- Professional conduct (Draper, 1996; McMahon, 1998).
- Accountability, for example Kitson (1997) argues that nurses need to determine the structure and function of nursing care in order both to demonstrate its value and to be able to influence and shape the broader issues in changes to the delivery of healthcare. Especially in the light of the increasing emphasis on practitioners of all healthcare disciplines providing evidence of the quality of care they provide contained within policy documents such as *A First Class Service* (Department of Health, 1998).

However, practitioners' and practice developers' perceptions varied from those in the literature. Practitioners interviewed described practice development as closely related to personal study and development. For nearly half (12 out of 25) the term was synonymous with training and attendance on courses. For most of the remainder continuing education was closely linked to improvements in practice that were driven by perceptions of what patients needed.

By contrast, practice developers tended to hold the view that the needs of individual practitioners were important but, in contrast with most of the practitioners that were interviewed, they emphasised that it was services as a whole that constituted the focus of practice development. One participant described the relationship as, 'not just about one individual person and their skills. . . . I think it's about practice at a macro level much more than a micro level' (focus group [FG] 9).[1] In all the focus group interviews it was apparent that the development of individuals was integral to, but also subordinate to, the development of patient care.

Transforming contexts and cultures of care

The emphasis on the development of patient care means that the nature of the transformation and the ways in which it takes place must be considered. Two main trends can be described. The first addresses the direction that changes in care should take and concerns the drive towards patient-centred models of care provision. The second reflects beliefs about the ways in which lasting change can best be brought about.

The increasing importance of the individual patient within healthcare is founded on both an emergent professional ideology within healthcare professions and on a 'customer care' model of consumerism that has developed within the NHS as a whole. Both trends challenge a historically dominant mode of organisation within the NHS characterised by bureaucratic and hierarchical organisation that resulted in task orientation and a lack of responsiveness to the needs of individuals. A major focus of development therefore is on the transformation of healthcare environments to ensure that they cater for the needs of individual patients (for example, Vaughan & Edwards, 1995; Graham, 1996; Kitson *et al.*, 1996; Ward *et al.*, 1998; Binnie & Titchen, 1999; Jackson *et al.*, 1999a). This demands an environment in which practitioners can make and act on decisions about the care given to individuals without being stifled by hierarchical models of reporting and approval. This in turn entails the development of knowledge, skills and decision-making in individuals and cultures that allow such attributes to be applied with regard to the safety and dignity of individual clients (McCormack *et al.*, 1999). Given the radical nature of the transformation being tackled the methods employed to effect such a change need to be carefully chosen. The dominant theme in the literature is for a model of change that achieves the attitudes and skills necessary for a more patient-centred form of care through the process of change itself.

Telephone interviewees recognised that practice development involved the development of an environment in which changes to practice were the norm and could be accepted. The practice developers also emphasised the need to get people to think differently about their work, for example talking about supporting risk-taking, valuing practitioners' ideas and 'realising capabilities that have been crushed' by bureaucratic models of organisation. For them practice development was associated with questioning the way in which practice takes place in order to attempt some change or improvement. Similarly, the policy agenda within the NHS clearly had an impact on perceptions of practice development issues. Practice developers talked about the need to incorporate national agendas within their work and acknowledged that at times these constituted 'top-down' drivers of change. Some practice developers talked of the necessity of adopting a multidisciplinary focus in their work. For some, the notion of unidisciplinary practice development for nursing alone was seen as 'obsolescent'. The necessity to think beyond the practice of one group and consider the developmental needs of all those whose work has an impact on patient care was evident in the shift from talk of nursing development units to practice development units (Williams *et al.*, 1993).

Practice development that is concerned with the development of one group alone may be limited in its potential for success. Making a difference to the experience of people receiving healthcare is likely to require work at a range of organisational levels involving people working within a number of disciplines (McCormack & Wright, 1999). The conceptualisation of practice development occurring at different levels (individual, team and organisational) was echoed by respondents in both sets of interviews. Within the focus groups in particular there were both explicit and implicit references to the necessity of working at a number of levels to transform the context of care.

What practice developers do

The literature identified a range of activities undertaken by practitioners concerned with practice development working in both internal (for example as practice development nurses within a Trust) and external (for example, working as an outside facilitator) roles. Based on a content analysis of the literature a list of 71 activities was drawn up. These terms were compared and analysed to arrive at six descriptive categories:

- Promoting and facilitating change
- Translation and communication
- Responding to external influences
- Education
- Facilitating the implementation of research into practice
- Audit and quality (including the development of policies and guidelines)

The practice developers who took part in the focus group interviews also described a wide range of activities. However, mapping them onto the headings above suggested a more discrete scope of activity. For the most part they talked about being concerned with promoting and facilitating change and communicating about the work with which they were involved. They talked relatively little about work concerned with getting research into practice or audit/quality activities. For this reason, only the first four activities listed above are discussed below.

Promoting and facilitating change

Activities within this category were concerned with supporting, raising awareness and helping create a culture to support change based on the perceptions and needs of the staff themselves. In two published accounts reference was also made to the needs of service users (Weir & Kendrick, 1994; Jackson *et al.*, 1999a), a theme that also emerged in two of the focus group interviews.

The dominant model of change agency within the literature is that which reflects normative re-educative theory (Bennis, 1991). Thus Weir (1995) talks of a change agent role with 'a professional rather than a managerial focus' that is concerned with the process of change as a means to develop individuals' skills and confidence as much as it is with achieving an outcome for its own sake. Weir positions the practice development nurse's role as 'working with and on behalf of directorate/clinical managers'. This is not a view that is shared by all practice developers. Within the focus group interviews quite polarised views were present concerning alignment with managerial structures. On the one hand there was the view that being involved with both practice development and management represented a conflict of interest and that the two functions should be distinct, each providing a foil for the other. On the other hand there was the view that practice development was integral to the 'business' of healthcare and so was part and parcel of the management and improvement of services.

The bulk of activities described by the practice developers in the focus group interviews involved aspects of promoting and facilitating change in practice. These could be focused on individuals, on teams or on larger groupings within the organisation. Two groups described the importance of working clinically. This could be used as a means of modelling practice (particularly where senior nurse posts incorporated practice development responsibilities). It was also described as a means of building credibility and as a 'bargaining' strategy, trading hours in practice in return for clinicians participating in an activity contributing to practice development such as searching literature or completing data collection tools. Working clinically could also be focused on working with individuals as a mentor or supporter, providing feedback and guidance on performance.

Another aspect of working with individuals was that termed 'counselling' by some practice developers. This involved being approached by clinicians about concerns that they had about issues in their clinical practice. Participants in the focus groups variously described this as being used as a 'sounding board', or as 'troubleshooting'. This area of activity, and that of working alongside individuals providing support and mentorship, could be said to overlap with the clinical leadership usually associated with ward leaders. However, there was also a sense of its relevance to practice development as a means of understanding clinician's perspectives on the issues that concerned them most. Participants acknowledged this duplication but argued that it was something looked for by clinicians and therefore as a valuable component of the practice development role: 'Practitioners use PD nurses as a "neutral ear", as sounding boards for problems they might have as a source of advice and support that is not shaped by line management. This is why practice development roles could not be combined with managerial roles' (FG8/419).

Practice developers talked about their role as gatekeepers to resources such as study days and courses, expertise within and outside their organisation and generating ideas for funding. Practice developers talked about a range of facilitative approaches including getting practitioners to think creatively and more broadly and helping them put their ideas into action. But they also saw their facilitative roles as being required at a variety of organisational levels. Participants frequently referred to their roles as being situated 'in the middle', working with practitioners but also with managers at middle and senior levels and increasingly with representatives from other healthcare occupations and user groups.

Translation and communication

People working in practice development roles both within and outside organisations describe a number of activities that suggest they are situated between top management and the practice area. Some activities could be characterised as top-down, such as interpreting and disseminating policy documents and information from an organisational level (Mallett *et al.*, 1997), while others, such as generating interest for project work at local level amongst managers and opinion leaders in the broader organisation (Marsh & MacAlpine, 1995; Abi-Aad & Raine, 1998; Jackson *et al.*, 1999b), can be seen as 'bottom-up'. These latter activities are seen as important components in planning for successful change. Additionally, activities around working on various representative groups and networking with other organisations are also described (Thomas & Ingham, 1995; Mallett *et al.*, 1997; Jeffries & Timms, 1998).

This area of work was talked about within the focus group interviews. As has been mentioned elsewhere practice development staff frequently see themselves as 'in between' managerial structures and clinical practice. Being seen and being known is therefore important to their work. Strategies employed ranged from 'being seen to go round and meet people' and 'smiling at everybody' to more formal activities such as representing nursing as a group in meetings with managers, members of other professions and service users.

Responding to external influences

There are external influences that, to a greater or lesser extent, have shaped the kind of work undertaken by healthcare organisations. Those who responded to Mallett and colleagues' survey (1997) indicated that external directions, such as policy documents, professional documents such as *The Scope of Professional Practice* (UKCC, 1992) and shifts in interprofessional boundaries, such as those resulting from the attempted reduction of the hours worked by junior doctors, all influenced how their role developed.

In the UK, the influence of government policy has been evident in the development of named nursing within *The Patients' Charter* (Department of Health, 1991), supervisory arrangements (Department of Health, 1993), and the development of dissemination networks (Department of Health, 1993) to name but three. However, as has been discussed above, the relationship between policy and the development of practice need not be one characterised by reaction to policy. The ideas and aspirations may be contained and developed within the policy environment, and indeed the policy environment can be used as a means for advancing practitioners' own agendas (Graham, 1996).

Practice developers acknowledged that policy documents could have a powerful effect on setting agendas for development work. Most of the groups saw responding to and working with policy agendas as part of their work. Clinical governance (Department of Health, 1998) particularly seemed to feature in their working lives. However, involvement with work derived from policy initiatives seemed to be characterised as something of a double-edged sword. On the one hand the fact that such initiatives were perceived as being imposed could be problematic. However, they were also seen as an opportunity to bring disciplines together to address issues.

Education

Descriptions vary as to the extent to which educational activities form part of practice development. The term professional development is frequently used to describe post-basic education which may or may not be associated with systematic changes in practice, and is a term that is frequently confused with practice development.

Mallett *et al.* (1997) suggest that the terms professional and practice development are distinct but can easily be taken as synonymous. They argue that professional development refers to the skills of the individual practitioner while practice development is about creating the conditions wherein such skills and knowledge can be applied. The confusion of the two terms is apparent in accounts such as that by Hanily (1995). Under the title of practice development Hanily describes the development and implementation of a training strategy based on the assumption that care would improve as a consequence of the provision of new knowledge. Others (for example, Kitson *et al.*, 1996) have challenged this view as over simplistic, neglecting as it does the complexity of change.

There seemed to be fewer references to educational activities by practice development staff interviewed within the focus groups than in the literature. In one focus group where practice developers were joint appointees between a university and a hospital there was a clear educational component to their work both in terms of a commitment to particular courses and in helping clinicians relate learning on taught courses to the practice area. But in most of the interviews, educational activities played little part in participants' discussions of what they did.

By contrast practitioners in the telephone interviews were more likely to say that practice development is closely related to personal study and development rather than changes to a service as a whole (Garbett & McCormack, 2001). In a number of organisations the term practice development was associated with groups who were concerned with both the co-ordination and provision of training as well as supporting change in the workplace. Where practice development nurses were present in clinical areas at least part of their perceived value was seen to be encouraging and supporting practitioners to follow particular courses of study. However, education was not necessarily seen as separate from practice and orientated only to the needs of the individual practitioner.

The attributes of practice development

Systematic approaches to practice development

The dominant trend in the literature is towards the presentation of practice development as systematic in nature. Nonetheless, it is most usually presented as a systematic process that engages with the 'messy' and context specific nature of the environment in which practice development takes place (Kitson *et al.*, 1996; Cutcliffe *et al.*, 1998; McCormack, 1998).

The importance of systematic approaches to practice development has been identified at a policy level, for example *Vision for the Future* (Department of Health, 1993) lays out the need for clearly specified goals, end points or outcomes and mechanisms for dissemination. Kitson & Currie (1996) surveyed practice development activity in one regional health authority. But while acknowledging that informal approaches to developing practice were not without value, they observed that without a systematic approach being taken there was little prospect of deriving a satisfactory account of how practice development might best be approached.

There are two broad areas of reasoning behind the idea that practice development should be systematic. The first concerns the argument that a systematic approach is more likely to result in a successful outcome (Marsh & MacAlpine, 1995; Vaughan, 1996). The second concerns the credibility of a systematic approach to external observers (Luker, 1997; McMahon, 1998) and the establishment of cost-effectiveness (McCormack *et al.*, 1999). However, interviewees differed in their opinion about the necessity of a systematic approach to practice development. For some, change in practice that occurs within a systematic framework was precisely the quality that differentiates practice development from the kind of attention to improving care that should be part and parcel of clinical practice. The logic of using systematic approaches was clearly articulated in the interviews. It seemed that practice developers accepted the adoption of systematic approaches as a strategy to meet particular aims (funding or other forms of support) and so as a kind of necessary evil. However, there were two main areas of discomfort with this position, one concerning the extent to which there was a mismatch between the demands of systematic approaches and the 'real world' of practice and another to do with the practical difficulties inherent in systematic approaches. In most of the interviews the view was expressed that formalising practice development had the effect of alienating practitioners. Moreover, formal structures were seen as stifling creativity and innovation. In most of the interviews there was a concern that systematic approaches to practice development risked missing out on work that the participants valued. Some participants described their work as reactive to issues that were arising in practice, hence the perception that formal approaches could hamper their ability to be responsive to the needs of practitioners. It was accepted that an approach to practice development that used no systematic frameworks to gather information could not account for progress. However, systematic approaches were also seen as inadequate at capturing all progress within practice development. For example, one participant claimed that, 'traditional systematic approaches do not capture all that happens, do not capture shifts in people's horizons when they are part of practice change' (FG8/318). Moreover, for some participants the lack of organisational strategic commitment to planning for practice development as well as limited or non-existent structures to support such work set up difficulties for systematic work.

Action research has been suggested by some as a potential means of addressing these problems (Manley, 1997; Binnie & Titchen, 1999). Its distinguishing features of being situational, collaborative, participatory and self-evaluative mean that it matches features of an inductive approach to bringing about change. In addition, its status as a research approach means that knowledge and theory generation also form part of its purpose, although some authors have suggested that practice development is no less concerned with contributing to the body of knowledge (Kitson *et al.*, 1996; Cutcliffe *et al.*, 1998). Value is placed on the potential of action research to address the gap between theory, research, and practice. This argument is supported by the experiences of nurses involved in NDUs who found that having researchers working alongside the clinical team had the effect of demystifying the research process (Vaughan & Edwards, 1995). Some argue that action research is congruent with the current emphasis on evidence-based practice, involving as it does the cycle of activity attributed to evidence-based practice of formulating clinical questions, finding solutions through appraisal of available evidence and implementing the findings (Nichols *et al.*, 1997; Wallis, 1998). However, the collaborative nature of the approach suggests that the outcome of such an endeavour is more likely to be successful in bringing about change (Nichols *et al.*, 1997; Wallis, 1998).

Facilitation

Kitson *et al.* (1998), considering the conditions that need to be in place in order for evidence-based practice to take place, suggest that the context of implementation and its facilitation are of equal importance to the nature of the evidence itself. They argue that features such as a lack of investment in individuals, poor leadership and lack of performance feedback indicate a context that is unlikely to foster successful change. By contrast, an environment in which people are valued, have a clear sense of what they are doing and have feedback about their performance is a more fertile environment for progress. Such an environment is more likely to be developed where individuals experience respect for their opinions and ideas, feel involved in changes to their work and where development reflects their individual needs than in a setting where such qualities are absent (Kitson & Currie, 1996; Manley, 1997; Binnie & Titchen, 1999).

In the telephone interviews practitioners talked about the facilitation that they experienced from staff in practice development posts in terms of receiving advice and support. One informant described how colleagues in practice development roles helped her over 'brick walls', that is to say they helped her deal with unfamiliar situations such as chairing meetings or finding information. Practice developers talked about a range of facilitative approaches including getting practitioners to think creatively and more broadly and helping them put their ideas into action. But they also saw their facilitative roles as being required at a variety of organisational levels.

Facilitation is associated with more than the successful completion of a single project. Rather it is an activity concerned with the development of individuals in groups in such a way as to help foster greater initiative, self-reliance, and motivation (McCormack, 1998; Titchen, 2001). The investment is therefore twofold; it is not only about achieving the goals of a particular project but also about equipping people with experience, skills and knowledge (Thomas & Ingham, 1995). Facilitation requires a range of qualities, skills, and abilities. For example, Titchen (2001), describing her critical companionship model, identifies openness, supportiveness, approachability, reliability, self-confidence, and the ability to think laterally and non-judgementally (see Chapter 7).

The consequences of practice development

Given the diversity of material identified it would be inappropriate and misleading to examine the consequences of practice development in terms of an aggregation of those outcomes contained in published work. However, on the basis of the discussion above we would venture that a number of consequences can be extrapolated from the purposes and attributes identified. These can be seen as concerned as much with process outcomes as they are with more traditional forms of clinical outcome. The evaluation of practice development is dealt with in greater depth in Chapter 5. The primary purpose of practice development is increased effectiveness in patient-centred care. Logically it can therefore be argued that a consequence of practice development should be to reflect that purpose. It is, however, difficult to always clearly demonstrate that impact.

As has been discussed above the pace and scope of change within the health service implies the need to help practitioners become more flexible and responsive in order to be able to adapt to and assimilate change. These are the intended outcomes of the approaches talked about in the practice development literature, by practice developers themselves and attested to by practitioners themselves. Adopting a facilitative approach also implies helping practitioners identify organisational factors that impede progress and helping them find ways around such barriers. Another consequence of practice development can therefore be construed as being concerned with promoting awareness of the impact of organisations on practice. The consequences associated with practice development are clearly congruent with the clinical governance agenda within the NHS at the present time. Clinical governance has been established to address the need to identify the activities involved in delivering high quality care to patients (Department of Health, 1998). Within clinical governance the need to recognise the contextual and situated nature of such a project is acknowledged. Practice development approaches explicitly address these concerns.

Qualities and skills

Relatively little attention had been paid in the literature to the qualities and skills required of people working in practice development roles when the study was carried out. Until recently the published information was derived largely from two personal accounts of roles (Thomas & Ingham, 1995; Weir, 1995) and from conclusions drawn by Kitson *et al.* (1996). Qualities described include those of being pragmatic, being a risk taker and being able to accept criticism. On a more ideological level, Weir (1995) and Thomas & Ingham (1995) emphasise the importance of a belief in the worth and value of people. In addition Weir describes the importance of gaining satisfaction from seeing others succeed. Thomas & Ingham (1995) describe the necessity of drive, commitment and patience. (Later in-depth work that looks in detail at roles and activities can be found in Chapters 4 and 7.)

Speaking to practice developers working in a range of different organisations and posts resulted in a rich description of the kinds of qualities and skills considered necessary to help develop practice. The qualities that they described bear close resemblance to those associated with the notion of transformational leadership (Manley, 1997; Antrobus & Kitson, 1999). They are concerned with helping colleagues develop ideas; helping them articulate and think

26

through ideas, but also feeding in knowledge, information and skills where necessary. There is consistent reference to understanding the experience of colleagues in practice as a starting point for changing it. Another strong dimension of these discussions was the tenacity and energy required to push ideas forward. The qualities that were talked about in the focus groups can be grouped under the following headings:

- *Affective* Practice developers talked about the need for energy, enthusiasm, optimism and having a positive outlook but also spoke with feeling about the need to be 'thick-skinned', to have a sense of humour, and to demonstrate honesty and patience.
- *Having vision* Participants talked about the importance of having vision to underpin practice development work.
- *Being motivated* This seemed to be an important component of participants' understanding of their work. They talked about the energy, enthusiasm and tenacity necessary to help change take place. One described it in graphic terms, 'you need this fire in your bum that keeps driving you' (FG5/140). Maintaining focus and impetus takes place against a backdrop of competing priorities that need to be understood and worked with.
- *Being empathic* The importance of understanding the impact that practice development has on people's lives was emphasised in three of the focus groups. Interviewees talked about the importance of being aware of the pressures acting on the professional and personal lives of practitioners and the impact that these might have on the kinds of activities for which they can spare the time and energy.
- *Experiential* The importance of being able to process and learn from experience was prized by many of the participants in the focus groups. Formal supervision relationships were seen as offering an opportunity to review and refine skills as well as maintaining a focus on the job at hand. Participants spoke about the importance of being aware of their limitations and their strengths.

Skills described in the literature range from clinical practice-based knowledge and skills (Kitson *et al.*, 1996) to those associated with bringing about change such as; leadership (Knight, 1994; Jackson *et al.*, 1999a); research skills; change management skills; problem solving skills; organisational analysis techniques; skilled interpersonal behaviour; decision-making skills; and facilitation skills (Kitson *et al.*, 1996). Marsh & MacAlpine (1995) have described similar themes in relation to the skills, knowledge and behaviour demonstrated by nurse managers in Nursing Development Units (Vaughan & Edwards, 1995).

Practice developers also talked about a range of skills that they considered central to their work. Once again these can be categorised under a range of headings:

- *Cognitive* Participants talked about the need for creativity, not only in problem solving, but also in finding novel ways of communicating with others about their work and, crucially, in finding resources. Similarly, they talked about the need to recognise and seize opportunities by thinking laterally. They also talked about the central importance of 'being curious'.
- *Political* Practice developers frequently describe themselves as 'being in the middle', they have access to various levels of managerial activity while also working with practitioners. While this could be a source of tension, it was also seen as one unique feature of a practice development role. Political awareness was seen as an important skill that underpinned the successful promotion of ideas and initiatives.
- *Communicative* Effectiveness at a political level was associated with an ability to communicate well. This involved being skilled at acquiring and processing information as well as being able to put arguments across. Practice developers talked about the need to 'tune in' to what they were being told by practitioners. By contrast practitioners who did not feel that they were listened to saw little value in the work of practice development staff.
- *Facilitative* There was a clear emphasis amongst practice developers that their work consisted of helping others articulate, develop and action their ideas.
- *Clinical* The emphasis placed on the importance of clinical skills varied between focus groups. In one area practice development activity was seen as being part of senior clinical roles. Consequently clinical skill was seen as an integral part of the work. By contrast, other practice developers who did not have a clinical component to their role talked of the need to 'market' their facilitative skills but recognised the importance placed on clinical credibility by practitioners. For some practitioners clinical skills were seen as being of central importance. Practitioners in the telephone interviews, who talked about the practice developer's skills as a practitioner, made the most enthusiastic accounts of practice development. While the perceived lack of clinical acumen was seen as affecting the ability of practice developers to do their job.

A definition of practice development

Arguably, the most comprehensive definition of practice development available when this study was conducted was provided by McCormack *et al.* (1999) who stated that:

> Practice development is a continuous process of improvement towards increased effectiveness in person centred care, through the enabling of nurses and healthcare teams to transform the culture and context of care. It is enabled and supported by facilitators committed to a systematic, rigorous continuous process of emancipatory change.
>
> (p. 256)

The definition above was largely supported by the concept analysis; however, we would argue that any definition needs to also reflect the importance of professional development for individuals involved in practice development. We would also argue that the importance of user perspectives should also be incorporated. We would therefore suggest the following revised definition:

> Practice development is a continuous process of improvement towards increased effectiveness in patient centred care. This is brought about by helping healthcare teams to develop their knowledge and skills and to transform the culture and context of care. It is enabled and supported by facilitators committed to systematic, rigorous continuous processes of emancipatory change that reflect the perspectives of service users.
>
> (Garbett & McCormack, 2002: 88)

Conclusion

In this chapter we have provided a summary of a study that was set up to clarify the concept of practice development. A concept development (Morse, 1995) was used to guide an analysis of the literature and data gathered from practice developers and practitioners who had been part of practice development activity. From this data a framework was developed that outlines the purposes, attributes and consequences of practice development. The purposes of practice development are described as increasing the effectiveness of patient care through the transformation of the context and culture of care. The attributes of practice development are that it is a continuous, systematic activity characterised by the facilitation of practitioners to help them explore and develop their own practice.

The intended consequences of practice development are, therefore, an improvement in patients' experience and the development of the capacity to explore and enhance practice amongst individuals, teams and organisations. The study described here has contributed to much of the subsequent (and parallel) work reported in the following chapters.

Note

1 Where direct quotes from the data are used the following terminology is used: FG denotes a focus group (FG1 is focus group 1 and so on), Int. refers to a telephone interview and similarly will be followed by a number; subsequent numbers (for example FG9/101 refers to the number given to the extract).

References

Abi-Aad, G. & Raine, R. (1998) Planning for action. *Nursing Times*, **94**(25), 46.

Antrobus, S. & Kitson, A. (1999) Nursing leadership: influencing and shaping health policy and nursing practice. *Journal of Advanced Nursing*, **29**(3), 746–53.

Bennis, W.G. (1991) Organisational development: its nature and perspectives. In: *Organisational Behaviour* (ed. A. Huczysnki). Prentice-Hall, London.

Binnie, A. & Titchen, A. (1999) *Freedom to Practice: The Development of Patient-centred Nursing*. Butterworth-Heinemann, Oxford.

Bolton, N. (1977) *Concept Formation*. Pergamon Press, Oxford.

Cutcliffe, J., Jackson, A., Ward, M., Cannon, B. & Titchen, A. (1998) Practice development in mental health nursing. *Mental Health Practice*, **2**(4), 27–31.

Department of Health (1991) *The Patients' Charter*. HMSO, London.

Department of Health (1992) *Health of the Nation*. HMSO, London.

Department of Health (1993) *A Vision for the Future*. HMSO, London.

Department of Health (1998) *A First Class Service: Quality in the New NHS*. The Stationery Office, London, p. 86.

Draper, J. (1996) Nursing development units: an opportunity for evaluation. *Journal of Advanced Nursing*, **23**(2), 267–71.

Dunning, M. (1998) Securing change: lessons from the PACE programme. *Nursing Times*, **94**(34), 51–2.

Garbett, R. & McCormack, B. (2001) The experience of practice development: an exploratory telephone interview study. *Journal of Clinical Nursing*, **10**(1), 94–102.

Garbett, R. & McCormack, B. (2002) A concept analysis of practice development. *Nursing Times Research*, **7**(2), 87–100.

References

Graham, I. (1996) A presentation of a conceptual framework and its use in the definition of nursing development within a number of nursing development units. *Journal of Advanced Nursing*, **23**(2), 260–6.

Hanily, F. (1995) A new approach to practice development in mental health. *Nursing Times*, **91**(21), 34–5.

Jackson, A., Ward, M., Cutcliffe, J., Titchen, A. & Cannon, B. (1999a) Practice development in mental health nursing: part 2. *Mental Health Practice*, **2**(5), 20–5.

Jackson, A., Cutcliffe, J., Ward, M., Titchen, A. & Cannon, B. (1999b) Practice development in mental health nursing: part 3. *Mental Health Practice*, **2**(7), 24–30.

Jeffries, E. & Timms, L. (1998) Sharing good practice: developing network forums. *Nursing Standard*, **12**(50), 33–4.

Kitson, A. (1997) Developing excellence in nursing practice and care. *Nursing Standard*, **12**(2), 33–7.

Kitson, A., Ahmed, L.B., Harvey, G., Seers, K. & Thompson, D.R. (1996) From research to practice: one organisational model for promoting research-based practice. *Journal of Advanced Nursing*, **23**(3), 430–40.

Kitson, A. & Currie, L. (1996) Clinical practice development and research activities in four district health authorities. *Journal of Clinical Nursing*, **5**(1), 41–51.

Kitson, A., Harvey, G. & McCormack, B. (1998) Enabling the implementation of evidence-based practice: a conceptual framework. *Quality in Healthcare*, **7**(3), 149–58.

Knight, S. (1994) An organisational approach . . . a model for nursing practice development. *Nursing Times*, **90**(41), 33–5.

Luker, K. (1997) Research and the configuration of nursing services. *Journal of Clinical Nursing*, **6**, 259–67.

McCormack, B. (1998) Caring for older people – enabling change in the 'messy' world of practice. *Journal of Nursing Care*, (Winter), 8–11.

McCormack, B. & Garbett, R. (2003) The characteristics, qualities and skills of practice developers. *Journal of Clinical Nursing*, **12**(3), 317–25.

McCormack, B. & Wright, J. (1999) Achieving dignified care through practice development – a systematic approach. *Nursing Times Research*, **4**(5), 340–52.

McCormack, B., Manley, K., Kitson, A., Titchen, A. & Harvey, G. (1999) Towards practice development – a vision in reality or a reality without vision? *Journal of Nursing Management*, **7**(2), 255–64.

McKenna, H. (1995) Skill mix substitutions and quality of care: an exploration of assumptions from research. *Journal of Advanced Nursing*, **21**(3), 452–9.

McMahon, A. (1998) Developing practice through research. In: *Research and Development in Clinical Nursing* (eds B. Roe & C. Webb). Whurr, London.

Mallett, J., Cathmoir, D., Hughes, P. & Whitby, E. (1997) Forging new roles . . . professional and practice development. *Nursing Times*, **93**(18), 38–9.

Manley, K. (1997) Practice development: a growing and significant movement. *Nursing in Critical Care*, **2**(1), 5.

31

Marsh, S. & MacAlpine, S. (1995) *Our Own Capabilities*. King's Fund, London.

Morse, J.M. (1995) Exploring the theoretical basis of nursing using advanced techniques of concept analysis. *Advances in Nursing Science*, **17**(3), 31–46.

NHSE (1996) *Promoting Clinical Effectiveness: A Framework for Action*. NHS Executive, Leeds.

Nichols, R., Meyer, J., Batehup, L. & Waterman, H. (1997) Promoting action research in healthcare settings. *Nursing Standard*, **11**(40), 36–8.

Rodgers, B.L. (1994) Concepts, analysis and the development of nursing knowledge: the evolutionary cycle. In: *Models, Theories and Concepts* (ed. J.P. Smith). Blackwell Science, Oxford.

Rolfe, G. (1996) *Closing the Theory–Practice Gap: A New Paradigm for Nursing*. Butterworth-Heinemann, London.

Thomas, S. & Ingham, A. (1995) The unit based clinical practice development role: a practitioner's and a manager's perspective. In: *Innovations in Nursing Practice* (ed. E. Rosser). Arnold, London.

Titchen, A. (2001) Critical companionship: a conceptual framework for developing expertise. In: *Practice Knowledge and Expertise in the Health Professions* (eds J. Higgs & A. Titchen), pp. 80–95. Butterworth-Heinemann, Oxford.

United Kingdom Central Council for Nursing, Midwifery and Health Visiting (UKCC) (1992) *The Scope of Professional Practice*. UKCC, London.

Vaughan, B. (1996) Developing nursing. *Nursing Standard*, **10**(15), 31–5.

Vaughan, B. & Edwards, M. (1995) *Interface Between Research and Practice*. King's Fund, London.

Walker, L.O. & Avant, K.C. (1995) *Strategies for Theory Construction*. Appleton & Lang, Norwalk, CT.

Wallis, S. (1998) Changing practice through action research. *Nursing Standard*, **6**(2), 5–14.

Ward, M.F., Titchen, A., Morrell, C., McCormack, B. & Kitson, A. (1998) Using a supervisory framework to support and evaluate a multiproject practice development programme. *Journal of Clinical Nursing*, **7**(1), 29–36.

Weir, P. (1995) Clinical practice development role: a personal reflection. In: *Innovations in Nursing Practice* (ed. E. Rosser). Arnold, London.

Weir, P. & Kendrick, K. (1994) Practice development: setting up networks to improve practice. *Nursing Standard*, **8**(41), 29–33.

Williams, C., Lee, D. & Lowry, M. (1993) Practice development units: the next step? *Nursing Standard*, **8**(11), 25–9.

3. *Practice Development*
Purpose, Methodology, Facilitation and Evaluation

Kim Manley and Brendan McCormack

Introduction

Practice development is recognised as a growing significant movement (Manley 1997a) but, until recently, it has been given little consideration in terms of its underlying theoretical concepts (Clarke & Proctor, 1999; McCormack *et al.*, 1999; Unsworth, 2000; Garbett & McCormack, 2002). Although some consider practice development an ambiguous concept (Clarke & Proctor, 1999), others imply that it primarily involves implementation and dissemination of research into practice (Kitson *et al.*, 1996). This narrow view of practice development holds that clinical effectiveness depends on practitioners using evidence from systematic reviews and meta-analysis to inform their practice (Haines & Jones, 1994). A broader view promotes practice development as all the activities necessary to achieve quality patient services and this includes nurturing innovation in practice settings (Knight, 1994; Manley, 1997a).

One certainty is that practice development is concerned directly with the world of practice and so it is not our intention to academicise it. However, we argue that effective practice development requires practice developers to be aware of and understand the assumptions underpinning the way they work; that the approaches used should be informed by their specific intended purposes; and that these approaches should be rigorous and systematic.

Practice developers, like all healthcare practitioners, are accountable for making clear the evidence base underpinning their decisions and actions. Evidence in this context includes explicit values and beliefs about purpose and means as well as understanding and insights from eclectic knowledge bases and different ways of knowing (Manley, 1997a). Values and beliefs underpinning the nature of practice development are the concern of practice development methodology, which in turn guides the methods and tools used, drawing parallels between methodology in practice development and research. 'Far from being merely a matter of making selections among methods, methodology involves the researcher [*and practice developer*] utterly – from unconscious worldview to enactment of that worldview' (Guba & Lincoln, 1989: 183).

The purpose of this chapter is to explore the methodology underpinning different approaches so as to encourage greater clarity about the processes and outcomes of effective practice development. Regardless of which methodology is used we argue that effective practice development involves rigorous, analytical thinking and systematic approaches (McCormack *et al.*, 1999). This chapter draws on the previous chapter, defining the concept of practice development, and introduces some perspectives on evaluation that will be explored in greater depth in Chapter 5.

Practivce development: purpose and means

Clarifying the purpose and means of practice development is fundamental to understanding what it is, as well as to the development of a common and shared vision (Manley, 2000a). If definitions include both purpose and means, then this will enable more tangible and meaningful understanding of complex concepts such as practice development. Two definitions allude to its purpose and means:

> Professional and practice development is a continuous process and, despite being inextricably linked, the two areas are distinct: the former is concerned with knowledge, skills and values and the latter with how these are used to provide good quality patient-focused care.
>
> (Mallett *et al.*, 1997: 38)

> Practice development is defined as a continuous process of improvement towards increased effectiveness in patient-centred care. This is brought about by helping healthcare teams to develop their knowledge and skills and to transform the culture and context of care. It is enabled and supported by facilitators committed to systematic rigorous continuous processes of emancipatory change that reflect the perspectives of service users.
>
> (Garbett & McCormack, 2002: 88)

The purpose of practice development in the first definition is 'good quality patient-focused care' and the means of achieving this is through *using* knowledge, skills and values developed through personal development. In the second definition the purpose is 'increased effectiveness in patient-centred care', and the means are through:

- developing knowledge and skills
- enabling nurses/healthcare teams to transform the culture and context of care
- skilled facilitation
- systematic, rigorous and continuous process of emancipatory change

Practice development draws on many different and diverse disciplines, which in turn enables all professional functions to be integrated for the benefit of patients (Manley, 1997b). It is a pre-requisite to clinical effectiveness, continuous quality improvement and development of a culture that facilitates the responsive and proactive action necessary for effective healthcare (Manley, 1997b). In a further refinement of our understanding of practice development, Manley (2001) argues for three additional characteristics to be made explicit:

- Practice development activities are directly targeted at practice and have an impact on how practitioners work with patients, discriminating it from personal development which may or may not indirectly impact on practice.
- Practice development includes using evidence in practice as well as generating evidence from practice. The knowledge base informing decision-making in practice development comprises:
  - policy
  - traditional propositional theory
  - local theory, i.e. concerning the specific context
  - personal theory encompassing professional craft knowledge (Titchen, 2000)
  - patient's personal knowing including their preferences
- The need for matched activity at the organisational and strategic interfaces to benefit activity at the client/patient interface (McCormack *et al.*, 1999).

The two definitions demonstrate how clarity of purpose and means may help in articulating what practice development is but they also suggest different means. These differences are presented as two worldviews of practice development each underpinned by different assumptions and linked to different methodologies. We have labelled them 'Technical practice development' and 'Emancipatory practice development' so as to parallel Habermas's (1972) different knowledge interests and Grundy's (1982) three modes of action research – both considered later in the context of practice development.

Central to methodology is the identification of assumptions, values and beliefs. Assumptions are usually unconscious, but by making assumptions conscious, explicit values and beliefs can be articulated (Schein, 1985; Manley, 2000a). The two worldviews are exaggerated here for the purpose of accentuating their differences, thus enabling readers to develop insight into their own position, to make sense of their own experiences, to identify the skills they may wish to develop, or to position their own organisation or department.

Technical and emancipatory practice development share some similarities even though they are different. Both focus on the purpose of achieving 'better' or 'best' services for users, regardless of the criteria used to judge this. The *raison d'être* of practice development is to improve some aspect of patient care or service directly. In a study using focus groups with practice developers, improvement was found to be a key reason for justifying the establishment of practice development roles in organisations (Garbett & McCormack, 2002). A direct focus implies that there is a desire to enable practitioners to change practice, rather than just their knowledge base, which is a more indirect focus. 'Better' and 'best' are placed in quotation marks because they may have different meanings to different people, reflecting the related debate about quality as a static benchmark versus an ongoing dynamic process (Berwick, 1989). Both the definitions used earlier focus on practice development as a continuous process (Mallet *et al.*, 1997; McCormack *et al.*, 1999). The criteria by which 'better' or 'best' service is judged (for example, person-centredness, continuity of care, cost-effectiveness, or evidence use from systematic reviews in practice, etc.) are derived from different sources in the two practice development approaches.

Differences in the purpose of practice development relate to whether there is deliberate attention to staff development and cultural change. Technical practice development of staff, if it occurs, is a *consequence* of practice development rather than a *deliberate* and *intentional* purpose. This is because practice development is considered a technical instrument for achieving the development of services to patients. Changing practice is seen as a technical process (Carr & Kemmis, 1986) consistent with Habermas's technical kind of knowledge (see below). Whereas, in emancipatory practice development, the development and empowerment of staff is deliberate and inter-related with creating a specific type of culture: termed a *transformational* culture (Manley, 2001). It is one where: quality becomes everyone's business; positive change becomes a way of life; everyone's leadership potential is developed; and where there is a shared vision, and investment in and valuing of staff (Manley, 2000a, b). The additional two purposes of emancipatory practice development are therefore, to:

- enable practitioners to become empowered to develop their individual and collective service;
- foster the development of an integrative (Kanter, 1983) and transformational culture (Manley, 2001).

All three purposes of emancipatory practice development are consistent with and reflect the influences of critical social science methodology. This methodology through the use of words such as 'transform' and 'emancipatory', and an explicit focus on context and culture are also evidenced in McCormack *et al.*'s (1999) definition of practice development.

Critical social science and practice development

Habermas (1972), a founder of critical social science, identifies three different kinds of knowledge but argues all are interwoven with human interest, being shaped by the human interest they serve. Human interest cannot be separated from knowledge because knowledge is not an outcome that can be separated from everyday concerns. He labels these three 'interests' as, *technical, practical* and *emancipatory.* Each is associated with different mediums and sciences.

Technical interest is about gaining technical knowledge that will enable greater skill and mastery over technical work activity. Such knowledge is derived from the natural sciences. In terms of practice development an example may be a nurse's concern for improving the care provided to patients with certain types of wounds. Practice development may result from becoming aware of the most effective intervention that will help the patient's wound to granulate. Practitioners may draw on technical knowledge derived from systematic reviews of evidence or meta-analysis based on randomised control trials that correlate the interventions with the outcomes of wound granulation and resolution. Habermas would argue that such technical knowledge serves a specific purpose but that it is not the only type of legitimate knowledge. Technical knowledge will be important in many clinical contexts. However, technical knowledge alone is insufficient in terms of improving practice. Technical interest can only lead to the development of technical evidence but practitioners need to be confident that such evidence is both valuable and relevant if it is to be used appropriately in practice.

In technical practice development the focus is on persuading practitioners to use technical knowledge as the mechanism for improving their patients' outcomes of care. (This may also be an outcome of emancipatory practice development, although the means would be different.) A strategic example of technical practice development may involve practice developers implementing a hospital strategy at clinical level. This strategy may have arisen from the work of senior people within the organisation, or be derived from government policy, for example, *clinical governance*. The goal is known and the focus is on achieving this, for example that clinical governance is implemented, rather than being concerned with how it is achieved. Staff, including, for example, specific practice development posts, may be considered the instruments through which such goals are achieved. This approach is frequently associated with 'top-down' change and deductive approaches to practice development (Kitson *et al.*, 1996). In its purest form the outcomes of such approaches are rarely sustainable. This is because there is no explicit concern with the process of developing practitioner ownership. Second, the social system or context within which evidence is being introduced is not recognised as an influencing factor on the uptake of evidence/innovation. The limited success in practice of this approach is evidenced by continuing concerns that practitioners do not use research evidence in their practice (Funk *et al.*, 1989; McGuire, 1990; Walshe, 1997; Dunn *et al.*, 1998; Kitson *et al.*, 1998), and practitioners' perceptions that strategy is imposed and complied with, rather than internalised and owned. Technical interest is therefore of value but alone is insufficient unless practitioners see its relevance and have developed a commitment to its ownership and use.

Practical interest is concerned with understanding and clarifying how others (e.g. patients, relatives, colleagues) see their world. The concept of *'knowing the patient'* (Jenny & Logan, 1992; Tanner *et al.*, 1993) – a concept described first in critical care nursing and now central to understanding nursing expertise (Manley & Garbett,

2000) – is an example of this focus. Practical interest generates *practical understanding*, which can inform and guide practical judgement. It is concerned with the medium of language and the hermeneutic or interpretive sciences such as phenomenology. In practice development and, as a step towards providing more personalised care, nurses may use such an approach to develop greater understanding of how individual patients 'see their world', or, through exploring experiences of a group of patients undergoing the same traumatic experience more relevant healthcare information can be provided which has been derived from an understanding of patients/clients' common concerns and experiences.

Although greater understanding of patients' and users' experiences may be achieved, this does not necessarily result in a change in the way nurses practise. For example, although a nurse may wish to develop more effective professional relationships with medical colleagues, and even though she may have become aware of why she is unable to assert herself and in which circumstances this occurs – action may not necessarily follow. It is this action component that is addressed by emancipatory interest.

Emancipatory interest is concerned with how self-reflection and self-understanding is influenced by social conditions. The medium here is *power* and the sciences are those of the critical sciences. As Carr & Kemmis assert:

> a critical social science will provide the kind of self-reflective understanding that will permit individuals to explain why the conditions in which they operate are frustrating and will suggest the sort of action that is required if the sources of these frustrations are to be eliminated.
>
> (1986: 136)

A single *critical theory* results from the process of critique undertaken by individuals or groups concerned with exposing contradictions in the rationality or justice of social actions. Such theories can arise from practical interest and also may transform consciousness (raise awareness), but not change practice (Carr & Kemmis, 1986). *Critical social science* goes beyond critique to include action from this raised awareness, rather than from coercion or habit. For example, a team of nurses may have an interest in changing the way that nursing is organised to reflect shared values and beliefs about providing continuity of care. In adopting a critical social science approach to practice development, the following would have occurred:

- critical reflection resulting in clarity about the values and beliefs held about nursing;
- recognition of any contradictions between the values and beliefs espoused (spoken about) and their actual practice;
- increasing awareness of the barriers within the workplace that prevent these values being practised;
- removing the barriers identified so as to practise in a way that is consistent with the values and beliefs espoused.

Technical practice development

When practice development is understood as a technical phenomenon then, as is also found in technical action research, the practice developer is perceived as an expert authority figure. That is, they know what has to be done, to what standard, and the criteria for success pre-exists in their mind (Grundy, 1982). It is the facilitator's ideas that direct a project, with the end point already in their mind (Grundy, 1982), such as, the implementation of clinical guidelines to ensure more effective care within a directorate, or developing the competence of practitioners in some new aspect of care to reduce waiting times. Staff are the instrument through which the outcome is to be achieved and therefore through which practice is to be improved. The danger here is that staff may be 'pawns' who are unconsciously manipulated for the facilitator's or organisation's ends (Grundy, 1982). Using two examples: implementing clinical guidelines (Example 1) and developing the competence of staff in a new area (Example 2), the focus of the practice developer and the outcomes evaluated in technical practice development are identified.

In Example 1 (clinical guidelines) the approach used by the practice developer would be deductive (Kitson *et al.*, 1996) and would focus on informing staff about a specific set of clinical guidelines in relation to their practice. This approach may include presenting formal sessions where the guidelines and evidence base underpinning them are outlined – thus attempting to develop practitioner's knowledge about what is and is not effective. This may be followed by the development of written standards and monitoring through audit.

In Example 2 the role of practice development would focus only on increasing an individual's competence in performing a specific task. The assumption in both these examples is that, armed with the technical skill and knowledge, practitioners will change the ways in which they practice. Yet there are many barriers to developing practice, not least the fact that situations everywhere are different, each setting poses greater or lesser barriers to implementation. Knowledge and skills acquired may not be realised in practice for a number of reasons, for example, the practice culture may not be conducive to developing practice. Although staff may identify with and plan to implement interventions on a study day or in a meeting, often when they return to their clinical areas a host of barriers frustrate them. Not least of these is that they are thrust back onto the same 'hamster-wheel' of activity where the burden of day-to-day care may provide little opportunity to implement new-found skills. As Grundy (1982) highlights, when working with staff in this way and depending on the facilitator's skill in inspiring, enthusing and gaining commitment from staff and expertise in the area, staff may take one of three actions:

- Reject the idea of the facilitator and refuse to work for its realisation
- Consent to work towards the goal
- Adopt the idea as their own

Where ideas are adopted as the practitioners' own, technical practice development may succeed in getting theoretical knowledge used in practice. But this is more a function of expertise in facilitation (Kitson *et al.*, 1998) together with mastery of technical knowledge. In summary, knowledge expertise alone is inadequate but facilitation skills associated with Habermas's practical and emancipatory interests are an influential factor. In technical practice development even if staff adopt ideas as their own, it is the practice developer who considers him/herself to be ultimately responsible for success or failure of a practice development initiative.

Earlier, it was proposed that practice development needs to be systematic and rigorous regardless of the approach. Evaluation is therefore integral to good practice development. As in other areas of practice development, the evaluation questions will be influenced by methodology with different questions being asked and different methods being used (McCutcheon & Jung, 1990). In technical practice development evaluation is guided by its underlying assumptions and the focus of evaluation would tend to be on numerical variables consistent with approaches to developing technical knowledge. The focus of evaluation in technical practice development is therefore measurement. Measures used may be as diverse as waiting time, length of stay, length of waiting lists, numbers of people cared for on trolleys in A&E, morbidity, mortality, nosocomial infection rates, cost-effectiveness, number of agency nurses used, number of complaints, amount of medication used etc. Alternatively, measures may involve the use of valid and reliable tools such as those concerned with measuring pain levels, wound granulation, quality of sleep, job satisfaction, quality of life, etc. This type of evaluation assumes correlation between independent (intervention) and dependent (outcomes) variables regardless of context.

Evaluation of the outcomes expected of technical practice development would thus be concerned with specific technical interventions and with demonstrating the impact of such interventions on the service or client care, showing that they made a difference. However good the evidence and however skilled the practice developer, the context, specifically the culture of care, may frustrate them. Culture and context is not a concern of technical practice development as it is assumed not to exert an effect. It is in this area that emancipatory practice development can augment technical practice development through addressing more directly issues that influence sustainability of change. Through working with fundamental assumptions held by practitioners about their work and the systems in which they practice, emancipatory practice development sets out to achieve sustainable action recognised in the workplace as consistent *utilisation* of technical and practical knowledge.

Emancipatory practice development

To achieve the three purposes of emancipatory practice development earlier outlined, the facilitator would work in a different way although this may include technical practice development to reflect specific stakeholders' needs. Emancipatory practice development focuses on the social system as well as the individual/group's own practice. Facilitators aim to help practitioners become aware of and freed from taken-for-granted aspects of their practice and the organisational systems constraining them. Facilitators foster a climate of critical intent through reflective discussion involving various 'ideas' of the group members and assist the group's enlightenment (increased awareness) through nurturing a culture which enables individuals and the group to act. Responsibility for action rests with the practitioners themselves (Grundy, 1982). This approach is consistent with critical social science, emancipatory practice development and, also, emancipatory action research (EAR), which, it is argued later, is synonymous. Emancipatory practice development may encompass technical interest, through group members sharing responsibility for identifying drivers such as pertinent policy, evidence and strategies. Through pursuing an interest in the external climate and broader social system in which care is provided, collective insight, understanding and ownership develop through the practitioners' own actions, rather than through the actions of others, thus enabling the first steps to be taken towards action from enlightenment. Emancipatory practice development does not pretend to overcome barriers that are beyond the influence of group members (for example limited financial resources and government influence). Instead emancipatory practice development enables group members to realise the influence they hold, how to use that influence most appropriately and effectively and to recognise aspects of decision-making that are beyond direct influence (although group members may be able to exert influence indirectly). Thus enlightenment in itself creates change through raised awareness, recognition of the power of influence, and understanding of the limitations on individual power in any organisational context. The facilitator is responsible for enabling a culture to develop where such enlightenment is possible – a culture of critique – and in addition its administrative organisation (Grundy, 1982). The facilitator may also have technical expertise to share but their contribution to the group is of no greater or lesser importance than that of other group members.

Evaluation within emancipatory practice development may encompass the same variables as technical practice development but in addition would also include personal/collective development, and the evaluation of culture. Evaluation processes would be transparent and underpinned by explicit values and beliefs that recognise that different types of knowledge are interwoven with the human interests they serve. Habermas proposes a more open focus on values, not as goals to be judged in terms of absolute truth, but for enabling the examination of the process of negotiation (Wuthnow *et al.*, 1984: 183). Such processes constitute the main work of practice developers using critical social science approaches.

Emancipatory practice development is concerned with the medium of power, so, when selecting evaluation approaches it is important to select those sharing similar premises and aims. Two particular approaches to evaluation are highlighted here as compatible with emancipatory practice development – Emancipatory Action Research (EAR) (Grundy, 1982) and 'fourth generation evaluation' (Guba & Lincoln, 1989). The links between practice development and action research are reflected in their similarity of purpose (Box 3.1).

All approaches to action research and practice development, whether focused on individuals or groups share the common

Box 3.1   Purposes of action research (Manley, 2000b).

- Develop practice, introduce a change, respond to a need or problem (Lewin, 1947; McNiff, 1988; Elliott, 1991; Whyte, 1991; Greenwood, 1994)
- Enable practitioners/participants to learn/develop/become empowered (Susman & Evered, 1978; Grundy, 1982; Whitehead & Foster, 1984; Kemmis & McTaggert, 1988; Greenwood, 1994)
- Contribute to or refine theory (Lewin, 1947; McNiff, 1988; Elliott, 1991; Whyte, 1991; Greenwood, 1994)

purpose of improving practice. The second purpose of action research (Box 3.1) is shared with emancipatory practice development but this purpose has only become deliberate since the influence of Susman and Evered (1978), and critical social science in the 1970s and 1980s when the limitations of technical knowledge were identified.

The third purpose of action research is most significant when considering evaluation in practice development. Critical social science has enabled traditional concepts of theory to be challenged. Traditionally, theory has been understood as descriptive, explanatory and predictive as derived from traditional science (Manley, 1997b) and technical interest, whereas in Habermas's *practical interest*, theory is derived from the interpretive sciences and is concerned with understanding. Theory in critical social science is that which informs action (called praxis) and reflexivity (a theorising spiral in practice), where personal theories evolve constantly from questioning one's action and then making changes which further inform personal theories. As with emancipatory action research, emancipatory practice development results in personal theory and through the vehicle of systematic evaluation it can also generate public theory and knowledge. Although initially evaluation of practice development may lead to the development of local theory (that is, theory relating to the local context) there may be elements of the theory that can be transferred to other contexts. These aspects can be considered *generalisable* in the sense that the same theory arises from different contexts.

There are a number of ways of thinking about how data from emancipatory practice development can be generalised. The first is that of 'community narrative' (Rorty, 1979). What Rorty argues is that the presentation of any findings should be recognisable in the form of a community narrative, i.e. that they reflect the values and norms of the community it represents. Thus judgements about the validity of the data will be made by the community on the basis of moral, societal, participatory, and democratic values (for example) that it holds. Thus it is essential for the practice developer to provide a detailed audit trail of steps, stages, processes and the relationship between these and outcomes. The second way of thinking about it is described by Richardson (1997) using the metaphor of a *crystal*. In using the metaphor of the crystal, Laurel Richardson makes the point that there are many ways of interpreting something. A crystal is a solid object (like a text!) but it can be turned many ways and in turning, it reflects and refracts light (multiple meanings) through which we can see whole parts (whole meanings) and 'particles' (feelings, connections and single elements of the data). Richardson's work provides some useful insights for practice development, as this issue of being able to extract important singular aspects of whole projects that can be transferred to other contexts is essential if practice development is to be useful to decision-makers. Finally, the idea of 'coherence' in the analysis and reporting of the evaluation is important. That is, can the reader/viewer see consistency in the representation, can they see that all voices have been represented fairly and can they see that the conclusions reached are evident in the data itself? House (1981) makes a compelling argument for the coherence of evaluation reports being an essential component in the degree to which audiences will perceive it as credible. Every evaluation, he says, must have a minimum degree of coherence, 'the minimum coherence is that the evaluation should tell a story. There must be either an explicit or tacit sequence of events (or more accurately interpretation of events) for the reader to use as a guide to valuing' (House, 1981: 102). So from this sense, good practice development (i.e. practice development that is systematic and rigorous) would also contribute to public knowledge and its refinement through evaluation. In technical practice development and technical action research the theory arising is considered explanatory and predictive in the traditional sense and does not encompass local or personal theory as reflected by praxis and reflexivity.

In summary, EAR can provide the guiding principles and framework for evaluation in emancipatory practice development with a focus on issues concerning power and inequity in the social system, raising consciousness and exploring the impact of the context on action. These include the constraining factors, which prevent individuals from developing their practice through their own action.

Guba & Lincoln (1989) provide a second practical evaluation strategy to inform practice development in their Fourth Generation

Evaluation approach. Fourth Generation Evaluation, a contemporary approach to evaluation, addresses the weaknesses inherent in earlier generations which focused first on *measurement*, then *description* and lastly, *judgement*. Weaknesses in these earlier generations include the limited consideration given to context, processes and the views of stakeholders. Fourth Generation Evaluation focuses on identifying stakeholders' concerns, claims and issues about the phenomena being evaluated, then reaching a consensus which is meaningful from these multiple perspectives. Stakeholders are defined as groups who, 'have something at stake in the evaluand – the entity being evaluated' (Guba & Lincoln, 1989: 51).

Guba & Lincoln (1989) highlight five reasons (Box 3.2) for involving stakeholders. These reasons reflect a similar concern for the impact of power as emancipatory practice development.

This evaluation approach also provides other benefits:

- promotes evaluation as co-operative, the evaluator works *with* people rather than *on* them, therefore providing a moral and authentic way of working;
- values the contributions made by stakeholders enabling them to learn about others' constructions;
- by involving stakeholders in the process means that they are more likely to develop ownership of subsequent change making the change process more successful.

There are also criticisms of Fourth Generation Evaluation in practice, specifically, the potential for misuse of power in two areas: evaluator and client privilege; and, the accountability mechanisms for

Box 3.2   Stakeholders (Guba & Lincoln, 1989).

Stakeholders:

- are groups at risk, because by definition they have a stake in what is being evaluated
- are open to exploitation, disempowerment, and disenfranchisement because the end product of evaluation is information. 'Information is power, and evaluation is powerful' (Guba & Lincoln, 1989: 52)
- are users of evaluation information
- can broaden the range of evaluative inquiry. 'When one does not know in advance what information is to be collected, it is literally impossible to design an inquiry that will provide it. Open-endness (an 'emergent' design) is called for' (Guba & Lincoln, 1989: 55)
- are mutually educated by the fourth generation process

reporting processes and action outcomes (Laughlin & Broadbent, 1996). However, through using Fourth Generation Evaluation with the processes of EAR these dangers can be minimised. EAR highlights the role of the facilitator in making such decisions open and transparent through accountability mechanisms (Grundy, 1982).

In summary, evaluation in emancipatory practice development may include technical evaluation approaches as this may reflect the concerns of specific stakeholders. In addition, emancipatory practice development will also need to reflect its two other purposes when evaluating – practitioner development and impact on culture. However, the processes of emancipatory practice development focus on these two areas as a mechanism for achieving sustainable change by developing a culture where practice development becomes integral to everyone's work sustained through the characteristics of a culture of critique.

Conclusion

This chapter has highlighted the methodological aspects underpinning practice development. It argues for clear understanding about the purpose of practice development with different purposes underpinned by different assumptions. It proposes that practice developers need to know the worldview in which they are operating as this has implications for the processes they use, their own enlightenment (as well as that of other practitioners), their facilitation approaches and evaluation focus. This chapter recognises not that one worldview of practice development is bad and the other is good, but that practice developers should knowingly be aware of the worldview they are working from, or where their organisation is positioned – it is naïve ignorance that needs to be challenged. Although it is acknowledged that much practice development has taken a technical focus in the past to serve a technical interest, it is argued that this is a narrow focus concerned with one set of stakeholder concerns. Emancipatory practice development is more sophisticated and is concerned with sustaining development and change as well as changing the culture of care more extensively to one truly reflective of the values underpinning the spirit of shared clinical governance. This approach, underpinned by the methodology of critical social science, recognises all key stakeholders' contributions and operates at a number of interfaces outlined further by McCormack *et al.* (1999). Knowing one's worldview as a practice developer will therefore influence the methods used, as methodology precedes methods. The key question for practice developers then is, how to enable others to become more effective in their learning and subsequent practice for the purpose of creating a learning organisation and culture that benefits users.

This chapter proposes that emancipatory practice development – a methodology underpinned by critical social science – is an approach that will achieve sustainable effects. It can transform both practitioners and their practice, as well as the culture and context in which care is provided, in addition to meeting the concerns of stakeholders who value only technical practice development.

References

Carr, W. & Kemmis, S. (1986) *Becoming Critical: Education, Knowledge and Action Research*. The Falmer Press, London.

Clarke, C. & Proctor, S. (1999) Practice development: ambiguity in research and practice. *Journal of Advanced Nursing*, **30**(4), 975–82.

Dunn, V., Crichton, N., Roe, N. & Williams, K. (1998) Using research for practice: a UK experience of the BARRIERS scale. *Journal of Advanced Nursing*, **27**, 1203–10.

Elliott, J. (1991) *Action Research for Educational Change*. Open University Press, Milton Keynes.

Funk, S.G., Tornquist, E.M. & Champagne, M.T. (1989) A model for improving the dissemination of nursing research. *Western Journal of Nursing Research*, **11**, 361–7.

Garbett, R. & McCormack, B. (2002) A concept analysis of practice development. *Nursing Times Research*, **7**(2), 87–100.

Greenwood, J. (1994) Action research: a few details, a caution and something new. *Journal of Advanced Nursing*, **20**, 13–18.

Grundy, S. (1982) Three modes of action research. *Curriculum Perspectives*, **2**(3), 23–34.

Guba, E.G. & Lincoln, Y.S. (1989) *Fourth Generation Evaluation*. Sage, Thousand Oaks, CA.

Habermas, J. (1972) *Knowledge and Human Interests*, trans J.J. Shapiro. Heinemann, London.

Haines, A. & Jones, R. (1994) Implementing findings of research. *British Medical Journal*, **308**, 1488–92.

House, E.R. (1981) *Evaluating with Validity*. Sage, London, Thousand Oaks, CA.

Jenny, J. & Logan, J. (1992) Knowing the patient: one aspect of clinical knowledge image. *Journal of Nursing Scholarship*, **24**(4), Winter, 254–8.

Kanter, R.M. (1983) *The Change Masters: Corporate Entrepreneurs at Work*. Unwin: London.

Kemmis, S. & McTaggart, R. (1988) *The Action Research Planner*. Deakin University Press, Geelong, Victoria, Australia.

Kitson, A.L., Ahmed, L.D., Harvey, G., Seers, K. & Thompson, D.R. (1996) From research to practice: one organisational model for promoting research-based practice. *Journal of Advanced Nursing*, **23**(3), 430–40.

Kitson, A.L., Harvey, G. & McCormack, B. (1998) Enabling the Implementation of evidence-based practice: a conceptual framework. *Quality in Healthcare*, **7**(3), 149–58.

Knight, S. (1994) An organisational approach. *Nursing Standard*, **90**(41), 33–5.

Laughlin, R. & Broadbent, J. (1996) Redesigning fourth generation evaluation. *Evaluation*, **2**(4), 431–51.

Lewin, K. (1947) Frontiers in group dynamics, II: Channels of group life. *Social Planning and Action Research Human Relations*, **1**, 143–53.

McCormack, B., Manley, K., Kitson, A., Titchen, A. & Harvey, G. (1999) Towards practice development – a vision in reality or a reality without vision? *Journal of Nursing Management*, **7**(2), 255–64.

McCutcheon, G. & Jung, B. (1990) Alternative perspectives on action research. *Theory Into Practice*, **29**(3), 144–51.

McGuire, J. (1990) Putting nursing research findings into practice: research utilisation as an aspect of the management of change. *Journal of Advanced Nursing*, **15**, 614–20.

McNiff, J. (1988) *Action Research: Principles and Practice*. McMillan Education, Basingstoke.

Mallett, J., Cathmoir, D., Hughes, P. & Whitby, E. (1997) Forging new roles . . . professional and practice development. *Nursing Times*, **93**(18), 38–9.

Manley, K. (1997a) Practice development: a growing and significant movement. *Nursing in Critical Care*, **2**(1), 5.

Manley, K. (1997b) Knowledge for nursing practice. In: *The Knowledge Base for Nursing* (ed. A. Perry) 2nd edn, Chapter 10. Arnold, London.

Manley, K. (2000a) Organisational culture and consultant nurse outcomes. Part 1: Organisational culture. *Nursing Standard*, **14**(36), 34–8.

Manley, K. (2000b) Organisational culture and consultant nurse outcomes. Part 2: Consultant nurse outcomes. *Nursing Standard*, **14**(37), 34–9.

Manley, K. (2001) *Consultant nurse: concept, processes, outcome.* Unpublished PhD thesis, Manchester University/RCN Institute, London.

Manley, K. & Garbett, R. (2000) Paying Peter and Paul: reconciling concepts of expertise with competency for a clinical career structure. *Journal of Clinical Nursing*, **9**(3), 347–59.

Manley, K. & McCormack, B. (2003) Practice development: purpose, methodology, facilitation and evaluation. *Nursing in Critical Care*, **8**(1), 22–9.

Richardson, L. (1997) *Fields of Play*. Rutgers University Press, New Jersey.

Rorty, R. (1979) *Philosophy and the Mirror of Nature*. Princeton University Press, New Jersey.

Schein, E.H. (1985) *Organizational Culture and Leadership*. Jossey-Bass, San Francisco, CA.

Susman, G.I. & Evered, R.D. (1978) An assessment of the scientific merits of action research. *Administrative Science Quarterly*, **23**, 582–602.

Tanner, C.A., Benner, P., Chesla, C. & Gordon, D.R. (1993) The phenomenology of knowing the patient, IMAGE. *The Journal of Nursing Scholarship*, **25**(4), 273–80.

Titchen, A. (2000) *Professional Craft Knowledge in Patient-centred Nursing and the Facilitation of its Development*. University of Oxford DPhil thesis. Ashdale Press, Oxford.

Unsworth, J. (2000) Practice development: a concept analysis. *Journal of Nursing Management*, **6**, 317–22.

Walshe, M. (1997) Perceptions of barriers to implementing research. *Nursing Standard*, **11**(19), 34–7.

Whitehead, J. & Foster, D. (1984) Action research and professional development. *Cambridge Action Research Network Bulletin*, No. 6. University of East Anglia Norwich.

Whyte, W.F. (ed.) (1991) *Participatory Action Research*. Sage, Newbury Park, CA.

Wuthnow, R., Davison Hunter, J., Bergesen, A. & Kurzweil, E. (1984) *Cultural Analysis*. Routledge, London.

This chapter is based on an article by Manley & McCormack (2003).

4. *Transformational Culture*
A Culture of Effectiveness

Kim Manley

Introduction

A key purpose of practice development is to transform the culture of care so that it becomes and remains patient-centred, evidence-based and continually effective within a changing healthcare context. This chapter focuses on what cultures are and on the characteristics of an effective workplace culture – defined as a 'transformational culture' (Manley, 1997a; 2001).

I have called such a culture 'transformational' because it changes its form and disposition, readily adapting and responding to a changing context. It is, however, based on fundamental core values that in turn enable individuals to develop their own potential, and their practice too. Such a culture nurtures and enables innovation through practitioner empowerment, practice development and a number of other workplace characteristics – all prerequisites to quality patient care.

Culture, contemporary healthcare and practice development

Culture has many meanings, but within the context of contemporary healthcare, culture and cultural change has a growing relevance. Savage (2000) suggests that culture is ubiquitous with the NHS and has become linked with the organisation of services and the provision of quality healthcare. Government policy alludes to this significance through *A First Class Service* (DoH, 1998) and *The NHS Plan* (DoH, 2000). The NHS Modernisation agenda has focused on new ways of working, leadership and the empowerment of front line staff – all processes linked to cultural change and a new NHS philosophy. The Kennedy report (2001) in highlighting lessons

learnt from the Bristol Royal Infirmary Inquiry illustrates extensively the role and impact of both NHS and team culture.

The concept analysis undertaken by Garbett & McCormack (2002)
endorses the centrality of culture to practice development. Culture
and context, together with skilled facilitation – a key practice development skill – are pivotal to the successful implementation and
actual use of evidence (see Chapter 6).

Flood (1994) argues that understanding culture and cultural
change may enable greater insight into how to reform healthcare.
Both Flood and Brown (1998) criticise the focus of many previous organisational studies has been on structural characteristics,
related in healthcare to what constitutes quality care, rather
than on 'ferreting out a model that explains the processes
whereby structure can affect quality of care' (Flood, 1994: 385). He
vehemently argues for the need to understand *how* organisational
factors promote better quality care suggesting that greater insight
into culture and cultural change may contribute to this
understanding.

What is culture?

In its simplest form culture can be understood as 'how things are
done around here' (Drennan, 1992: 3). However, culture is complex
as is reflected by the lack of consensus in its definition. Some argue
that organisational culture is best understood as a metaphor which
acts as an organising tool to help understand complex entities in
relation to each other, and as a powerful way of communicating
ideas (Smircich, 1983; Morgan, 1986). From this perspective every
aspect of an organisation is part of its culture and cannot be understood as separate from it – culture is not an objective tangible or
measurable aspect of an organisation; organisations *are* cultures
(Pacanowsky & O'Donnell-Trujillo, 1982: 26). This view is also proposed by Bate (1994) who promotes an understanding of culture·
from the anthropological view in contrast to the engineering, traditional scientific perspective, where culture is viewed as one of a
number of sub-components which can be replaced. Meek (1988)
argues for the inappropriateness of treating culture as a variable
that can be manipulated. Others consider culture as a set of psychological predispositions called 'basic assumptions' (Schein, 1985:
9) that members of an organisation possess, and which tend to cause
them to act in certain ways. These assumptions, the deepest
manifestations of culture, are linked to values and beliefs, and ultimately behaviour norms.

A single organisational culture or multiple subcultures?

Organisational culture has in the past been assumed as singular and pervasive, monolithic and integrative, but all organisations have multiple cultures usually associated with different functional groupings or geographical locations (Gregory, 1983; Louis, 1986; Kotter & Heskett, 1992; Bolan & Bolan, 1994). Subcultures are now recognised as prevalent within work settings (Louis, 1986: 135).

Corporate culture refers to values and practices shared across all groups in an organisation, at least within senior management (Kotter & Heskett, 1992). Anthony (1994) challenges the use of 'corporate culture', suggesting instead that this reflects the culture that organisations (and therefore probably senior executives) want to portray for the purpose of influencing public relations or employee motivation, and that this may not be the actual culture experienced. Anthony's distinction is 'between the espoused version of culture and the real, between the proposed and the descriptive, between what should be and what is' (1994: 3).

He proposes that corporate culture reflects the espoused form and organisational culture, the culture that is. According to Hofsteede *et al.* (1990) previous literature does not often differentiate between the values of founders and significant leaders, and the values of the bulk of the organisation's members.

Organisations also possess internal interest groups or constituencies whose members have identifiable common interests that they try to promote. Such constituencies may be differentiated by departmental, hierarchical boundaries or, 'more generally, by clusters of members that share distinct values and interests' (Goodman & Pennings, 1977: 148). So, an organisation comprises multiple subcultures, each with their own agenda and perspective (Gregory, 1983; Van Maanen & Barley, 1985). Bolan and Bolan (1994) argue that the concept of organisational culture needs to be dismantled to reflect the underlying group cultures. They introduce the concept of 'idioculture' to overcome the implication that 'subculture' is derived from organisational culture, when in fact organisational culture may be derived from the interaction of subcultures.

Idiocultures can serve as building blocks to organisational culture, and interactions between idiocultures can create organisational culture (Bolan & Bolan, 1994). This is achieved through shared meanings about a cultural element passing from one idioculture to another. My own research demonstrated this clearly with the unit culture influencing the hospital's culture (Manley, 2000b; 2001).

When thinking about culture in relation to the workplace, factors such as the content, group and relationship as well as the source of culture, the penetration and direction of culture need to be considered (Louis, 1986). To date, culture research has focused mainly on content. Schein (1985) identifies the content culture researchers have typically addressed, from the more concrete to the more abstract:

- *Artefacts* These are the tangible and more superficial aspects of culture – verbal, behavioural and physical artefacts.
- *Perspectives* These are the socially shared rules and norms, the solutions to common problems encountered by members.
- *Values* These form the evaluation base by which members judge situations, and are often stated in philosophies and mission statements.
- *Assumptions* These are the tacit beliefs that members hold about themselves and others, their relationships with others, and the nature of the organisation in which they live.

When exploring workplace culture Van Maanen & Barley argue:

> If we wish to discover where the cultural action lies in organizational life, we will probably have to discard some of our tacit (and not so tacit) presumptions about organizational (high) culture and move to the group level of analysis. It is here where the people discover, create, and use culture, and it is against this background that they judge the organization of which they are part.
>
> (Van Maanen & Barley, 1985: 51)

In relation to healthcare, it is pertinent to ask then, which culture is most influential on the experience of patients and users? The level at which patients interface with and experience care is commonly at the unit, ward, team or service level, rather than at the organisational level.

The role of values, beliefs and assumptions

Values and beliefs, and/or attitudes, assumptions, norms and shared meanings are pivotal to many definitions of workplace culture by writers and researchers regardless of whether the focus is organisational, idiocultural, or anthropological (Lorsch, 1986; Morgan, 1986; Denison, 1990; Kotter & Heskett, 1992; Williams *et al.*, 1993; Brown, 1998). Within these definitions, values and beliefs contribute to shared meanings, understandings and expectations which are tacit and distinctive to a particular group and passed on to new members (Louis, 1980). Values and beliefs may be implicit or explicit; they underpin the way things are done within any cultural focus. They reflect the deep manifestation of workplace culture and are part of its cognitive substructure (Brown, 1998), whereas symbols and artefacts such as logos or mission statements are more superficial manifestations (Lundberg, 1985; Schein, 1985). For Hofsteede *et al.* (1990), values are at the deepest level of culture and are shared by people in a group. They tend to persist over time, even when membership of the group changes (Kotter & Heskett, 1992). Values determine what people think *ought* to be done and are inextricably linked with moral and ethical codes, whereas beliefs are what people think is true or not true, for example that devolved decision-making produces greater commitment and job satisfaction. Beliefs and values are interrelated because it is difficult to separate values from their believed effect. It is difficult to know if values are valued for their own sake or because of the belief that they have a specific effect. Beliefs can become taken for granted and accepted as an accurate description of how the world works. They are then described as basic assumptions, accepted as true and held unconsciously. Basic assumptions involve beliefs, interpretations of beliefs plus values and emotions (Schein, 1985). Changing culture at a deep level is difficult because values are often invisible, whereas group behavioural norms, being more visible, are easier to change (Kotter & Heskett, 1992).

Basic assumptions can be understood as accepted truths that are held unconsciously and are taken for granted. Basic assumptions involve beliefs, interpretations of beliefs plus values and emotions (Brown, 1998).

A case study

Within my own research I operationalised the role of the consultant nurse over many years within an intensive care and nursing development unit (ICU/NDU). Early developmental work focused on making values and beliefs explicit through the use of values clarification. This informed the development of a shared vision; guided subsequent, strategic direction and development of an infrastructure of shared governance and primary nursing; and guided actions in everyday as well as unfamiliar situations. I used the processes of critique and reflection (Grundy, 1982; Carr & Kemmis, 1986) to facilitate staff:

- to identify contradictions between espoused culture and culture-in-practice
- to live and act out their values and beliefs

The espoused values and beliefs were distilled from the unit's stated philosophy and early publications (Manley, 2001). These reflected the centrality of patients and their families to the work of the unit. There was a focus on quality of care and the need to work constantly to improve this. The values and beliefs espoused were not just about patients, but also concerned:

- *staff* – that they should be cared for, supported and enabled to develop
- *change* – that staff are involved in change, foster innovation, develop the research base to their practice, and recognise the continuous nature of change
- *ways of working*:
  - open exchange of views and opinions
  - reflecting and challenging
  - teamwork and learning from others
  - participation through active involvement and taking responsibility which enables sustainable change

I later found these values to be similar to those identified by other researchers as contributing to effective organisations, namely, people values (Gregory, 1983), and a concern for key stakeholders (Baker, 1980; Kotter & Heskett, 1992); respect for all employees at all levels (Peters & Waterman, 1982), aspiring to excellence and the importance of the *customer* (Peters & Waterman, 1982; Kotter & Heskett, 1992); and teamwork (Baker, 1980).

Other characteristics of effective workplace cultures were espoused in the unit's philosophy and publications: the conviction that shared values and beliefs result from participative approaches (which are specifically linked to sustained change); the importance of learning, adaptability and continuous improvement (Denison, 1990; Kotter & Heskett, 1992); and a focus on continuous improvement in response to a changing health climate.

The unit's espoused mission, philosophy and publications clearly articulated the values and beliefs of the staff, and these are typical of effective cultures within the literature. However, espoused values and beliefs are frequently not experienced in practice (Kilman *et al.*, 1986; Anthony, 1994; Brown, 1998). Where the espoused culture is reflected in the culture-in-practice, then a strong culture is said to be present, one where there is consistency, a clear mission (Denison, 1990), and penetration across the cultural group being examined (Louis, 1980).

The actual culture-in-practice, in contrast to the espoused culture identified above, was derived from the experiences of staff and returners (a small group of nurses who left the unit and then returned within a period of two to three years) and emerged spontaneously from unstructured interviews.

The significance of values and beliefs was recognised by staff in that they frequently mentioned them in the points they made. The predominance of specific values and beliefs were experienced by the returners – a group particularly aware of contrasts (Louis, 1980). Returners identified values and beliefs that continued to be evident when returning after two to three years; their perception was accentuated by working in other units with different cultures. Congruency between values and beliefs espoused, and those practised were substantiated by insiders and concerned six areas:

- *The primacy of the patient* Staff followed a patient-focused philosophy, technical care being considered an accessory to patient-centred care rather than its central focus. The early work on values clarification within the unit led to the implementation of the organisational approach of primary nursing. This approach focuses on the nurse developing a therapeutic relationship with the patient and family, and promoting continuity of care (Manley *et al.*, 1996; Manley *et al.*, 1997).

- *Providing support to staff* Providing mutual and reciprocal support was evidenced in practice between all staff. Staff felt valued and respected. Respect for staff is central to effective workplace cultures (Peters & Waterman, 1982; Baker, 1980) and evident as influential within 'magnet hospital' research (Kramer, 1990).

- *Devolved decision-making in relation to both patient care and unit activity* Devolved and decentralised decision-making is a characteristic of primary nursing, implemented to reflect the values and beliefs held by staff about nursing (Manley *et al.*, 1997). The culture of the unit was perceived as one where participative approaches underpinned every aspect of unit activity. This culture was achieved by enabling staff to contribute to decision-making in all areas and this in turn was reflected by an openness to different ideas and a commitment to innovation. Inter-team projects provided a formal infrastructure for enabling all staff to be involved in the unit's direction, developments and shared governance. This covered quality, research, finance, marketing, education, and off-duty rostering. This enabled a marked focus on team working generally.

- *Openness to suggestions/involvement of everyone* The culture was perceived to be participative, drawing on everyone's contribution, regardless of the individual staff member's level of grade or experience. But also encouraged was 'giving an opinion' and individuals were not afraid to speak their minds even if this challenged the status quo. The antithesis of this is a 'harmonious team' (Johns, 1992) where individuals preserve a façade of harmony for fear of rocking the boat, and where conflict is avoided or suppressed. The harmonious team works against the giving and receiving of feedback and the development of authentic, reciprocal and mutual relationships. This is because it tries to avoid conflict, despite, the fact that conflict can be beneficial to both individuals and organisations (Cavanagh, 1991). In harmonious teams practitioners attempt to cope with work through ownership, by preventing individuals from sharing feelings, by avoiding conflict and by seeking support from colleagues, rather than through mutual and shared methods of working (Johns, 1992). Janis's (1972) 'groupthink' and Street's (1995) 'tyranny of niceness' are similar concepts. 'Groupthink' may therefore be a greater risk in groups where there are shared value systems, unless these values encompass ways of working which preserve adaptability in relation to a changing context. This latter feature endorses the dialectical principle that progress and development is dynamic and only occurs by constantly challenging, querying, criticising and breaking down parts of existing practice with the aim of reconstructing a new alternative which is believed not to contain the 'deficiencies and errors that can be identified with existing ones.' (Mogensen, 1997: 434). Denison (1990) recognises that consistency in values and beliefs can often oppose adaptability, but the presence of both is apparent in effective cultures. A therapeutic team (Benner, 1984; Johns, 1992) is the opposite of the 'harmonious' team: it reflects the healthy management of conflict, where new ideas can be raised and team members can be direct. The ability to challenge the status quo is essential for the focus on continuous improvement and for maintaining external adaptability (Denison, 1990) – or 'strategic appropriateness' – where the culture fits the environment (Kotter & Heskett, 1992).

- *Education and personal development* The fifth value emerging as recognised by co-researchers was that of education and personal development – necessary prerequisites for continuing adaptability. Education and development were valued and staff perceived more was invested in them, than they had ever experienced elsewhere.
- *The role of nursing* Nursing was seen within the unit to have a specific and deliberate contribution to make and was valued as something special, distinguishing the NDU from other ICUs.

This examination of espoused values and beliefs on the one hand, and those experienced in practice on the other, suggest that the culture-in-practice was congruent. Specific configurations of values are evident about person-centredness, providing support, enabling development, encouraging active participation and ensuring devolved decision-making.

Although there was evidence of shared meanings and a common mission, which provides an internalised system of control, such mechanisms can work against an effective workplace culture if they fail to recognise the need to respond to a changing environment. Continued challenge, and the recognition of different staff's opinions, are measures which go some way towards preventing this from occurring.

Sufficient evidence is provided to demonstrate the presence of all four of Denison's (1990) hypotheses characteristic of effective workplace cultures, namely:

- a sense of mission, which impacts on effectiveness by providing both meaning and direction;
- consistency, as reflected in the match between dominant belief systems and actions taken;
- adaptability which influences effectiveness through both internal flexibility and external focus;
- involvement within the unit culture which has an impact on effectiveness through both informal and formal structures.

Impact of the culture

The impact of this culture was particularly noticeable to the returners who identified appreciable changes between leaving and returning to the unit. Returners remarked on the paradox of being familiar with the culture even though many of the staff were different. This familiarity may be accounted for by the presence of a strong culture sustained during their period of absence. Dramatic changes were noted on their return across five areas:

- Increased amount of teaching and education – staff were perceived as taking responsibility for planning and auditing teaching events within the unit.
- The amount of development undertaken by everyone.
- Much greater involvement in developmental work, particularly by the more junior staff. Also initiatives and innovations previously talked about when they left were now up and running.
- The impact on teamwork.

• The differences in individuals, namely, their increased commitment and their willingness to take responsibility, which in turn was linked to being and feeling involved and empowered.

Involvement results in a shared common purpose and means of achieving that purpose (Denison, 1990; Brown, 1998), producing greater commitment (Denison, 1990) and high employee motivation (Levine, 1995; Brown, 1998). This is achieved through using practices that employees find more rewarding (Denison, 1990; Kotter & Heskett, 1992; Levine, 1995) and is associated with professional self-regulation rather than external control (Khandwalla, 1974) leading to the taking of greater responsibility.

Magnet hospital research demonstrates how increased role definition is associated with greater collegial working and autonomy, reflected in greater self-determination within the professional role (McClure *et al.*, 1983). The same research demonstrated a shift of power to nurses because staff became more confident in their own competencies and their values, which would no longer let them accept situations where they did not have a voice. Evidence is therefore provided, by the returners, of some of the changes which they perceived were linked to the culture. These included a sense of commitment and responsibility, of energy and excitement, as well as a sense of control: all characteristics or consequences of empowerment (Fay, 1987; Gibson, 1991; Rodwell, 1996).

Impact of culture on recruitment and retention

The culture of the unit was also linked to a positive influence on the recruitment and retention of staff. Many insiders had some knowledge of the unit prior to joining it, as agency nurses, through friends, or as course nurses who had chosen to work within the unit on completion of their course. Alternatively, recruited staff had read unit publications and were attracted to the values and beliefs espoused therein about nursing.

Recruitment and retention of nurses is linked to job satisfaction, but also to productivity and effectiveness, which can be compromised by continued staff instability (Hinshaw & Atwood, 1984). The practice of primary nursing enabled more meaningful relationships with patients to be formed and provided opportunities for increasing autonomy and responsibility, which subsequently influenced job satisfaction (Manley *et al.*, 1996).

The ICU/NDU therefore demonstrated a strong culture. Attributes of cultures linked with successful performance are also present,

namely: shared values and practices; staff feeling valued and supported as key stakeholders (Denison, 1990; Kotter and Heskett,
1992); participative and decentralised approaches (Cotton *et al.*,
1988; Ichniowski *et al.*, 1996); a focus on education and development
consistent with the attributes of learning organisations (Senge,
1990). A positive effect on recruitment and retention was also noted
in those magnet hospitals which demonstrated similar values
(Kramer, 1990; Aiken *et al.*, 1997).

This case study has provided some evidence to suggest that the
culture established within the NDU was transformational. First, the
culture of the NDU can be considered as strong. Values and beliefs
were consistently held in practice, the culture-in-practice was congruent with the espoused culture, and a specific combination of
values was evident.

In relation to facilitating cultural change, the contribution of two
processes has been recognised. The first is the use of values clarification to guide ways of working, future direction and the development of a common vision. The second is the role of highlighting
contradictions between espoused values and practice, thus enabling
an espoused culture to become a culture-in-practice. Such processes
had been actively and deliberately pursued. In addition, although
a strong culture has been demonstrated, it is known that a strong
culture alone is insufficient. A further specific configuration of
values focusing on 'whole systems' ways of working was also
evident. Features include participation, devolution, valuing individuals and promoting leadership at all levels, as well as adaptability and strategic appropriateness consistent with research on
organisational culture in commercial organisations and magnet
hospitals.

Finally, a number of outcome indicators have been alluded to
which support the link between effective cultures and outcomes.
These outcome indicators included a positive impact on recruitment
and retention, something also demonstrated in magnet hospital
research. There were also more traditional management quality
indicators, such as, reduced complaints and accident rates. The
informal feedback provided through relatives was positive and cost
comparisons were also favourable. Other outcomes relate to the
influence the unit had on the remainder of the organisation, sharing
and disseminating practices that have worked within the unit, and
also influencing the organisation's own culture. Outcomes for individual practitioners and the way they worked are summarised in
Chapter 5.

Transformational culture

The notion of transformational culture is a construct that describes the nature of an effective culture. It comprises three components, staff empowerment, practice development and a number of other workplace characteristics. It is proposed that the three outcomes are synonymous with a culture where effective (quality) patient care is delivered. Each has identified cultural indicators.

This understanding of what a transformational culture is for healthcare has emerged from a synthesis of the literature and an action research study linked to 12 years of researching how to enable staff to develop the quality of their service for patients through the role of a consultant nurse (Manley, 1997a; 2000a, b; 2001). The achievement of this culture is associated with key processes, contextual factors, as well as the knowledge, skills and expertise of a consultant nurse, as illustrated within Fig. 4.1 and Table 4.1. Although the framework relates to the consultant nurse role, it can be argued that the framework has relevance for all those interested in developing and sustaining a culture of effectiveness.

The cultural indicators developed have been informed by literature focusing on:

- corporate or organisational culture;
- nursing, health and education literature on staff empowerment and practice development;
- magnet hospital research.

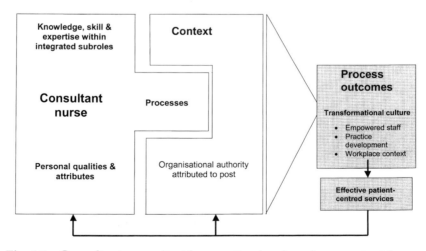

Fig. 4.1 Consultant nurse (insider practice developer): conceptual framework highlighting the relationship between outcomes (Manley, 2001).

Table 4.1 The consultant nurse's knowledge, skills, attributes and processes (NB the columns are not intended to be read across).

Knowledge, skills & expertise in integrated subroles ('know-how' & 'know that')	Personal qualities & attributes	Processes
Nursing practice as a generalist/specialist Research & evaluation in practice Practice development and the facilitation of structural, cultural and practice change Education & learning in practice Consultancy: clinical to organisational Management, leadership & strategic vision	Being patient-centred Being available, accessible, generous & flexible Being enthusiastic Being self-aware and attuned to others Being a collaborator and a catalyst Having a vision for nursing and healthcare Being a strategist and demonstrating political leadership Academic criteria	*Transformational leadership processes* Developing a shared vision Inspiring and communicating Valuing others Challenging and stimulating Developing trust Enabling *Processes of emancipation* Clarifying & working with values, beliefs & assumptions challenging contradictions Developing critical intent of individuals and groups Developing moral intent Focusing on the impact of the context/system on structural, cultural and practice change as well as on practice itself Using self-reflection and fostering reflection in others Enabling others to 'see the possibilities' Fostering widening participation and collaboration by all involved *Practising expertly in practice as a practitioner, researcher, educator, consultant and practice developer* Role modelling Facilitating individual, collective and organisational learning Facilitating change, practice and service development

Table 4.2 The components of a transformational culture and related cultural indicators.

Components of transformational culture	Cultural indicators
Staff empowerment	Continuing development of practice and self-knowledge Altered ways of working through self-knowledge Practitioners are self-energising and self-organising Staff have a clear sense of purpose Practitioners communicate freely, question, challenge and support each other Practitioners take responsibility for developing own practice and introducing innovation Formal & informal systems that foster critical thinking are evident
Practice development with its focus on developmental work patient-centredness and quality services	Patient-centred care is designed around the needs, concerns and experiences of patients/users Activity is focused directly on practice and how knowledge & skills are used in practice Activity at the patient/client interface matches activity at organisational and strategic interfaces Changes are evident within individuals and culture Teams are enabled to develop knowledge and skills The focus is on emancipatory change Evidence used to inform decision-making is drawn from policy (local to global), propositional knowledge, personal knowledge, craft knowledge, local theory and patient's own personal knowledge Evidence is also generated from practice through systematic and rigorous approaches at individual and collective levels
Workplace context	Quality is everyone's concern Espoused values & beliefs are realised in action A strategic fit between the environment, local, national, global policy (strategic appropriateness) Positive change is a way of life, constantly addressing & anticipating changing healthcare needs through adaptability & flexibility, internally and externally Decision-making is transparent, participative and democratic Staff participation is fundamental to the infrastructure & reflected in a spirit of shared governance A focus on developing the leadership potential of all staff All stakeholders are of value

Cultural indicators

The cultural indicators for each of the three components of a transformational culture are summarised in Table 4.2.

Espoused values and beliefs realised in action

Differences between espoused culture and the culture in-practice as experienced by employees accounts for the reason why so many organisational cultures appear confused and contradictory (Kilman & Saxton, 1983; Kilman *et al.*, 1986; Anthony, 1994; Brown, 1998). The potential power of an aligned and motivated group is relevant to a large number of institutions, as strong cultural norms make an organisation efficient (Kotter & Heskett, 1992). This is because everyone knows what is important and how things are done, which enables them to respond rapidly (Wallach, 1983). Strong cultures are influential in contributing to efficiency but are not necessarily always appropriate. Strong cultures can have powerful consequences, either positive or negative, as a strong set of values may not accommodate a changing environment (Kotter & Heskett, 1992). The case study above highlights a culture where the values espoused matched those experienced and this was linked to positive outcomes.

Leaders have been identified as expert in the promotion and protection of values (Peters & Waterman, 1982) with virtually all the best performing companies having a well defined set of guiding beliefs (usually in qualitative rather than quantitative terms). Excellent organisations have been linked with the specific values. Magnet hospitals in the United States, considered to provide a high quality of service, have also been found to have similarity with Peters and Waterman's criteria (Kramer & Schmalenberg, 1988a, b). Magnet hospitals embody 'a set of organizational attributes that nurses find desirable (and are also conducive to better patient care)' (Aiken *et al.*, 1994: 771). These organisational attributes appear similar to those found in effective organisations. The environment is supportive of staff and learning; a common mission is evident – that of providing quality patient care; individual nurses are valued as key stakeholders; and the presence of flexible work processes is suggested. In a follow-up study of magnet hospitals (Kramer & Hafner, 1989) further work was undertaken on core values. Four common values resulted:

- Respect for one another
- Competence and scholarship
- Quality of care through:

- creativity and innovation
- autonomy at the front line
- competence
- pride in self and work

- Cost-effectiveness

Kramer (1990) identified one hospital that valued 'hardiness', which was perceived as needed for dealing with change, uncertainty and creativity – an interesting finding, as adaptability has been identified as highly significant in cultures which sustain their effectiveness (Denison, 1990; Kotter & Heskett, 1992). Other values identified seem to capture mainly beliefs about how quality patient care is achieved rather than fundamental values. McClure *et al.* (1983), however, acknowledge, the importance of having a 'total picture' similar to Khandwalla's (1974) 'gestalt' as being a more potent determinant of effectiveness than single interventions.

The importance of enabling espoused values to become realised in practice, and the processes necessary to achieve this are not mentioned in magnet hospital research, neither is insight provided about the processes necessary to enable hospitals to become a magnet hospital.

Magnet hospitals are therefore considered to illustrate similar attributes to Peters & Waterman's (1982) companies of excellence (Kramer & Schmalenberg, 1988a, b) and this led to the claim that: 'An institutional culture with a set of basic core values is essential. It is necessary for hospitals to do a serious evaluation of what their core values are and how these core values are created and instilled' (Kramer & Schmalenberg, 1988b: 17).

Culture, then, is used explicitly for the first time in relation to magnet hospital research, whereas the importance of developing a value system shared by all employees for the purpose of maintaining stable nursing staffing was identified in 1983:

> Organisational values as determinants of organizational behaviour must therefore be considered in any hospital that seeks to maintain a stable nursing staff. A value system that is shared by all participants, from members of the board to every employee, may be one of the most crucial requirements for sound management in the changing health care agency of the future.
>
> (McClure *et al.*, 1983: 101)

Strategic appropriateness: fit with the environment

To be effective a culture must not only be efficient (the contribution made by strong cultures) but appropriate to the needs of the organisation and employees (Wallach, 1983). Kotter & Heskett (1992) introduce the concept of the 'strategically appropriate culture'. The theory proposes that cultures which fit with the environment, business or other appropriate organisation perform relatively better than those that do not. That is, only those that are contextually or strategically appropriate will be associated with excellent performance. The better the fit the better the performance. This theory is widely supported (Burns & Stalker, 1994; Schein, 1995).

The key concept in this theory is 'fit' (Kotter & Heskett, 1992). Gordon (1986) argues that there is not a 'one-size-fits-all' winning culture that works well anywhere, rather a culture is only good if it fits the context. Different contexts may need different cultures, or different cultures may serve different functions (Handy, 1993).

The context is constantly changing in healthcare, and similarly healthcare cultures may become dysfunctional if not dynamic. Hence the role of practice development, as a continuous process, must be both sensitive and adaptive to changes in local, national and global policy, local population profiles, and community trends (McCormack *et al.*, 1999).

Positive change as a way of life: internal and external adaptability and flexibility

A positive approach towards change is associated with adaptability and flexibility internally and externally, reflected often through innovation. Adaptive culture theory proposes that only cultures that can help workplaces anticipate and adapt to environmental change will be associated with superior performance over a long period (Denison, 1990; Kotter & Heskett, 1992).

Denison (1990) states that non-adaptive cultures are bureaucratic, people are reactive, risk averse, uncreative, and information flows slowly and with difficulty through the organisation. Whereas an adaptive culture:

> entails risk-taking, trusting, and proactive approach to organisational as well as individual life. Members actively support one another's efforts to identify all problems and implement work solutions. There is a shared feeling of confidence: the members believe, without a doubt, that they can effectively manage whatever new problems and opportunities will come their way. There is widespread enthusiasm, a spirit of doing whatever it takes to achieve organizational success. The members are receptive to change and innovation.
>
> (Kilman, 1986: 356)

Kanter (1983) argues that this kind of culture values and encourages entrepreneurship which in turn can help adaptation by allowing it to identify and exploit new opportunities. Kotter & Heskett (1992) stress leadership rather than entrepreneurship is the force for change, arguing that the primary function of leadership is to produce change and if the culture encourages this there will be a great deal of risk-taking, use of initiative, communication and motivation as the aim is to produce a culture that can deal with a changing world – all characteristics of transformational leadership.

Developing leadership potential of all staff

The single most visible factor that distinguishes successful cultural change is competent leadership in both commercial organisations (Kotter & Heskett, 1992; Schein, 1995) and magnet hospital research: 'When all is said and done, probably the one essential *sine qua non* of a culture of excellence is the quality of the leadership' (Kramer, 1990: 43).

Although ideas and solutions that become embedded in a culture can originate from an individual, or a group, at the bottom of the organisation or the top, in the firms with strong corporate cultures, these ideas were often associated with a founder or other early leaders who articulated them as a 'vision', a 'business strategy', a philosophy or all three (Kotter, 1990). However, in magnet hospitals decentralised and flattened management structures enabled power to be vested in the staff that are interacting with patients.

Bate (1984) argues vehemently that leadership is not an individual but a collective activity, with limitations on what any one person may achieve because culture is a social not an individual phenomenon. It is a system of collective enterprise, which spreads throughout the organisation. This view of culture is consistent with the concept of transformational leadership (Kouzes & Posner, 1987), an approach which fosters leadership potential at all levels of the organisation with everyone using processes underpinned by the same values necessary for successful cultural change. It is proposed that through using these processes, and participative and facilitative methods, together with a context of shared values and beliefs, a transformational culture can be collectively achieved, one that promotes effectiveness, and is adaptable and strategically appropriate.

The role of leadership, then, in achieving cultural change is indisputable, with successful leadership being defined as the ability to bring about sustained cultural change (Allen & Kraft, 1987). Thus the leadership approach needs to encompass the development of the leadership potential of all staff.

All key stakeholders are valued

The purpose and direction of leadership in the most highly performing organisations is linked to cultures that place a high value on all key stakeholders – not just customers, and leadership at all levels. Kotter & Heskett's (1992) research showed consistent findings through focusing on and caring about key stakeholders, whoever they were.

Valuing everyone's contribution is a transformational leadership characteristic; providing opportunities through formal participation is another. Bellman (1998) in her action research study of nurse-led change highlighted the importance of ensuring stakeholder feedback as a strategy for promoting nurse empowerment.

Staff participation is fundamental

Formal mechanisms to enable staff participation are proposed as the foundation of a transformational culture. Approaches, however, need to be whole systems and owned by staff to achieve positive outcomes, rather than short term or tokenistic (Cotton *et al.*, 1988; Wagner, 1994).

Increased innovation, increased responsibility and autonomy are manifestations of whole systems approaches or workplace cultures which foster comprehensive involvement and participation of staff (Khandwalla, 1974; Cotton *et al.*, 1988; Levine, 1995). They are also evident in the decentralised approaches of magnet hospitals (McClure *et al.*, 1983; Aiken *et al.*, 1998), and in those workplace cultures which are considered highly effective (Denison, 1990; Kotter & Heskett, 1992).

Shared governance and the provision of quality services has been linked to the empowerment of nurses (Thrasher *et al.*, 1992; Geoghegan & Farrington, 1995; Mitchell & Brooks, 1999) and is a formal system of organisation where practitioners – rather than managers – participate in, and are responsible for, the decision-making which influences and governs clinical practice (Manley, 1998). It is an accountability model which requires decision-making to occur at the point of care (Porter O'Grady, 1994), and is concerned with all components of patient care (Scott, 1999). Shared governance is associated with certain values and beliefs (Manley, 1998), but the term 'clinical governance' promoted by government policy linked with clinical effectiveness (DoH, 1997), and increasing individual accountability (DoH, 1998), tends to emphasise structures (Manley, 1998). Nevertheless, the RCN argue that clinical governance is about helping clinical staff to continuously improve quality and safeguard standards of care (RCN, 1998; 2000).

Decision-making is transparent, participative, and democratic

Decision-making would be transparent, open to challenge, involvement and debate, but also arising from a process of critique manifested in a readiness to share rationales for decision-making.

Quality is everyone's concern

A transformational culture is one where all staff take responsibility for the quality of service they provide through continuing to maintain their own effectiveness. The quality of the service provided individually and collectively to users would therefore be everyone's concern and reflected in their daily work.

Staff empowerment

Staff empowerment is the second component of a transformational culture. Five cultural indicators were derived from: Fay's (1987) definition of empowerment and two concept analyses (Gibson, 1991; Rodwell, 1996). These indicators were evident in my own research (Manley, 2001). Empowerment is understood as an enabling and motivating resource (Fay, 1987); it is both a process and an outcome (Gibson, 1991).

Continuing development of self-knowledge

A focus on continual development as a process and outcome of staff development is linked specifically to continually increasing one's self-knowledge, articulated in critical science as enlightenment (Fay, 1987), 'consciousness-raising' (Habermas, 1972), or 'conscientisation' (Freire, 1972).

Evidence that self-knowledge has developed (Fay, 1987) would arise from practitioners' own perceptions of how their self-knowledge had changed them, as individuals and practitioners, and the way they worked.

Central to critical social theory are the problems that arise in everyday life and the acknowledgement that barriers need to be removed if problems are to be solved (Carr & Kemmis, 1986). This requires transformed social action that arises from enlightenment (Fay, 1987). This occurs when practitioners freely commit to action; are involved in a democratic process where they can speak openly and freely; where their action is authentic with self-deception minimised through group critique; and, where decision-making is guided by rational arguments for different courses of action, not by considerations of power.

Continuing development due to increased self-knowledge results in empowerment (Fay, 1987). Enlightenment, an antecedent to empowerment, involves identifying taken for granted aspects in everyday life, working through consciousness-raising to make them obvious (Mezirow, 1981; Fay, 1987). Emancipation follows (Fay, 1987), and is realised in action which is informed and meaningful, and based on critical insights, reflection and dialogue (Stevens, 1989), not 'wishful thinking' (description of reflection and enlightenment without action) (Freire, 1972). Processes that are associated with fostering enlightenment, emancipation and action competence (Mogensen, 1997) are those of critical reflection (Carr & Kemmis, 1986), social critique (Habermas, 1979), critical thinking (Mogensen, 1997), perspective transformation (Mezirow, 1981), 'guided structured reflection' (Johns, 1995), clinical supervision (Manley & McCormack, 1997) and action learning (McGill & Beaty, 1997) which aim to develop self-knowledge (Fay, 1987) and understanding about the structures that constrain action (Habermas, 1979). Habermas (1974) considers self reflection or 'reflexivity' a characteristic of being human, one which enables a capability for developing insight into one's history as individuals and members of society, as well as ways of changing this course. The processes used to foster enlightenment and emancipation are the processes of enablement (Fay, 1987) rather than command, or 'power over' (Hawks, 1991).

The critique of theoretical concepts, fundamental values, interest-based elements, power, dominance, oppression, and conflict can lead individuals to feel pessimistic and powerless to resist or change the systems in which they work (Mogensen, 1997). Giroux (1988) therefore argues for the need to generate knowledge that enables people to become empowered through seeing the possibilities – a language of possibility, a vision of what is possible or how things can be. Critical thinking encompasses such visionary thinking and thus the ability to imagine alternatives and propose possible courses of action (Mogensen, 1997). Critical thinking and emancipation are inextricably linked; both may lead to transformation at different levels (Mogensen, 1997). At the individual level this may manifest itself in changed attitudes, values and behaviour; at the structural level, this may be seen in changed social, political and organisational structures.

Emancipation, then, is found when groups or individuals act from empowerment through new found self-understanding, radically altering their social arrangements (Carr & Kemmis, 1986; Fay, 1987).

Radically altered ways of working through self-knowledge
Within the earlier case study, staff radically altered their ways of working through self-knowledge, demonstrated through the

development of an infrastructure that enabled staff's values and beliefs about nursing and participation to be realised. The organisational approach led to small team working which resulted also in greater support for staff and paved the way for focusing on team function and effectiveness, a core component of learning organisations (Senge, 1990).

The inter-team projects arose from values and beliefs about staff, their participation and individual responsibility and had enabled an infrastructure of shared governance to evolve, one that reflected a shared responsibility and accountability for providing services to patients through formal decentralisation and whole systems approaches to participation (Cotton *et al.*, 1988; Wagner, 1994). Radical restructuring of clinical practice has resulted from similar changes in nurses' understandings and actions in other action research studies (Street, 1995; Bellman, 1998).

Self-energising and self-organising practitioners

From the case study, evidence that practitioners were self-energising, and organised themselves (Fay, 1987) was seen in practitioners' own descriptions of greater confidence, self mastery, enthusiasm, a sense of pride, and seeing the possibilities for their own contribution as an individual and as a nurse (Manley, 2001), and also in having a vision of nursing, something not experienced before. All contributed to a positive sense of self-esteem, hope and excitement. These are consequences of empowerment (Gibson, 1991; Rodwell, 1996) accounted for by the attributes – freedom to make choices and accepting responsibility (Rodwell, 1996) – for developing their own practice and introducing innovation. Such attributes require a context where democratic ways of working pervade.

A sense of mastery is a factor in Gibson's (1991) empowerment model in relation to client–nurse relationships. Rodwell (1996) recognises positive self-esteem as a consequence of empowerment. Personal mastery is about the ability to continually deepen and clarify one's own personal vision and learning (Senge, 1990), an active process requiring commitment to lifelong learning. It is linked to becoming aware of one's own 'mental models' (for example, values, beliefs and personal theories), and how they influence one's decision-making, similar to Mezirow's construct of perspective transformation – the product of his reflective process (Mezirow, 1981), or as a component of critical thinking (Mogensen, 1997).

Personal mastery and mental models relate to knowing one's vision and how one makes decisions that continually evolve

72

reflexively through learning. Both are prerequisites to developing a learning organisation (Senge, 1990). The processes that enable self-mastery and knowing one's mental models are those that focus on increasing self-awareness, enlightenment and raising consciousness. These processes focus not just on how individuals act but also the impact of the system on how one acts – a tenet of critical social science. Social systems contribute to dominant processes and power structures and critical social science highlights how such systems inhibit action and greater effectiveness (Carr & Kemmis, 1986). Critical social science fosters the identification of the factors and power dynamics that frustrate action and increase awareness of how as individuals we act in response. Only then can individuals move towards empowerment and emancipation through action (Fay, 1987). Formal or informal systems of clinical supervision (RCN, 1999), action learning, or accessing the help of a critical companion (Titchen, 2000), or a critical friend (Carr & Kemmis, 1986) can all help individuals and groups to achieve such change through mechanisms that foster personal critique, provide high challenge and high support, and reduce self-deception (Habermas, 1974).

New sense of purpose, and knowing that purpose

A renewed sense of purpose suggests empowerment (Fay, 1987). This can be reflected by practitioners implementing their own ideas, taking more responsibility and being more autonomous in their work. Such changes have also been present in studies examining 'whole systems' approaches to participation (Ichniowski *et al.*, 1996), reflected in formal structures of participation rather than just paying 'lip-service' (Wagner, 1994).

Practitioners communicate freely, question and challenge each other

Evidence that staff's opinions are valued and welcomed, and that staff can communicate freely (Harden, 1996) is a key indicator. Waterman (1994) noted that where nurses perceived they had the power to change practice, they were more successful. In the first study of magnet hospitals McClure *et al.* (1983) also demonstrated a shift in the balance of power related to nurses' increasing confidence and competence.

For Fay (1987), power has both negative and positive connotations. As Freire (1972) points out the characteristics of oppressed groups stem from the ability of dominant groups to identify their norms and values as the right ones in subordinate groups. This is recognised where nurses perceive they lack autonomy, accountability and control over their own profession (Harden, 1996).

73

Oppression is achieved through domination that is most complete, when it is not recognised (Freire, 1972), for example where ideology serves to hide the interests of the dominant groups themselves (Harvey, 1990).

Essentially then people cannot *be* empowered, they have to empower themselves (Gibson, 1991). Emancipated nurses enable emancipated patients (Newham & Howie, 1996).

Practice development

Practice development is the third component of a transformational culture. It can be understood as eclectically drawing on diverse disciplines, thus providing the mechanism for integrating all professional functions for the benefit of patients (Manley, 1997b). It is a prerequisite to clinical effectiveness, continuous quality improvement and development of a culture that facilitates the responsive and proactive action necessary for effective healthcare (Manley, 1997b). Practice development therefore concerns all the activities necessary to achieve quality patient services and also includes the nurturing of innovation in the practice setting (Knight, 1994; Manley, 1997a).

There are nine cultural indicators for practice development, six derived from the concept analysis undertaken by Garbett & McCormack (2002) and expanded further elsewhere (Manley, 2001) (see Chapter 3):

- A focus on emancipatory change
- Changes are evident within individuals and culture
- Needs of service users are the focus of continuous developmental work
- Patient care designed around the needs, concerns and experience of the patient
- Teams are enabled to develop knowledge and skills
- Systematic and rigorous processes of investigation, action and evaluation

Three further cultural indicators of practice development include (Manley, 2001):

- a direct focus and impact on practice – rather than focusing on professional development which may or may not indirectly impact on practice;
- the use of diverse but transparent sources of evidence to inform decision-making in practice and which also involves generating evidence reflexively from practice. These are drawn from:

- research-based evidence which would encompass technical, practical and emancipatory knowledge constitutive interests (Habermas, 1974);
- client preferences and their personal knowing;
- clinical judgement/expertise evident in personal knowing and craft knowledge (Titchen, 2000), and praxis reflexively achieved through processes such as structured reflection, critical dialogue;
- local theory – reflecting the characteristics of the specific context and its impact on practice;

- the need to match organisational and strategic activity with activity at the patient/client interface (McCormack *et al.*, 1999).

A culture is described as transformational because it results from transformation processes evident within transformational leadership and emancipatory processes (Table 4.1). Additionally, transformation culture also describes the key attribute of continuous positive change and adaptation internally and externally in response to a changing environment – a discriminating factor essential for sustained effectiveness. Formal participatory mechanisms, a strong culture with a set of specific values around patient-centredness, development of leadership potential in all staff, and a valuing of all key stakeholders, staff empowerment and practice development would also be present.

Cultural change processes

> The pursuit of cultural change is deemed to be synonymous with the pursuit if excellence and therefore of unquestioned utility.
> (Anthony, 1994: 4)

Major cultural change does not happen easily or quickly (Kotter & Heskett, 1992). There is little agreement about how long cultural change takes except that it takes years rather than months (Williams *et al.*, 1993). It is a slow process that can be assisted rather than controlled (Anthony, 1994).

Transformational leadership is argued as influential in developing a transformational culture, but so too, is the use of specific processes such as: values clarification (Warfield & Manley, 1990; Manley, 1992); formal systems for critique and reflection; and the facilitation of others through role modelling and facilitation in the workplace (Table 4.1).

Schein (1985) proposes that an organisational leaders' beliefs can be transformed into collective beliefs through the medium of values and that eventually such values become basic assumptions because they may be seen to work reliably and then become taken for granted. The specific mechanisms through which leaders achieved action (Kotter, 1990) have been identified as:

- Creating a perceived need to change
- Clarifying their vision of what change was needed
- Challenging the status quo but marshalling evidence to support this
- Communicating a new vision in words and deeds
- Motivating many others to provide the leadership to implement the vision

Phillips and Kennedy (1980) demonstrated that leadership in excellent companies was more about success in instilling values than having a charismatic personality. However, other researchers argue that leadership is more than this, it is about facilitating the type of culture that people want to work in (Ichniowski *et al.*, 1996). As Bate (1994) states, leaders cannot control or manipulate the culture – they can only initiate, influence and shape the direction as it emerges. Cultural leadership is about 'helping to create or develop a particular way of life (form) and way of living (process) for an organisation and its members' (Bate, 1994: 237).

Summary

The focus on culture has led to the exploration of a new area of literature, that concerns workplace culture. Transformational culture is presented here as a new construct comprising a number of attributes derived from research undertaken on organisational and corporate culture in commercial settings, but enhanced by similar findings found in magnet hospitals and my own research at the unit level. Magnet hospital research has begun to recognise the role of culture but its impetus has mainly been on organisational structure as a variable in relation to nursing outcomes such as retention of staff, and latterly, indicators of effectiveness. Later magnet hospital research has recognised a number of similar attributes to Peters and Waterman's work on excellent companies. However, the criticisms of Peters and Waterman's work, as for other theories promoting strong cultures, and specific combination of values, is that this does not guarantee sustainability of an effective culture. The work of Denison (1990) and Kotter & Heskett (1992), in particular, has recognised the additional attributes that are required. These are the maintenance of a close fit with the environment – termed 'strategic appropriateness', and also, adaptability. Consequently I have argued that the attributes which characterise transformational culture are practice development, staff empowerment and the following workplace characteristics:

- Shared values and practices
- Adaptable, reflected by the presence of a learning culture
- Strategically appropriate
- Value stakeholders (this includes customers and employees)
- Value effective leadership at all levels – a characteristic of transformational leadership (Kouzes & Posner, 1987)

In effective cultures, staff will be empowered and practice develops to enable a constant fit between the environment and the culture to be maintained through adaptability and learning.

One of the attributes of effective cultures is the valuing of leadership at all levels. This is a characteristic of transformational leadership which focuses on creating a culture where everyone can be a leader (Manley, 1997a). To create such a culture requires leadership in the initiation phase and thereafter. Bate reminds us that 'culture is socially created, socially maintained and socially transformed' (Bate, 1994: 239) and that:

> It follows that all leaders can do is create the conditions for the potential energy and momentum already present in the system to be released, and then try to do something constructive with it. Their role is therefore not one of manipulation but facilitation, not because this is ethically more correct (which it certainly is), but because it cannot be otherwise.
>
> (Bate, 1994: 244–5)

References

Aiken, L.H., Sloane, D.M. & Klocinski, J.L. (1997) Hospital nurses' occupational exposure to blood: prospective, retrospective, and institutional reports. *American Journal of Public Health*, **87**(1), 103–7.

Aiken, L.H., Sloane, D.M. & Sochalski, J. (1998) Hospital organisation and outcomes. *Quality in Health Care*, **7**, 222–6.

Aiken, L.H., Smith, H.L. & Lake, E.T. (1994) Lower medicare mortality among a set of hospitals known for good nursing care. *Medical Care*, **32**(8), 771–87.

Allen, R.F. & Kraft, C. (1987) *The Organizational Unconscious*. Human Resources Institute, Morristown, NJ.

Anthony, P. (1994) *Managing Culture*. Open University, Buckingham.

Baker, E. (1980) Managing organizational culture. *Management Review*, July, 8–13.

Bate, P. (1994) *Strategies for Cultural Change*. Butterworth-Heinemann, Oxford.

Bellman, L. (1998) *Exploring Nurse-led Change and Development in Clinical Practice Through Critical Action Research*. Unpublished PhD thesis, Cranfield University School of Management.

Benner, P. (1984) *From Novice to Expert: Excellence and Power in Clinical Nursing Practice*. Addison-Wesley, Menlo Park, CA.

Bolan, D.S. & Bolan, D.S. (1994) A reconceptualization and analysis of organizational culture: the influence of groups and their idiocultures. *Journal of Managerial Psychology*, **9**(5), 22–7.

Brown, A. (1998) *Organisational Culture*, 2nd edn. Financial Times/Pitman Publishing, London.

Burns, T. & Stalker, G.M. (1994) *The Management of Innovation*. Oxford University Press, Oxford.

Carr, W. & Kemmis, S. (1986) *Becoming Critical: Education, Knowledge and Action Research*. London, The Falmer Press.

Cavanagh, S.J. (1991) The conflict management style of staff nurses and nurse managers. *Journal of Clinical Nursing*, **16**(10), 1254–60.

Cotton, J.L., Vollrath, D.A., Froggatt, K.L., Lengnick-Hall, M.L. & Jennings, K.R. (1988) Employee participation: diverse forms and different outcomes. *Academy of Management Review*, **13**(1), 8–22.

Denison, D. (1990) *Corporate Culture and Organizational Effectiveness*. John Wiley, New York.

Department of Health (DoH) (1997) *The New NHS: Modern, Dependable*. HMSO, London.

Department of Health (DoH) (1998) *A First Class Service: Quality in the New NHS London*. The Stationery Office, London.

Department of Health (DoH) (2000) *The NHS Plan*. The Stationery Office, London.

Drennan, D. (1992) *Transforming Company Culture*. McGraw-Hill, London.

Fay, B. (1987) *Critical Social Science: Liberation and Its Limits*. Polity Press, Cambridge.

Flood, A.B. (1994) The impact of organizational and managerial factors on the quality of care in health care organizations. *Medical Care Review*, **51**(4), 381–428.

Freire, P. (1972) *Pedagogy of the Oppressed*. Herder & Herder, New York.

Garbett, R. & McCormack, B. (2002) A concept analysis of practice development. *Nursing Times Research*, **7**(2), 87–100.

Geoghegan, J. & Farrington, A. (1995) Shared governance: developing a British model. *British Journal of Nursing*, **4**(13), 780–3.

Gibson, C.H. (1991) A concept analysis of empowerment. *Journal of Advanced Nursing*, **16**, 354–61.

Giroux, H.A. (1988) *Teachers as Intellectuals: Toward a Critical Pedagogy of Learning*. Critical Studies in Education series. Bergin & Garvey, Granby, MA.

Goodman, P.S. & Pennings, J.M. (1977) *New Perspectives on Organizational Effectiveness*. Jossey–Bass, San Francisco, CA.

References

Gordon, G. (1986) The relationship of corporate culture to industry sector and corporate performance. In: *Gaining Control of the Corporate Culture* (eds R.H. Kilmann, M.J. Saxton & R. Serpa), pp. 103–25. Jossey-Bass, San Francisco, CA.

Gregory, K.L. (1983) Native-view paradigms: multiple cultures and culture conflicts in organizations. *Administrative Science Quarterly*, **28**, 359–76.

Grundy, S. (1982) Three modes of action research. *Curriculum Perspectives*, **2**(3), 23–34.

Habermas, J. (1972) *Knowledge and Human Interests*, trans J.J. Shapiro. Heinemann, London.

Habermas, J. (1974) *Theory and Practice*, trans J. Viertel. Heinemann, London.

Habermas, J. (1979) *Communication and the Evolution of Society*, trans T. McCarthy. Beacon Press, Boston.

Handy, C. (1993) *Understanding Organisations* (4th edn). Penguin, Harmondsworth.

Harden, J. (1996) Enlightenment, empowerment and emancipation: the case for critical pedagogy in nurse education. *Nurse Education Today*, **16**, 32–7.

Harvey, L. (1990) *Critical Social Science*, Unwin Hyman, London.

Hawks, J. (1991) Power: a concept analysis. *Journal of Advanced Nursing*, **16**, 754–62.

Hinshaw, A.A. & Atwood, J.R. (1984) Nursing staff turnover, stress and satisfaction: models, measures and management. In: *Annual Review of Nursing Research* (eds H.H. Werley & J.J. Fitzpatrick), vol. 1, pp. 133–53. Springer, New York.

Hofsteede, G., Nneuijen, B., Ohayv, D. & Sanders, G. (1990) Measuring organizational cultures: a qualitative study across twenty cases. *Administrative Science Quarterly*, **35**, 286–316.

Ichniowski, C., Kochan, D.L., Olson, C. & Strauss, G. (1996) What works at work: overview and assessment. *Industrial Relations*, **35**(3), 299–333.

Janis, I.L. (1972) *Victims of Groupthink*. Houghton Mifflin, Boston.

Johns, C. (1992) Ownership and the harmonious team. *Journal of Clinical Nursing*, **1**(2), 89–94.

Johns, C. (1995) Achieving effective work as a professional activity. In: *Towards Advanced Nursing Practice: Key Concepts for Health Care*. (eds J.E. Schober & S.M. Hinchliff), pp. 252–80. Arnold, London.

Kanter, R.M. (1983) *The Change Masters: Corporate entrepreneurs at work*. Unwin, London.

Kennedy, I. (Chairman) (2001) *Learning from Bristol: The Report of the Public Inquiry into Children's Heart Surgery at the Bristol Royal Infirmary 1984–1995*. Department of Health, London.

Khandwalla, P.N. (1974) Mass output orientation of operations technology and organizational structure. *Administrative Science Quarterly*, **19**, 74–97.

Kilman, R.H. (1986) Five steps for closing culture gaps. In: *Gaining Control of the Corporate Culture* (eds R.H. Kilmann, M.J. Saxton & R. Serpa), pp. 351–69. Jossey-Bass, San Francisco, CA.

Kilman, R.H. & Saxton, M.J. (1983) *The Kilman-Saxton Culture Gap Survey.* Organization Design Consultants, Pittsburgh, PA.

Kilman, R.H., Saxton, M.J. & Serpa, R. (1986) *Gaining Control of the Corporate Culture.* Jossey-Bass, San Francisco, CA.

Knight, S. (1994) An organisational approach. *Nursing Standard,* **90**(41), 33–5.

Kotter, J.P. (1990) *A Force for Change: How Leadership Differs from Management.* Free Press, New York.

Kotter, J.P. & Heskett, J.L. (1992) *Corporate Culture and Performance.* The Free Press, New York.

Kouzes, J.M. & Posner, B.Z. (1987) *The Leadership Challenge.* Jossey-Bass, San Francisco, CA.

Kramer, M. (1990) The magnet hospitals: excellence revisited. *Journal of Nursing Administration,* **20**(9), 35–44.

Kramer, M. & Hafner, L. (1989) Shared values: impact on staff nurse job satisfaction and perceived productivity. *Nursing Research,* **89:38**(3), 172–7.

Kramer, M. & Schmalenberg, C. (1988a) Magnet hospitals: institutions of excellence, Part 1. *Journal of Nursing Administration,* **18**(1), 13–24.

Kramer, M. & Schmalenberg, C. (1988b) Magnet hospitals: institutions of excellence, Part 2. *Journal of Nursing Administration,* **18**(2), 11–9.

Levine, D.I. (1995) *Reinventing the workplace: how business and employees can both win.* Brookings Institution, Washington, DC.

Lorsch, J.W. (1986) Managing culture: the invisible barrier to strategic change. *California Management Review,* **28**(2), 95–109.

Louis, M.R. (1980) Organizations as culture-bearing milieux. In: *Organizational Symbolism* (eds L.R. Pondy, P.J. Frost, G. Morgan & T.C. Dandridge) JAI press, Greenwich, CT.

Louis, M.R. (1986) Sourcing workplace cultures: why, when, and how. In: *Gaining Control of the Corporate Culture* (eds R.H. Kilmann, M.J. Saxton & R. Serpa), pp. 126–36. Jossey-Bass, San Francisco, CA.

Lundberg, C. (1985) On the feasibility of cultural intervertions in organisations. In: *Organisational Culture* (eds P.J. Frost, L.F. Moore, M.R. Louis), pp. 169–85. Sage, Beverly Hills, CA.

McClure, M., Poulin, M., Sovie, M. & Wandelt, M. (1983) Magnet hospitals: attraction and retention of professional nurses. *American Academy of Nursing: Taskforce on Nursing Practice in Hospitals,* Kansas City.

McCormack, B., Manley, K., Kitson, A., Titchen, A. & Harvey, G. (1999) Towards practice development – a vision in reality or a reality without vision? *Journal of Nursing Management,* **7**(2), 255–64.

McGill, I. & Beaty, L. (1997) *Action Learning.* Kogan Page, London.

Manley, K. (1997a) A conceptual framework for advanced practice: an action research project operationalising an advanced practitioner/consultant nurse role. *Journal of Clinical Nursing,* **6**(2), 179–90.

Manley, K. (1997b) Practice development: a growing and significant movement. *Nursing in Critical Care,* **2**(1), 5.

Manley, K. (1998) Shared clinical governance. *Nursing In Critical Care,* **3**(2), 57–8.

References

Manley, K. (2000a) Organisational culture and consultant nurse outcomes. Part 1: organisational culture. *Nursing Standard*, **14**(36), 34–8.

Manley, K. (2000b) Organisational culture and consultant nurse outcomes. Part 2: consultant nurse outcomes. *Nursing Standard*, **14**(37), 34–9.

Manley, K. (2001) *Consultant nurse: concept, processes, outcomes.* Unpublished PhD thesis, University of Manchester/RCN Institute, London.

Manley, K., Cruse, S. & Keogh, S. (1996) Job satisfaction of intensive care nurses practising primary nursing and a comparison with those practising total patient care. *Nursing in Critical Care*, **1**(1), 31–41.

Manley, K., Hamill, J.M. & Hanlon, M. (1997) Nursing staff's perceptions and experiences of primary nursing practice in intensive care four years on. *Journal of Clinical Nursing*, **6**, 277–87.

Manley, K. & McCormack, B. (1997) *Exploring Expert Practice (NUM 65u).* MSc Nursing module: Distance Learning. RCN Institute, London.

Meek, V.L. (1988) Organizational culture: origins and weaknesses. *Organizational Studies*, **9**(4), 453–73.

Mezirow, J. (1981) A critical theory of adult learning and education. *Adult Education*, **32**(1), 3–24.

Mitchell, M. & Brooks, F. (1999) Balancing nurse empowerment with improved practice and care: an evaluation of the impact of shared governance. *Nursing Times Research*, **4**(3), 192–200.

Mogensen, F. (1997) Critical thinking: a central element in developing action competence in health and environmental education. *Health Education Research: Theory and practice*, **12**(4), 429–36.

Morgan, G. (1986) *Images of Organization.* Sage, Thousand Oaks, CA.

Newham, C. & Howie, A. (1996) Reflection on a patient receiving high frequency oscillatory therapy. *Nursing in Critical Care*, **1**(1), 31–41.

Pacanowsky, M.E. & O'Donnell-Trujillo, N. (1982) Communication and organizational culture. *The Western Journal of Speech Communication*, **46**(Spring), 115–30.

Peters, T.J. & Waterman, R.H. (1982) *In Search of Excellence.* New York, Harper & Row.

Phillips, J.R. & Kennedy, A.A. (1980) Shaping and managing shared values. *McKinsey Staff Paper*, December.

Porter O'Grady, T. (1994) Whole systems, shared governance: creating the seamless organisation. *Nursing Economics*, **12**(4), 187–95.

Rodwell, C.M. (1996) An analysis of the concept of empowerment. *Journal of Advanced Nursing*, **23**, 305–13.

Royal College of Nursing (RCN) (1998) *RCN Information: guidance for nurses on clinical governance.* RCN, London.

Royal College of Nursing (RCN) (1999) *Realising Clinical Effectiveness and Clinical Governance Through Clinical Supervision.* Radcliffe Medical Press Ltd, Oxford.

Royal College of Nursing (RCN) (2000) *Clinical Governance: How Nurses can get Involved.* RCN, London.

Savage, J. (2000) The culture of 'culture' in National Health Service policy implementation. *Nursing Inquiry*, **7**(4), 230.

Schein, E.H. (1985) *Organizational Culture and Leadership*, 2nd edn. Jossey-Bass, San Francisco, CA.

Schein, E.H. (1995) Process consultation, action research and clinical inquiry: are they the same? *Journal of Managerial Psychology*, **10**(6), 14–19.

Scott, I. (1999) Clinical governance: an opportunity for nurses to influence the future of healthcare development. *Nursing Times Research*, **4**(3), 170–6.

Senge, P.M. (1990) *The Fifth Discipline: The Art and Practice of the Learning Organisation*. Doubleday Currency, New York.

Smircich, L. (1983) Concepts of culture and organizational analysis. *Administrative Science Quarterly*, **28**, 339–58.

Stevens, P.E. (1989) A critical social reconceptualization of environment in nursing: implications for methodology. *Advances in Nursing Science*, **4**(1), 56–68.

Street, A. (1995) *Nursing Replay*. Churchill Livingstone, Melbourne.

Thrasher, T., Bossman, V.M., Carroll, S., *et al.* (1992) Empowering the clinical nurse through quality assurance in a shared governance setting. *Journal of Nursing Care Quality*, **6**(2), 15–19.

Titchen, A. (2000) *Professional Craft Knowledge in Patient-centred Nursing and the Facilitation of its Development*. University of Oxford DPhil thesis. Ashdale Press, Oxford.

Van Maanen, J. & Barley, S.R. (1985) Cultural organization: fragments of a theory. In: *Organizational Culture* (ed. P.J. Frost), pp. 31–53. Sage Publications, Newbury Park CA.

Wagner, J.A. (1994) Participation's effects on performance and satisfaction: a reconsideration of research evidence. *Academy of Management Review*, **19**(2), 312–30.

Wallach, E.J. (1983) Individuals and organizations: the cultural match. *Training and Development Journal*, February, pp. 29–36.

Warfield, C. & Manley, K. (1990) Developing a new philosophy in the NDU. *Nursing Standard*, **4**(41), 27–30.

Waterman, H. (1994) *Meaning of visual impairment: developing ophthalmic nursing care*. Unpublished PhD thesis, University of Manchester, Faculty of Medicine, Manchester.

Williams, A., Dobson, P. & Walters, M. (1993) *Changing Culture, New Organisational Approaches*, (2nd edn.) Institute of Personnel Management, London.

5. Evaluating Practice Developments

Brendan McCormack and Kim Manley (with a contribution from Val Wilson)

Introduction

In this chapter we aim to explore a variety of approaches to evaluating practice developments. The chapter will include consideration of appropriate methodologies that are consistent with how practice development is talked about and understood in this book. The chapter does not provide a list of data collection methods as details of these are provided in most research methods textbooks that are freely available. However, it has already been identified that 'participation' is central to practice development work and thus working with participatory principles will be explored from the perspective of data collection. The chapter will primarily focus on the meaning of 'effectiveness' in a practice development context and how it works at individual, team, organisational and strategic levels. The chapter will end with the development of an 'evaluation checklist' for practice development.

What is evaluation?

Evaluation is said to refer to the everyday occurrence of making judgements of worth. Making evaluative judgements is a normal part of our everyday lives. For nurses, making evaluative judgements is central to being a professional and reflective practitioner (Schön, 1991). The development of nursing theories made explicit the role of the nurse in evaluating the effectiveness of patient care and is a core component of the 'nursing process'. Among nurses who demonstrate expertise in their practice, evaluation is integral to everyday decisions and actions. It is deeply interwoven with 'knowing the patient'; a 'holistic practical knowing' that constantly influences the nurse's judgements; a sense of saliency (that is, an ability to determine what is pertinent in a situation linked to the most relevant action); but always within a patient–nurse relationship that preserves the dignity and personhood of the patient.

We engage in such evaluation in our everyday personal and professional lives. However, when we think about practice development, we recognise that for the most part, we are engaged in a formalised programme of activities, with the purpose of increasing effectiveness in patient-centred practice, i.e. a programme of development work. Evaluation in this context is more than the making of everyday judgements, but instead implies the systematic utilisation of scientific methods and techniques for the purpose of making an evaluation of the 'worth' of a programme (Wortman, 1983), demonstrating progress towards achieving specific objectives, or as a basis for learning about the refinements required in the processes used. One of the earliest definitions of the term 'evaluation' is that of Suchman (1967), who defined evaluation as 'a method of determining the degree to which a planned programme achieves the desired objective'.

As Nolan & Grant (1993) point out, whilst this definition appears deceptively simple, it rests on the assumption that all evaluations have stated objectives, that the steps to achieving the objectives are clear and that the effectiveness of these steps can be measured. However, even more important is the naïvety of assuming that stated objectives are realistic and achievable. In practice development work, it is important that a programme is realistic in itself before any evaluation is established. With this in mind, contemporary evaluation literature has challenged Suchman's original definition and embraces many perspectives that broadly aim to determine the value (or worth) of a programme, including the achievement of intended and unintended outcomes; intended and unintended consequences; and benefits to individuals and communities (Wortman, 1983; Guba & Lincoln, 1989; Simons, 1996; Owen & Rogers, 1999; Kushner, 2000). Owen & Rogers (1999) therefore describe the objects of an evaluation as: negotiating an evaluation plan; collecting and analysing evidence to produce findings; and disseminating the findings to intended audiences, for use in describing or understanding a programme or making judgements and/or decisions related to that programme. In embracing this description, Owen & Rogers suggest that evaluators have expanded the range of questions asked in an evaluation to include questions about:

- What is needed?
- What are the components of this programme and how do they relate to each other?
- What is happening in this programme?
- How is the programme performing on a continuous basis?
- How could we improve this programme?
- How could we repeat the success of this programme elsewhere?

(Owen & Rogers, 1999: 3)

Whilst there appears to be common agreement in contemporary evaluation literature that evaluation designs need to embrace a range of questions (such as those listed above), there remains a tendency for 'objective truth' to dominate evaluation methodology (House, 1993; Sharp & Eddy, 2001) with the emphasis on seeking what is 'fact' and 'true' in any programme of work. Thus experimentation and control of factors that can impact on outcomes continues to be seen as the most accurate way of determining the worth of a programme. However, many authors (Guba & Lincoln, 1989; Stake, 1994; Simons, 1996; Pawson & Tilley, 1997; Kushner, 2000) argue that this objectivity fails to capture the range of perspectives that comprehensive evaluation requires nor indeed does it reflect the range of stakeholder values implicit and explicit in an evaluation design. Guba & Lincoln (1989) argue that no evaluation is value-free, as values are reflected in the theory that may underpin the evaluation, in the interpretations that the evaluator and others bring to the inquiry, and in the methodology adopted to answer the evaluation question(s). They suggest that the values of the evaluator (and of those who influence him or her, especially funders, sponsors, professional peers and those from whom information is solicited) inevitably enter the design of the evaluation in connection with the whole series of decisions involved in its designing, conducting and monitoring. Indeed, Guba & Lincoln (1989) argue that evaluations *always* take place against a background of certain values, that is to say, a programme of work is usually carried out in a specific context that has both implicit and explicit values associated with it. This assertion is especially important to practice development, as all practice development takes place in a practice context. McCormack *et al.* (2002) in a concept analysis of 'practice context' identified the sub-elements of leadership, culture and evaluation as being particularly important. Each of these has a particular set of stated or unstated values, depending on the particular context. Thus it can be argued that for an evaluation to be comprehensive, logical and inclusive, arguments about the merits (or

Box 5.1 Evaluation questions.

> 1. Whether it works.
> 2. Why it works.
> 3. For whom it works.
> 4. Under what circumstances it works.
> 5. What has been learnt to make it work?

otherwise) of quantitative versus qualitative methodologies are superfluous and instead, evaluation designs need to embrace a range of methods that can be grouped within quantitative or qualitative methodologies, but which more importantly can adequately answer the stated evaluation question(s). Thus the only true judgement of 'worth' of a programme is the quality of the evidence provided (Owen & Rogers, 1999) and whether the evidence collected answers the evaluation question(s) asked. Redfern (1998) asserts, the primary purpose of any evaluation framework should be to answer four essential questions about programmes/actions/interventions (Questions 1–4: Box 5.1) and, we would argue that in the context of practice development work, a fifth question is also important (Question 5: Box 5.1).

These five questions are important in the context of practice development, for three reasons. First, as has already been articulated, developments in nursing practice are often criticised for being unsystematic, non-rigorous and with little evidence to support their transferability (Kitson & Currie, 1996). Focusing on these five questions would enable the adoption of a systematic approach to the development work and its evaluation. Second, if practice development activities are to contribute to the evidence base of nursing practice, then nurses should be able to review the evidence base underpinning the practice developments before adopting the developments in their own practice. This of course is an issue of transferability of evidence but it is also an argument for the need for rigour in practice development designs. Third, answering the questions 'under what circumstances does a particular development work?' and 'what has been learnt to make it work?' enables the consumer of a practice development report to make judicious decisions about the applicability of the practice to their own particular context. This is different to being able to 'systematically review' research evidence, but is instead an argument for practice developers to make explicit the 'audit trail' (the decisions, actions and processes) of their development work and a 'thick' description (Geertz, 1973) of the practice development context. Such descriptions enable nursing teams to make decisions about the usefulness (or not) of the development work or its underpinning principles to their particular practice context. Quinn-Patton (1997) presents a detailed approach to what he terms 'utilization-focused evaluation'. He argues that the worth of any evaluation activity is the utility of the results to 'real people in the real world'. Quinn-Patton (1997: 20) asserts that 'evaluations should be judged by their utility and actual use; therefore, evaluators should facilitate the evaluation process and design any evaluation with careful consideration of how everything that is done, from beginning to end, will affect use'. The fifth question is focused on this objective, as learning from the activities that enabled or hindered the development is a key part of the rigour of practice development programmes.

Whilst not wishing to engage in a 'paradigm war' about methodologies, it is certainly true that after agreeing the question(s) for evaluation, decisions about the evaluation design are key to how useful the evaluation results are. Thus, in the next part of this chapter, we will outline four popular methodological approaches to evaluation in practice development work. We do not in any way want to suggest that these are the only approaches to evaluation, but they do represent a broad range of methodologies that are in common use and which are illustrated in practice examples, in later parts of this book.

Methodological approaches in common use

Action research

Action research integrates evaluation through a 'spiral of interrelated cycles involving planning, acting, observing and reflecting which are systematically and self-critically implemented', the second of three criteria constituting an action research project (Grundy & Kemmis, 1981). As the name implies action research is concerned with 'action' and 'research' but also the process of 'collaboration' which varies in degrees according to the type of action research practiced. The 'action' component itself may be perceived in different ways. At one extreme, 'action' is viewed as the researcher's action or intervention as in technical action research, and collaboration may be limited to reconnaissance and assistance with diagnosing a need for action or using a specific intervention. The evaluation aspect will be concerned with judging the effectiveness of the intervention in this type of situation. Whereas at the other extreme, approaches focus on the everyday 'actions' of practitioners and communities who are researching their own practice as practitioner-researchers, with collaboration fundamental to every activity including evaluation, and opportunities for participation are always widened as more people become involved (Grundy, 1982).

Action research can be classified in as many different ways as research can itself, and is underpinned by the same philosophically different worldviews about the nature of reality and truth as other approaches to research (Grundy, 1982; McCutcheon & Jung, 1990). One approach to action research informed by the emergence of critical social science (see Chapter 3) is known as emancipatory action research (EAR) (Grundy, 1982) and is associated by its proponents with achieving sustainable change that is not dependent on key facilitators. This is because it aims to help practitioners develop ownership through becoming aware of the way they practice, the context influencing it, developing their own self-knowledge, and acting on this. EAR is well suited to practice development because it not only integrates evaluation as a key process, and contributes to public knowledge and understanding (in common with other approaches to research), but also aims to develop practitioners and practice at the same time (Manley, 2001).

Within the context of EAR the meaning of 'emancipation' is about helping practitioners to free themselves from the things they take for granted in their everyday practice as well as the context in which they work. An example of these 'taken-for-granted' aspects is reflected in the metaphor of the 'hamster-wheel of busyness' experienced by many practitioners at some time, be that themselves or observed in others. On this 'hamster-wheel' the goal of the moment is to keep going, doing the same things day in and day out without questioning the 'what we do' or the 'how we do it' because both are taken for granted and often habitual – there is no time to think! For the practitioner this is often experienced as an incessant demand for their work, within insufficient resources and staff, leading to feelings of powerlessness and disempowerment. EAR is concerned with, for example, helping practitioners either as individuals or groups to get off this hamster-wheel by enabling them to first become aware that they are on one, and its consequences, and then, to think about what they are trying to achieve, their priorities and the actions they need to take to change how they work and what they do. Integrated with this process is the development of the practitioners' own theories, which describe and explain what they do, why they do it, how they do it and the consequence of these. These 'personal' theories are constantly refined and revised through use, constant reflection and critique – this phenomena is called 'Praxis' which conjures up a picture of practitioners moving through continuous cycles of action, reflection on this action and its consequences, evaluation, and refinement of their theories, which then inform next actions. But how is it specifically used and where does one start?

EAR is normally concerned with 'social practice susceptible to improvement through deliberate strategic action' – the first criteria of action research projects (Grundy & Kemmis, 1981). This is linked to asking 'how' questions, for example, how do I/we develop a common vision about something, and then evaluate it? The 'something' could be as broad as a Trust-wide practice development strategy or unit shared governance, or, more narrowly, as a system of self-medication, clinical supervision, or patient-held health records.

The third and final criteria for action research projects is, 'involvement of those responsible for practice in each moment of activity, widening participation as the project involves or affects others, and maintaining collaborative control of the process' (Grundy & Kemmis, 1981). As a facilitator of EAR, there are a number of challenges, and these are presented as 'how' questions, reflecting that the individual facilitator will also be researching their own facilitation practice within the project:

- How do I enable a common vision to develop about our strategic direction?
- How do I facilitate critique and reflection about ideas and strategies used?
- How do I enable group members to contribute freely to the critique and not be inhibited by the power of my position/title or the status of others?

The challenge for those using action research in terms of evaluation falls into two areas. The first is concerned with enabling the decision trail arising from the 'spiral of interrelated cycles involving planning, acting, observing and reflecting which are systematically and self-critically implemented' (Grundy & Kemmis, 1981) to be transparent. This can be achieved through ongoing and systematic documentation, analysis and verification of data arising from the project, be that data concerning the decision-making processes themselves, or data concerning the phenomena being implemented and evaluated. Formal project management groups and processes may also serve the dual function of engaging key stakeholders as well as challenging the quality of the decision trail.

The second challenge is related to the first, and is about enabling others to judge the appropriateness of any claims resulting. For

Box 5.2   Criteria for judging the quality of action research.

- It should succeed in bringing the situation to life but (at the same time) bring out its aims and emergent themes (methodological, professional, personal, developmental). In other words it should make explicit the points of interest it potentially shares with the reader (Clarke *et al.*, 1993).
- It should be credible and established by the voice of the researcher being made public (Tickle, 1995). It should also be authentic in the action research process.
- It should include the researcher's values and beliefs (Tickle, 1995).
- It should use reflexive critique: how the researcher has influenced the research process through questioning claims and relating it closely to the experiences in which it is grounded by fully showing its foundations (Winter, 1989).
- It should highlight tensions and contradictions (Clarke *et al.*, 1993).
- It should demonstrate a sense of responsibility (Clarke *et al.*, 1993).
- It should discuss how data was collected and analysed (Clarke *et al.*, 1993).

action research there are a number of criteria that need to be satisfied and these are illustrated in Box 5.2. These should be considered in conjunction with the criteria used to judge constructivist inquiry (Box 5.3).

Titchen (1995) states that providing evidence of trustworthiness in action research is demanding, time-consuming and formidable. She highlights the difficulty of balancing tests of rigour with taking forward action, and developing and renegotiating ground rules for each situation. Other challenges she acknowledges include time constraints that may impede the processes of trustworthiness and issues affecting participants' validation of interpretations, such as memory lapses. She particularly emphasises the boldness required by participants to challenge a researcher's interpretation – but recognises this is more likely to occur if the action research has been truly collaborative.

Titchen (1995) makes three conclusions in relation to issues of validity (trustworthiness) based on her experiences of action research in nursing.

1. Valid knowledge can be generated through action research but the final test is the degree to which other practitioners are guided in their own practice from this knowledge. This is similar to Lincoln & Guba's (1985) concept of transferability.

Box 5.3 Criteria for judging naturalistic/constructivist inquiry (after Lincoln & Guba, 1985; Stringer, 1999).

Credibility is established by the following processes:

- **Prolonged engagement** with participants
- **Triangulation** of information from multiple data sources
- **Member checking** – to enable members to check and verify the accuracy of information recorded
- **Peer debriefing** processes to enable research facilitators to articulate and reflect on research procedures

Transferability is established by

- Describing the means for applying findings to other contexts
- Providing thick detailed descriptions that enable others to identify similarities with other settings
- Enabling audiences to see themselves/their situations in accounts presented

Dependability and confirmability are achieved by

- Providing an audit trail
- Clearly describing the processes of collecting and analysing data
- Providing a means for the audience to refer to raw data

---

2. Validation processes are integral to the collaborative nature of action research that involves participants reflecting on and evaluating their work before deciding future action.
3. Ensuring validation processes are carried out with integrity requires a high level of researcher skill and sensitivity.

   Valid action research is an ethical enterprise which rests on the researchers' honesty, trustworthiness and integrity. Conducting tests of rigour requires self-discipline and high-quality awareness; awareness of their values, bias and effect on the realities being studied.

   (Titchen, 1995: 47–8)

   The nature of validity and trustworthiness in action research is therefore interrelated with a concern for ethics.

In conclusion, emancipatory action research provides a whole framework for developing practice and practitioners that includes in-built evaluation, as well as contributing to theory, knowledge and understanding. In addition it promotes a 'way of being' which seeks to be authentic, open and ethical, and which acknowledges the potential impact of power, be that from the context, or the persons facilitating the research.

Fourth generation evaluation

Guba & Lincoln (1989) do not use the term action research in their book *Fourth Generation Evaluation*, although there are similarities in its processes to emancipatory action research. Guba & Lincoln start with the premise that the major purpose of evaluation is to 'refine' and 'improve' as well as 'judge', whereas improving a situation is one of the purposes of action research, refinement and judgement are incorporated within the action research cycle. The values under-pinning Fourth Generation Evaluation are similar to those of criti-cal social theory, with its focus on the nature of power relations, as well as emancipatory and empowering processes:

> Where the effort to devise joint, collaborative, or shared con-structions solicits and honors the inputs from many stakeholders and affords them a measure of control over the nature of the eval-uation activity. It is therefore both educative and empowering, while also fulfilling all the usual expectations for doing an eval-uation, primarily value judgements.
>
> (Guba & Lincoln, 1989: 184)

However, education and empowerment are portrayed as conse-quences or benefits of stakeholder involvement, rather than a primary intention. The primary intention of Fourth Generation Evaluation is evaluation. However, action research from a critical social science perspective differs from Fourth Generation Evalua-tion in that action (emancipation) from education and empower-ment is the primary intention, together with developing practice and contributing to theory.

Carr & Kemmis's (1986) criticism of the interpretive/construc-tivist paradigm within which Fourth Generation Evaluation is located, is that, although understanding and 'subjective meanings' are enhanced, action is not guaranteed, whereas in the critical social theory approach, the researcher/evaluator has the role of partici-pating in the development of knowledge, which is 'comprehended as social and political action which must be understood and justi-fied as such' (Carr & Kemmis, 1986: 152). Further, the aim of criti-cal science is to transform practice compared with the aims of positivism, which is explanation and prediction; or, interpretivism, which is understanding (Carr & Kemmis, 1986: 156). Action researchers using the critical science worldview 'aim to transform the present to develop a different future' (Carr & Kemmis, 1986:

183). This is achieved through providing 'a way of participating in decision-making about development' (Carr & Kemmis, 1986: 162). Group decision-making is a matter of principle rather than technique and essential to authentic social action (Carr & Kemmis, 1986).

Fourth Generation Evaluation particularly highlights the processes involved in drawing on stakeholders, whereas the central tenet of action research, underpinned by critical social science, is the emancipation of practitioners and the transformation of practice. It is proposed therefore that Fourth Generation Evaluation (Guba & Lincoln, 1989) is a methodology that can be used on its own or assimilated within an action research approach. The benefits it offers to evaluating practice development are that it:

• can be integrated into everyday project facilitation;
• enables a focus on different stakeholders' groups, their concerns, claims and issues;
• facilitates mutual education and understanding between different stakeholder groups.

Fourth Generation Evaluation is so called because it emerges from three previous generations of evaluation approaches. These have focused in turn on measurement, description and judgement (Guba and Lincoln, 1989). Each generation is deemed to have addressed the criticisms of its predecessor, but all three have flaws, summarised as:

• a tendency towards managerialism – 'their susceptibility to managerial ideology' (1989: 51);
• a failure to accommodate value pluralism – they presume value consensus;
• over-commitment to the scientific paradigm of inquiry – that is to say under-pinned by an assumption that a single verifiable truth can be discovered.

Even if these flaws could be overcome, Guba and Lincoln consider there to be compelling arguments to focusing on stakeholder claims, concerns and issues as the basis of what they term the Fourth Generation approach to evaluation. They highlight five reasons for involving stakeholders (Box 5.4).

Stakeholders are defined as groups who, have something at stake in the evaluand – (i.e. the entity being evaluated) (Guba & Lincoln, 1989: 51). The entity being evaluated in the context of practice development may include:

- implementation processes for establishing structures and systems, such as shared governance, recognition/accreditation processes for competence, expertise, career progression;
- the structures, systems and initiatives themselves in relation to their impact on a number of stakeholders or resources.

Stakeholders are classified as agents, beneficiaries and victims as outlined in Box 5.5. Involving stakeholders can also have other benefits depending on one's values. First, evaluation is promoted as something that is co-operative (Heron, 1981) where the evaluator works *with* people rather than *on* them. Second, through valuing the contributions of all stakeholders, understanding the constructions of others is enabled. Third, by involving stakeholders in the process they are more likely to develop ownership of subsequent changes, making the facilitation of change more successful.

The implications of using this approach then involves identifying and working with key stakeholder groups. Stakeholder inputs are defined as their claims, concerns, and issues and these arise from constructions that a stakeholder group have formulated reflecting their particular experiences, circumstances and values (Guba & Lincoln, 1989). Deliberate activity would require an opportunity to

Box 5.4 Reasons for involving stakeholders (Guba & Lincoln, 1989).

- They are groups at risk, because by definition they have a stake in what is being evaluated.
- They are open to exploitation, disempowerment and disenfranchisement because the end product of evaluation is information. 'Information is power, and evaluation is powerful' (1989: 52).
- They are users of evaluation information.
- They can broaden the range of evaluative inquiry: 'When one does not know in advance what information is to be collected, it is literally impossible to design an inquiry that will provide it. Open-endness (an "emergent" design) is called for' (1989: 55).
- They are mutually educated by the fourth generation process.

Box 5.5 Classification of stakeholders (Guba & Lincoln, 1981).

Agents	Beneficiaries	Victims
Producers, users implementers of evaluand	Profit from using evaluand	Negatively affected by use of evaluand or its failure

Box 5.6   Claims, concerns and issues.

Claims

A claim is any favourable assertion about the evaluand and its implementation
Example: 'Discussing what we mean by practice development is helping me to contribute to developing our vision.'

Concerns

A concern is any unfavourable assertion about the evaluand and its implementation
Example: 'I can't visualise how the evaluation strategy and the practice development strategy all fits together with what I do in everyday practice.'

Issues

Issues are questions which reflect what any 'reasonable person' might be asking about the evaluand and its implementation
Example: 'What strategies can I/we use to gain commitment for this work, from others who are not here today?'

---

explore and capture stakeholders' concerns, claims and issues, described and illustrated in Box 5.6.

These concerns, claims and issues are then:

1. Shared with other stakeholder groups thus enabling mutual understanding and to agree the focus of the evaluation
2. Used to enable concerns and issues to formally and transparently be surfaced and addressed, normally through an action research type mechanism. Also claims to be celebrated and acknowledged
3. Used to capture the implementation journey, through their analysis at different points during the journey.

In its purest form, each stakeholder group's concerns, claims and issues are introduced to other groups for comment, refutation or agreement and this leads to exploration of unresolved items and re-negotiation between stakeholders with all stakeholders in possession of the same level of information (Koch, 1994).

The role of the evaluator is to facilitate this process, termed a 'hermeneutic dialectic' process, which in its purest form may be seen as a very 'ideal' and extreme process that can continue indefinitely. The practice developer may therefore need to inject a dose of realism in terms of how many and which stakeholder groups are included in the process, as well as for how long they continue the negotiation. This therefore involves making decisions that need to be transparent. Similar issues can exist for the facilitator of the hermeneutic dialectic process as for the facilitator of emancipatory action research, in relation to power issues and its potential for misuse. As Laughlin & Broadbent (1996) argue this is because the facilitator/evaluator may be 'quite possibly the only person who has moved extensively between participants, stakeholders, and respondents and, therefore has the benefit of having heard a more complete set of constructions than anyone else'. However, this danger can be minimised if collaborative responsibility rests with a number of co-researchers rather than with one person, and if combined with a disciplined verification of the data resulting.

So, although Fourth Generation Evaluation has its critics, some of these criticisms can be overcome by using its principles as a tool within, for example, an action research framework. The great strength of the Fourth Generation Evaluation approach is the recognition of the need to engage with the many different stakeholders that exist when participating in practice development. This approach must also recognise the different needs of the various stakeholders, which in turn may influence the type and range of evaluation indicators used. It also provides a valuable mechanism for raising concerns and issues to be addressed – a process that contributes to achieving a more open culture combined with the potential for greater mutual understanding of different groups' concerns.

Realistic evaluation

Pawson & Tilley (1997) developed the methodology of 'realistic evaluation'. They argue that in the history of evaluation research, the philosophy of positivism has dominated the agenda. They argue that evaluation research has been greatly influenced by the desire to demonstrate causal relationships between systems and outcomes. In experimental design the aim is to demonstrate a 'cause and effect' relationship and whilst confounding factors can be controlled in a laboratory setting, Pawson & Tilley argue that such control is not possible in social settings. The philosophy of realism, in contrast, attempts to take account of those explanatory elements in the social world that are overlooked by experimentation.

Pawson & Tilley (1997) argue that thus far in evaluation research methodology a stark contrast has been made between the naturalists' (positivists) desire to control contextual factors that might impinge on the identification of causal relationships and the constructivists' desire to negotiate a shared reality (Guba & Lincoln, 1989). A constructivist approach to evaluation is shaped by a relativist philosophy whereby there is no fixed meaning of 'truth' and the participants in the social world being studied negotiate all versions of truth among key stakeholders. Constructivist evaluation adopts the hermeneutic approach of interpretation whereby it is the way that participants see events that matters and not those of the evaluator/researcher. Through prolonged periods of data collection (observation and questioning) the evaluator establishes the concerns, claims and issues of all stakeholders and through a 'forum' (a process of democratic decision-making) arises at a shared reality. Pawson & Tilley are critical of this methodology because of its relativist traits and its naïvety. They argue that the approach is predicated on assumptions of democracy and equality that are rarely found in organisations and thus in attempting to reject a positivist approach, lose some essential principles in evaluation research, i.e. those of understanding the relationship between elements 'as they exist' (realism) and not as we might like for them to exist (constructivism). From a realist perspective, the context of the evaluation can neither be denied nor reconstructed to reflect a shared reality:

> One of the useful lessons we learn from the pragmatists is that policy making and programme development are part of a vast intersection of ideas and interests. . . . The social world consists of more than the sum of people's beliefs, hopes and expectations.
>
> (Pawson & Tilley, 1997: 22–23)

What Pawson & Tilley argue is that the social world consists of asymmetries of power (also the focus of emancipatory action research and Fourth Generation Evaluation) and that these asymmetries allow some people to advance their ideas whilst others have theirs constrained.

Realistic evaluation tries to outline the relationship between *mechanisms* (M), the *context* (C) within which the mechanisms exist and the resulting *outcomes* (O) from the functioning of the mechanisms in a given context, i.e. the M, C, O relationship. In evaluating a development programme (for example, the development of a patient-led drug administration system), Pawson & Tilley argue that this is essentially an evaluation of a social system. Social systems consist of the interplay between individuals and institution, of agency and structure and of micro- and macro-social processes. The methodology of realistic evaluation as outlined by Pawson and Tilley operates within five concepts:

- *Embeddedness* The inbuilt assumptions about a wider set of social rules and institutions that underpin social actions. This means that (for example) a statutory training activity (e.g. drug administration) is understood as such because we take for granted its place within the social organisation of the hospital.
- *Mechanisms* Social interventions, such as a specific practice change, work, not because of isolated variables, but by the weaving together of resources such as facilitation, and reasoning such as shared decision-making, rather than viewing them as isolated variables.
- *Contexts* All social interventions have to take account of prevailing contextual conditions as they are usually introduced into prevailing contexts. These contextual conditions are crucially important when explaining the successes and failures of social programmes. Context does not simply mean geographical, spatial or institutional location, but also includes established rules, norms, values and inter-relationships that influence (enhance or inhibit) a social programme.
- *Regularities* The explanation of social patterns, associations, and outcomes. Regularities are explained as the relationship between mechanisms and contexts and their impact on the goal of the social programme.
- *Change* The way in which social programmes can grow and develop is determined by the interrelationship between regularities, mechanisms and contexts. For example, people in an organisation may have limited knowledge about the context (e.g. decision-making structures) and regularities (e.g. code of professional conduct) within which a social intervention works and thus changes made may have unanticipated and unpredictable consequences.

Evaluation programmes adopting a realist methodology operate within 'the realist evaluation cycle' where there is interplay between theory generation, hypothesis testing, observation and programme specification (Fig. 5.1).

The realist evaluation cycle enables the development of an evaluation framework that moves from describing the elements of the programme in detail in order to identify 'hypotheses' that can be subjected to further testing (evaluation). In the Royal College of Nursing's 'Expertise in Practice Project' (RCN, 2003) the recognition process for enabling expertise to be accredited had to be developed

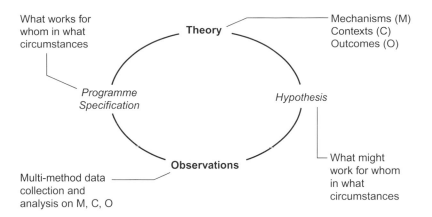

Fig. 5.1 The realistic evaluation cycle (Reprinted by permission of Sage Publications Ltd, from Pawson & Tilley, 1997).

and described in detail before it could be used in practice to test out whether it was useful in capturing and recognising expertise and evaluating its impact. This is a useful illustration of a realistic evaluation cycle. Pawson & Tilley argue that before a programme can be thoroughly evaluated in terms of identifying what works, for whom and in what circumstances, then the elements of the programme need to be described. The Royal Hospitals Trust Clinical Careers Framework provides a useful case study of realistic evaluation being used to guide the 'staging' and evaluation of a programme (Box 5.7). The focus of the activity is that of describing the relationships between the mechanisms for change, the key elements of the context that might impact on any development activity and explaining the relationships between patterns and associations in the programme. Thus, this stage of the evaluation aims to explain the relationship between mechanisms and contexts and their impact (outcomes) on the goal of the social programme in order to predict 'what *might* work for whom and in what circumstances', i.e. hypothesis generation. The identification of these hypotheses forms the agenda for stage 2 of the evaluation cycle, whereby the use of multi-methods of data collection enables the testing out of the hypothesis in order to identify 'what works for whom and in what circumstances. This, Pawson & Tilley describe as 'programme specification' – that is, a detailed description and analysis of the programme that details the relationships between mechanisms, context and outcomes.

Box 5.7   Realistic evaluation: a case study.

The Royal Hospitals Trust, Belfast is developing an integrated professional and practice development framework, known as the REACH Project

1. Aim of the programme:

For every nurse in the Trust to have a clinical career pathway that will include:

i.   A work-based learning contract
ii. Participation in facilitated reflective practice
iii. Support to develop nursing practice through critical inquiry and practice development frameworks
iv. An Annual Review of progress with attributes
v.   Accreditation of learning achieved

2. Components of REACH

REACH comprises five elements:

- **The attributes framework:** this framework describes areas of activity that are focused on the delivery of patient-centred care.
- **Appraisal system:** Entry into the framework will be through a first appraisal with a named clinical leader and regular reappraisal.
- **Work-Based Learning Contract:** Following the initial appraisal discussion, the participating nurse will be required to develop a learning contract.
- **Learning Sets:** Learning sets will be established across directorates to support participants and develop the knowledge, skills and expertise of mentors.
- **Formal learning opportunities:** as provided by universities and training institutions.
- **Portfolio of learning and development for accreditation** Each participant will develop a portfolio of evidence, incorporating their continuous assessment of development and learning needs, evidence of achievement in attributes and reflection on the impact of learning and development activities on practice.

3. Expected outcomes

i.   Competent and confident practitioners
ii. Practice development and education with measurable outcomes
iii. Clinical and career pathways for all grades of nurses
iv. Recognition and value of staff regardless of academic or clinical pathway through the availability of a variety of options for the accreditation of lifelong learning

Box 5.7 *Continued*

4. Evaluation of the programme

Stage 1: Theory generation and hypothesis definition (6 months)
During this stage, the mechanisms, contexts and outcomes will be described. Pawson & Tilley (1997) argue that theories are concerned with the identification and explanation of regularities, that is, describing the relationship between mechanisms, context and outcomes. Thus, this stage of the project is exploratory in nature with the aims of:

i.   Making sense of the way in which REACH operates in the Trust
ii. Generating theories (hypotheses) about the framework that could be subjected to further testing and development.

Stage 2: Programme Specification (18 months)
During this stage, the hypotheses generated in stage 1 will be tested out in order to understand the relationships between the mechanisms, contexts and outcomes developed. In order to achieve the aims of the study a combination of both qualitative and quantitative research methods will be employed. Pawson & Tilley (1997) argue that a realistic evaluation design requires the use of a range of data collection methods in order to explore the M, C, O relationship. In this study, methods include:

- One-to-one interviews with participants at three-monthly intervals throughout their period of participation will be conducted.
- Records of learning sets will be standardised and these thematically analysed for evidence of learning.
- Reflective discussions will be held with mentor and participants together in order to develop an understanding of the shared experience of participation.
- An evaluation of the 'costs' of the project will be undertaken, by costing the hours of work inputted by participants, mentors and facilitators. Infrastructure costs will also be evaluated.
- Review of portfolio evidence at six-monthly intervals for evidence of changes in practice; developments in knowledge; advancement in skill and expertise.

Layers of evaluation in practice development

Throughout this book we explore practice development at a variety of levels. Consistent with the conceptual framework developed by McCormack *et al.* (1999), we have emphasised practice development occurring at an individual patient level, that is, the primary focus of practice development is on becoming increasingly effective in patient-centred practice. This is of course an issue for individual nurses, as the essence of being patient-centred is the quality of the relationship between individual nurses and patients. However, McCormack *et al.* (1999) identified the importance of practice development being embraced at a variety of levels in order for therapeutic patient-centred relationships to be sustained in practice. Table 5.1 identifies the four levels we have defined and the primary emphasis of practice development work at each level.

In order to illustrate the operationalisation of these levels of work, below are detailed examples of practice development work and its evaluation in which we are engaged. We do not suggest that these levels are separate to each other, and in much practice development work activities focus on some or all of these levels in an integrated programme of work. McCormack *et al.* (1999), Clarke & Wilcockson (2001), Graham (1996) and Manley (2001) argue that for practice developments to be sustained, then all of these levels need to be considered in an integrated programme of development work. The examples below are illustrative only and the chapters in Part 2 of this book provide more detailed case studies of similar work in progress.

Table 5.1 Levels of practice development and primary emphases in PD work.

Practice development levels	Primary emphasis in practice development work
Corporate/Strategic	Creating a Trust-wide culture of effectiveness that is patient and person-centred, evidence-based, and constantly interacts with a changing context
Service/Organisational	Creating a learning culture to enable the sustaining of developments in practice through learning in and from practice
Team	Developing team structures and processes that enable practice developments to occur that are supportive of patient-centred approaches to practice
Individual	Empowering individual practitioners to develop therapeutic patient-centred relationships with patients and evidence-based care

Evaluation at a corporate/strategic level

The need for corporate and strategic frameworks to optimise the potential of practice development activity at the patient interface (McCormack *et al.*, 1999; Manley, 2001) was the impetus for the RCN Institute to establish a programme of support to help NHS Trusts (both acute and primary care) to develop Trust-wide practice development and integral evaluation strategies. Two of these NHS Trusts, are the focus of later chapters.

The programme of support is achieved through an outsider–insider partnership, the outsider, a member of the RCNI's practice development function, and the insider, either the internal lead co-ordinator of the Trust's practice development activity or a group of facilitators sharing a co-ordination function. Through working together with key stakeholder groups, a Trust-wide vision and strategy results from clarifying values and beliefs about the purpose of practice development and how to achieve it. Subsequently, the vision leads to strategic objectives that provide an integrating framework for both corporate and local action, an evaluation framework, and a programme of evaluation activity which enables and integrates evaluation at all levels: Trust, directorate, unit/ward and individual. This creates the potential for achieving 'joined-up' working across the organisation, enabling valuable resources to be used effectively and efficiently, yet acknowledging that every context is different.

A shared vision is sought through engaging colleagues locally, facilitating seminars and road shows, making presentations, using Trust websites, as well as presenting ideas for critique through clinical governance mechanisms, the steering group of key stakeholders, and presentations to the executive Trust board.

The development of the evaluation strategy is an integral part of a collaborative action research study that starts by asking, 'How do we develop, implement and evaluate a Trust-wide practice development strategy?' Progress in the study is achieved through monthly workshops with co-researchers and a programme of continuing activity accountable to a steering group and shared governance structures.

The evaluation strategy is derived from the vision, through identifying related evaluation questions, specifically 'what' questions. The vision centres around the purposes of practice development, for example; providing patient-centred and evidence-based care, creating a culture of effectiveness, introducing practice development processes, so examples of evaluation questions resulting include:

- What impact is the practice development strategy having on patients' experiences and patient outcomes?
- What impact is the practice development strategy having on the quality of evidence used in everyday practice?
- What impact is the practice development strategy having on the workplace culture experienced by staff and patients?
- What impact are practice development processes having on individuals, the work of colleagues and practice?

Evaluation questions are themed to construct the evaluation framework and linked to data collection methods selected. Before methods can be identified, continuing workshops help co-researchers to begin to explore what data might already be available, as well as any data omissions, for answering the evaluation questions.

NHS Trusts collect large amounts of data, but rarely is this accessed by practitioners, or presented in a meaningful form so that practitioners can be alerted to less obvious changes that may need to be made to improve services for patients. In the NHS Trusts involved in the programme so far, patient stories, staff stories and cultural assessment per se, linked to evaluating leadership and facilitation expertise, did not previously feature Trust-wide. These methods have been selected by co-researchers for exploring the evaluation questions in tandem with exploring how Trust-wide data routinely collected can be made more useful to practitioners and contribute to a portfolio of evidence for informing each local area's practice development focus and direction.

In addition to answering the evaluation questions data collection serves several equally important purposes for practice developers, providing:

- impetus for immediate local action through local action plans;
- a way of engaging all staff in addressing issues which require action through involving them in obtaining or using the data, or through feedback mechanisms;
- development of staff in using tools and data that will assist them in continuous development of their practice and service;
- feedback and opportunities for discussion with others about what constitutes a quality service for patients;
- feedback on progress towards achieving the vision at both local, directorate and trust level.

Developing a Trust-wide evaluation strategy in itself does not take much time; however, the preparation involved to achieve the strategy does. Due to the action research nature of the overall project, there has been the need to work closely with co-researchers to help them develop the skills and confidence necessary to use evaluation methods not experienced before. Workshops using a number of creative learning methods such as interactive freeze-framed dramatisations have enabled skills to develop in using these methods, as well as the development of clear research protocols from the practitioners' own learning and practice – praxis in its purest form!

The workshops have concentrated on the principles of informed consent and unstructured interviewing approaches, developing patient story protocols, staff story protocols, observation of care, 360° feedback, tools for evaluating understanding and use of evidence-based practice, as well as how to analyse the data arising, how to verify it, what to do with it, and how to give and receive feedback on the findings resulting. Analysis at different levels enables action plans to result for individual units/wards, directorates as well as the Trust as a whole.

Whilst staff are developing key research and evaluation skills, these skills in themselves enable individuals to develop their practice. So, for example, learning to interact with a patient in a way that enables them to tell their story is a vital skill in enabling staff to 'see the world through the patient's eyes' and to realise patient and person-centredness every day. Another example of how developing the Trust evaluation strategy is interwoven with developing practice itself is apparent in learning how to give feedback on the findings arising. These skills help co-researchers, and all involved to increase and improve the giving and receiving of feedback in their daily practice. This has the effect of beginning to change the culture both locally and across the Trust to one where the giving and receiving of open, direct and supportive feedback can begin to become the norm.

Developing Trust-wide evaluation strategies and implementing them requires considerable support from Trusts as well as commitment and perseverance from practitioners. However, they benefit, in that all their efforts and mechanisms to improve practice can be integrated at a local level with the skills necessary to help all staff to become more effective, through the framework and common vision provided by the practice development strategy. In both the Trusts alluded to, the long and continuing journeys which commenced as 'bolt-on' projects were considered a good thing to do, have begun to deliver what they promised – with the subsequent result that the practice development strategy and its evaluation are becoming mainstay Trust activity. Thus the Trust-wide frameworks necessary to enable practice development facilitators, practitioners and other staff to integrate practice development and evaluation at local level in their everyday practice are gradually being put in place.

Evaluation at a service level

Following a period of negotiation and relationship building, a programme of development was initiated by the Lead Cancer Nurses and the Directors of Nursing in Belfast City Hospital and St James' Hospital, Dublin. Their vision, as the two major cancer centres on the island of Ireland was to collaborate on a programme of development that would empower clinical leaders to create sustainable practice developments. The University of Ulster was approached to provide external facilitation to the programme and lead the evaluation of the work. After a number of meetings between the centres involved in the programme, including the 24 clinical leaders who would be participating in the work, four aims of the programme were agreed:

1. develop the leadership potential of clinical leaders of cancer services in both hospitals through a programme of work-based and action learning;
2. develop the practice development knowledge, skills and expertise of clinical leaders in the two organisations;
3. organise a programme of development activities that will be initiated, implemented and sustained by clinical leaders participating in the programme of work;
4. evaluate the processes and outcomes of the work from the perspectives of the participants and their colleagues.

In order to determine the effectiveness of the programme in meeting these aims, two evaluation questions were agreed:

1. Does a programme of work-based and action learning enable clinical leaders in two cancer services to be more empowered to develop practice?
2. Do the learning and development processes used emancipate clinical leaders from the taken-for-granted assumptions in everyday practice and the systems in which they work in order to create change?

A programme of work extending initially over two years was agreed and centred around three 'action cycles'. Action cycle 1 focused on working with the clinical leaders and the lead nurses to establish a shared vision for cancer nursing in both centres. This cycle was facilitated through a range of visioning workshops that incorporated the use of artistic processes in developing a vision as well as more formalised processes such as that of Manley (1997). Clinical leaders facilitated visioning exercises with their clinical teams over a six-month period until a shared vision for cancer nursing was agreed.

Action cycle 2 focused on evaluating the context of care delivery and planning practice changes. This cycle centred on evaluating the context of practice in the two centres in order to design a programme of practice developments. Each participant was 'trained' in the use of a variety of data collection methods and organised into sub-groups to collect 'baseline' information. The same data was collected in all clinical areas (n = 14) across the two cancer centres. Two hundred and sixty three informants (members of the multidisciplinary team, patients, relatives and carers) participated in focus groups and individual discussions, observed practice and completed questionnaires. The data collected was analysed collaboratively by participants in small groups and through facilitated workshops.

Action cycle 3 focused on maximising the leadership potential of clinical leaders. This was done through 'action learning sets' (two groups of 12 who met for one day each month for 18 months), leadership workshops, skills workshops (e.g. conflict management) and supported by individual leadership learning contracts. All learning sets were tape-recorded and process evaluation notes maintained.

A project advisory group was established made up of key stakeholders internal to the participating centres and from 'policy' perspectives in Ireland. As the project progressed, participants and the advisory group identified the need for specific areas of external evaluation. As a result an external evaluator was recruited to undertake reflective conversations and focus groups with programme participants and other key stakeholders.

The analysis of data was undertaken at three levels.

Analysis to inform individual learning contracts

Participants analysed specific data (e.g. 360° feedback questionnaires) to inform their own development as identified in individual learning contracts.

Analysis to inform practice developments

This data was analysed by project participants and the external facilitator through 'data analysis workshops'. The emphasis was on evaluating the 'baseline data' of individual practices and planning changes to the way services are delivered across clinical areas and participating sites.

Analysis to inform overall project

This data was analysed by the external facilitator and the external evaluator in collaboration with project participants, in order to provide information about overall project processes and experiences, and project outcomes.

Overall project processes and experiences

i. Individual development and experiences
   - Reflective reviews undertaken during action learning sets
   - Analysis of provisional objectives/learning contracts
   - Individual reflective conversations (undertaken by external evaluator) following initial analysis of action learning data to identify evidence of change/development
ii. Group processes and experiences
   - Focus groups (undertaken by external evaluator) – analysis of audio recordings
   - Analysis of audio recordings of action learning sets (jointly undertaken by external facilitator and external evaluator)
   - Action learning processes

Project outcomes

- Pre- and post-implementation evaluation of action plans
- Analysis of action learning data – outcomes for individuals
- Individual reflective conversations (undertaken by external evaluator) – outcomes for individuals
- Interviews with other stakeholders (undertaken by external evaluator) – outcomes for teams and organisations

Evaluation at a team level
(*Val Wilson*)

This section describes the evaluation of a practice development research project being undertaken over 18 months with a team of nursing staff working within a special care nursery in Melbourne, Australia.

The aim of the project is to extend the practice development knowledge and skills and expertise of nursing staff within the special care nursery. The project is also working with staff to develop their ability to critically challenge practice and continuously improve the quality of care delivered to patients and families.

The activities of the project focus on working with nursing staff to develop a programme of practice development activities that are initiated, implemented and sustained by them. Each aspect of the practice development work is being evaluated from the perspectives of both active and non-active participants. The terms 'active' and 'non-active' are used to distinguish those staff that are leading on particular parts of the project work and those who are supportive but not actively participating in the work.

The project is underpinned by three evaluation questions:

1. Does implementation of practice development strategies influence the development of the individual nurse as well as clinical practice?
2. What, if any, practice development strategies work, for whom do they work and in what circumstances do they work?
3. Does the use of practice development strategies assist nurses to realise their espoused values in practice?

The project is put into operation through four development cycles. These are: getting to know staff and understanding the culture of the unit; developing a shared vision and implementing practice development strategies; planning practice changes using emancipatory action research principles; and maximising opportunities to challenge practice. Participants in the project have adopted a variety of roles, including, action learning group participants (7); nursing staff actively involved in practice development strategies (half the staff); co-researchers; lead researcher (Val).

Methodologically, the project is located within an emancipatory action research framework and underpinned by the principles of realistic evaluation. Thus, data is collected from/through all activities that involve action and evaluation. This includes: an information session on practice development and related strategies; values clarification exercises; pre- and post-evaluation of the culture of practice within the unit; and workshops (e.g. introduction to action learning and creative approaches to achieving evidence-based practice (EBP)). Specific practice development activities include:

- Action Learning Group
- High Challenge/High Support in clinical decision-making
- Case study presentations incorporating EBP
- Reflective practice
- Emancipatory Action Research (EAR) processes

The data analysis focuses on four levels:

- *Analysis to inform individual and team learning*
  Data from interviews held with participants and non-participants before, during and after implementation will highlight changes in the learning culture and development of nursing staff.

- *Analysis to inform the development of practice*
  Data analysis is undertaken by the researcher outlining the culture. Baseline observational data is discussed with nursing staff who have added to the data and analysis through an in-depth interview process.
- *Analysis of individual EAR projects*
  Data from each project will be analysed by participants with the assistance of the researcher.
- *Analysis to inform the overall project*
  Data will be analysed by the researcher in collaboration with participants and will focus on:
  - Overall project process and experiences for individual nursing staff, including learning and development achieved and changes in individual practices;
  - Participants' journeys through action learning identified through achievement/non-achievement of 'action points';
  - Analysis of observational, interview and reflective journal data, defining what changes if any have been made in the culture of the unit.

The project intends to produce data that will inform these different levels of stakeholder need and typically outcomes will focus on outcomes for the clinical unit as a whole, outcomes for individuals and practice change outcomes.

Evaluation at an individual level

The individual level of evaluation includes both the individual's evaluation of their own practice, as well as the evaluation of others' practice. This level of evaluation is strengthened if it draws on multiple sources of evidence, thus enabling triangulation. Although this also applies to other evaluation levels, when evaluating one's own development it is important to be particularly aware of the danger of self delusion (Habermas, 1972). So what evidence can be used to demonstrate the impact of practice development on the effectiveness of individual practitioners?

Within an action research study that set out to operationalise the role of the consultant nurse through using practice development processes (Manley, 2001), a number of outcomes resulted demonstrating the impact on individuals and their work. These outcomes listed in Box 5.8 were derived from a number of different data sets including the perceptions of the practitioners themselves, the perceptions of others (insiders and outsiders), and analysis of publications, notes and action plans.

Box 5.8 Impact on individual practitioners of practice development processes operationalised through a consultant nurse role (Manley, 2000, 2001).

Impact on individual practitioners

- Greater enthusiasm which helped to achieve more
- Felt more confident through being provided with opportunities for involvement
- Felt more involved and empowered
- Saw the possibilities for their own contribution as an individual and nurse
- Developed a vision for nursing and achieved a patient-centred approach
- Felt part of a team
- Had someone to help with the development of new ideas
- Had a clinical career pathway to progress along for the first time

Impact on individual's work and how they worked

- Improved patient care through:
  - Direct benefits to patients from primary nursing reviews
  - Providing more individualised, comprehensive and better follow-up care for patients
  - Providing more up-to-date and research-based care
- Role development
- Increased commitment to, and involvement in developmental work
- Increased willingness to take responsibility for their own work
- How practitioners approached their work
  - Practitioners found that they thought and practised differently
  - Challenged practice and used research
  - Began using the same processes as the consultant nurse

The consultant nurse evaluated her own effectiveness in facilitating others by moving constantly through action research cycles, which involved drawing on data from structured reflection, peer supervision notes, action plans, research notes, unstructured interviews, focus groups and 360° analysis. Reflective reviews at six-monthly intervals and analysis of action learning set processes and outcomes are also methods used to demonstrate the impact of practice development processes on an individual's practice.

Individuals may show how they develop greater effectiveness by collating practice – based evidence compiled into a portfolio that can be judged against practice standards and competency frameworks. One such project, the RCN Expertise in Practice Project (RCN, 2003) has enabled participants as co-researchers to research their own practice expertise and through this process, to demonstrate: their expertise against attributes derived from the literature; the impact of being part of the project on themselves; and the impact of their expertise on others, patients and the service. Sources of practice evidence were drawn from critical reflections, observation of practice, user narratives, 360° feedback and testimonials as well as creative expressions.

A portfolio of evidence can be used by practitioners to evaluate any aspect of their practice, be that to show for example, how they have become more effective, how they have incorporated a range of different sources of evidence into their practice, how they have developed their leadership skills, or how they have become more patient-centred.

The conceptual framework derived from the consultant nurse work above (Manley, 2001) identified the link between practice development processes and staff empowerment amongst other characteristics. Indicators of staff empowerment can be used as an evaluation tool at both the individual and organisational level to demonstrate impact of practice development processes and programmes on individuals (see also Chapter 4).

An evaluation checklist for practice development

It is important to be clear about the decisions underpinning the design of a practice development evaluation framework. Below is listed a series of questions that we believe need to be explored/ answered as a part of the overall design of practice development programmes. Considering these questions should facilitate the design of a systematic approach to evaluation.

1. **Values, beliefs, purpose**
   - What are the beliefs and values about practice development held by the commissioners of the work?
   - As a practice developer, what are your beliefs and values about practice development?
   - What is the purpose of the practice development?
   - What are the intended outcomes?
   - What are the anticipated outcomes?

2. Stakeholders

- Who are the stakeholders involved?
- What do the commissioners of the work and other stakeholders want from an evaluation? i.e. what expectations do they have of the evaluation?
- Whose agenda(s) dominate?

3. Roles

- What is your role? i.e. practice developer integrated with lead evaluator or one or the other?
- What is your role in the organisation?
- What is your role in the practice development programme?

4. Engagement and widening participation

- Can the potential enthusiasts and potential blockers be identified?
- What needs to be done to gain participation?

5. Support mechanisms

- How will you balance your time in order to balance action and evaluation?
- Do you need to take time to negotiate issues of power in the programme and how this will be managed?
- How will you build in time for reflection into the programme?
- How will mechanisms for support for programme participants be built into the programme?

6. Evaluation design

- What are your evaluation questions?
- What is the most appropriate evaluation design?
- What skills are needed to undertake the evaluation and are these readily available?
- What data will be collected?
- What are the ethical implications of your evaluation approach?

7. Time frames, monitoring and resources

- Are time-lines planned realistically, taking account of time needed for planning and negotiation?
- How will participation be continuously increased in the programme and how will this be accounted for in the evaluation?
- How will evaluation data be used to help with maintaining momentum?
- What resources are available to enable evaluation?

8. **Accountability mechanisms and management of conflict**
    - How will conflict be managed?
    - Given the available time, what can be realistically achieved?
    - What ownership do you have over the evaluation findings?
    - To whom are you accountable for the evaluation strategy and its achievement?
    - What mechanisms will enable you to monitor progress?

Conclusion

This chapter has presented a detailed discussion of evaluation in the context of practice development. Previous chapters in this book have highlighted the importance of a systematic approach to practice development. Having a clear evaluation strategy to underpin or integrate with the development work is central to being systematic. We have presented a variety of approaches, methodologies and frameworks for evaluating practice developments at a variety of levels in the organisation. However, whilst all of these frameworks provide useful approaches to frame evaluation designs, we would argue that the most important factor is 'clarity of purpose' of practice development work. When the purpose of the practice development work is clear, determining the most appropriate evaluation approach is also easier. It is essential, however, that the evaluation approach is thought through at the outset of the practice development, even if the intended outcomes aren't clear!

References and further reading

Ayer, A.J. (1964) *The Concept of a Person and Other Essays*, Macmillan & Co Ltd, London.

Carr, W. & Kemmis, S. (1986) *Becoming Critical: Education, Knowledge and Action Research.* The Falmer Press, London.

Clandinin, D.J. & Connelly, M.F. (1996) Personal experience methods. In: *Handbook of Qualitative Research* (eds N.K. Denzin & Y.S. Lincoln.) pp. 413–27. Sage, Thousand Oaks, CA.

Clarke, C. & Wilcockson, J. (2001) Professional and organizational learning: analysing the relationship with the development of practice. *Journal of Advanced Nursing*, **34**(2), 264–72.

Clarke, J., Dudley, P., Edwards, A., Rowland, S., Ryan, C. & Winter, R. (1993) Ways of presenting and critiquing action research reports. *Educational Action Research*, **1**(2), 490–1.

Collier, J. Jnr (1967) *Visual Anthropology: Photography as a Research Method.* Holt, Rinehart & Winston, New York.

References

Eisner, E. (1991) *The Enlightened Eye: Qualitative Inquiry and the Enhancement of Educational Practices*. Macmillan, New York.

Fay, B. (1987) *Critical Social Science: Liberation and Its Limits*. Polity Press, Cambridge.

Geertz, C. (1973) Thick description: toward an interpretative theory of culture. In: *The Interpretation of Cultures* (ed. C. Geertz). Basic Books, New York.

Graham, I. (1996) A presentation of a conceptual framework and its use in the definition of nursing development within a number of nursing development units. *Journal of Advanced Nursing*, **23**(2), 260–6.

Grundy, S. (1982) Three modes of action research. *Curriculum Perspectives*, **2**(3), 23–34.

Grundy, S. & Kemmis S. (1981) Educational action research in Australia: the state of the art. Paper presented at the Annual Meeting of the Australian Association for Research in Adelaide. Cited by S. Grundy (1982) Three modes of action research. *Curriculum Perspectives*, **2**(3), 23–34.

Guba, E.G. & Lincoln, Y.S. (1981) *Effective Evaluation*. Jossey-Bass, San Francisco, CA.

Guba, E.G. & Lincoln, Y.S. (1989) *Fourth Generation Evaluation*. Sage, Thousand Oaks, CA.

Habermas, J. (1972) *Knowledge and Human Interests*, trans J.J. Shapiro. Heinemann, London.

Heron, J. (1981) Philosophical basis for a new paradigm. In: *Human Inquiry: A Sourcebook of New Paradigm Research* (eds P. Reason & J. Rowan). Wiley, Chichester.

House, E.R. (1981) *Evaluating With Validity*. Sage, London, Beverly Hills, CA.

House, E.R. (1993) *Professional Evaluation: Social Impact and Political Consequences*. Sage, London.

Kitson, A. & Currie, L. (1996) Clinical practice development and research activities in four district health authorities. *Journal of Clinical Nursing*, **5**(1), 41–51.

Koch, T. (1994) Beyond measurement: fourth-generation evaluation in nursing. *Journal of Advanced Nursing*, **20**(6), 1148–55.

Kushner, S. (2000) *Personalizing Evaluation*. Sage, London.

Laughlin, R. & Broadbent, J. (1996) Redesigning fourth generation evaluation: an evaluation model for public-sector reforms in the UK. *Evaluation*, **2**(4), 431–51.

Lincoln, Y.S. & Guba, E.G. (1985) *Naturalistic Inquiry*. Sage, Newbury Park, CA.

McCormack, B. (2001) *Negotiating Partnerships with Older People: A Person-centred Approach*. Ashgate, Aldershot.

McCormack, B. (2002) Getting research into practice: the meaning of 'context', *Journal of Advanced Nursing*, **38**(1), 94–104.

McCormack, B., Illman, A., Culling, J., Ryan, A. & O'Neill, S. (2002) Removing the chaos from the narrative: preparing clinical leaders for practice development. *Educational Action Research: An International Journal*, **10**(3): 335–52.

115

McCormack, B., Manley, K., Kitson, A., Titchen A. & Harvey, G. (1999) Towards practice development – a vision in reality or a reality without vision? *Journal of Nursing Management*, **7**(2), 255–64.

McCutcheon, G. & Jung, B. (1990) Alternative perspectives on action research. *Theory Into Practice*, **29**(3), Summer, 144–51.

McNiff, S. (1998) *Arts-Based Research*. Jessica Kingsley, London.

Manley, K. (1997) Operationalising an advanced practice/consultant nurse role: an action research study. *Journal of Clinical Nursing*, **6**(3), 179–90.

Manley, K. (2000) Organisational culture and consultant nurse outcomes. Part 2: consultant nurse outcomes. *Nursing Standard*, **14**(37), 34–9.

Manley, K. (2001) *Consultant nurse: concept, processes, outcome*. Unpublished PhD thesis. University of Manchester/RCN Institute, London.

Manley, K. & McCormack, B. (2003) Practice development: purpose, methodology, facilitation and evaluation. *Nursing in Critical Care*, **8**(1), 22–9.

May, R. (1994) *The Courage to Create*. W.W. Norton and Co., New York.

Nolan, M. & Grant, G. (1993) Service evaluation: time to open both eyes. *Journal of Advanced Nursing*, **18**(9), 1434–42.

Owen, J.M. & Rogers, P.J. (1999) *Program Evaluation – Forms and Approaches*. Sage, London.

Pawson, R. & Tilley, N. (1997) *Realistic Evaluation*. Sage, London.

Quinn-Patton, M. (1997) *Utilization-Focused Evaluation*. Sage, London.

Redfern, S. (1998) Evaluation: drawing comparisons or achieving consensus? *Nursing Times Research*, **3**(6), 464–74.

Richardson, L. (1997) *Fields of Play*. Rutgers University Press, New Jersey.

Royal College of Nursing (RCN) (2003) *Expertise in Practice Project: Final Report*. RCN, London.

Schön, D.A. (1991) *The Reflective Practitioner: How Professionals Think in Action*. Avebury, Aldershot.

Sharp, A. & Eddy, C. (2001) Softly, softly catch the monkey: innovative approaches to measure socially sensitive and complex issues in evaluation research. *The Canadian Journal of Program Evaluation*, **16**(2), 87–99.

Simons, H. (1996) The paradox of case study, *Cambridge Journal of Education*, **26**(2), 225–40.

Simons, H. & McCormack, B. (2002) Arts based inquiry – the challenges for evaluation. Paper presented at the annual Conference, United Kingdom Evaluation Society, The Art of Evaluation: Artistry, Discipline, and Delivery. South Bank Centre, London, 12–13 December.

Stake, R.E. (1972) An approach to the evaluation of instructional programs (program portrayal versus analysis). Paper delivered at the annual meeting of the American Educational Research Association, Chicago, April. Extracts reprinted in: *Beyond The Numbers Game: A Reader in Educational Evaluation* (eds D. Hamilton, D. Jenkins, C. King, B. MacDonald & M. Parlett) (1977). Macmillan Educational, London.

Stake, R.E. (1994) *Case Studies. Handbook of Qualitative Research* (eds N.K. Denzin & Y.S. Lincoln). CA Publications, Newbury Park, CA.

References

Stake, R.E. (1995) *The Art of Case Study Research*. Sage, London.

Stake, R.E. & Kerr, D. (1994) *Rene Magritte, constructivism and the researcher as interpreter*. Paper presented to the Annual Meeting of the American Educational Research Association, New Orleans, LO.

Stringer, E.T. (1999) *Action Research*, 2nd edn. Sage Publications: Thousand Oaks, CA.

Suchman, E.A. (1967) *Evaluative Research*. Russell Sage Foundation, New York.

Tickle, L.(1995) Testing for quality in educational action research: a terrifying taxonomy? *Educational Action Research*, **3**(2), 233–7.

Titchen, A. (1995) Issues of validity in action research. *Nurse Researcher*, **2**(3), 39–51.

Winter, R. (1989) *Learning From Experience: Principles and Practice in Action Research*. The Falmer Press, London.

Wortman, P.M. (1983) Evaluation research: a methodological perspective. *Annual Review of Psychology*, **34**(2) 223–60.

This chapter originally appeared in Manley & McCormack (2003). Reproduced with permission.

6. Research Implementation
Evidence, Context and Facilitation – the PARIHS Framework

Jo Rycroft-Malone

Introduction

It is 30 years since Briggs (1972) called for nursing to be research based. Despite this declaration there remains a general consensus in the literature that research-based nursing is still not a reality. It could be concluded that the use of research is easier to promote than to achieve, with much of the literature identifying why nurses do not use it, rather than how and when they do. Whilst nurses have a clear responsibility to offer care to patients that is based on the best available research evidence, this presents a number of challenges that do not have simple solutions. Much practice development activity begins from the perspective of research utilisation, with an explicit emphasis on addressing practice context issues that act as barriers to the use of research as well as developing practices that are based on research evidence. Thus, considering approaches to research implementation is a legitimate component of practice development and indeed, constitutes a significant agenda for practice developers.

This chapter begins by outlining the political context that places an onus on nurses to deliver care based on research. The demands and complexities involved in getting research into practice are then discussed and the Promoting Action on Research Implementation in Health Services (PARIHS) framework introduced as a means to consider the many factors influencing the uptake of evidence into practice.

118

The policy context

Evidence-based healthcare has evolved against a background of rising health costs, a management ethos of 'doing things right' and a drive for quality improvement. It has emerged as one of the dominant themes of practice, management and education within the National Health Service (NHS) in the United Kingdom. Muir Gray (1997) argues that in the twenty-first century, every healthcare decision will have to be based on a systematic appraisal of the best available evidence, which of course includes research. As such, mounting pressure is being exerted to ensure that the delivery of care is evidence-based and clinically effective with recent policy statements including:

> The Government is determined that the services and treatment patients receive across the NHS should be based on the evidence of what does and does not work and what provides best value for money.
>
> (DoH, 1997a)

The setting up of the National Institute for Clinical Excellence (NICE), the proliferation of national guidelines, protocols and systematic reviews and the advent of clinical governance is visible confirmation of an increasing emphasis on an NHS founded on evidence of what works. Furthermore, the aim of the NHS Research and Development strategy is to 'create a knowledge-based health service in which clinical, managerial and policy decisions are based on sound information about research findings and scientific developments' (DoH, 1997b). So, the expectation from government is that nurses (alongside their multidisciplinary colleagues) will be basing their practice on the best available evidence, including research.

However, as Hunt (1996) points out, whilst evidence-based healthcare remains 'flavour of the month', the idea of basing care on available research knowledge has featured in nursing literature and policy for over 30 years. Nursing policy documentation consistently emphasises the role of research in informing nursing, midwifery and health visiting practice (e.g. DoH, 1999; 2000). For example, *Making a Difference* clearly states that: 'Practice needs to be evidence based. Research evidence will be rigorously assessed and made accessible. Nurses . . . need better research skills to translate research findings into practice' (DoH, 1999).

Whilst there is no ambiguity in this intention and some progress has been made, nurses and nursing have still failed to realise the full potential of their contribution. In recognition of this, recommendations, in the form of a strategy document, have been made for strengthening the nursing contribution to undertake research *and* support nurses' use of research (DoH, 2000). Clearly the level of support that is provided to addressing the recommendations will be crucial to determining the successful implementation of this strategy and thus of nurses' contribution to this important activity. Meanwhile the message is clear – nurses should be using research in their practice. The challenges that this message presents, however, are considerable and complex. If it were straightforward, the production of research evidence, perhaps in the form of guidelines, followed by an education or teaching package would lead to an expectation that practitioners would automatically integrate them into their everyday practice. But we know that this is not the case, and often practice lags behind what is known to be current best practice.

The challenges and complexities of using research in practice

Much of the research exploring why nurses might not use research in practice has focused at the level of the individual practitioner and identified obstacles and barriers to utilisation (e.g. Hunt, 1981; Funk *et al.*, 1991; Rogers, 1994, 2000; Nolan *et al.*, 1998; Parahoo, 1999; Thompson *et al.*, 2001a; McCaughan *et al.*, 2002). In parallel, models and frameworks that have been developed to encourage nurses' use of research in practice focus on the role that individuals play in the process (e.g. Titler *et al.*, 1994, Burrows & McLeish, 1995). As a result emphasis has been placed on helping nurses to find and critically appraise research evidence in the hope that this will influence its transfer into practice (e.g. *Making a Difference*, DoH, 1999). However, despite all these efforts and considerable investment, for the most part, research is still not used routinely in practice. The question then remains, why is this the case?

The broad answer to this question is that getting research into practice is a complex process, which requires more than a focus on addressing individual influencing factors. Addressing the education of individual nurses by for example enhancing their critical appraisal skills is unlikely to affect their ability to use research in practice, moreover it is unrealistic to expect it to do so. The individual nurse cannot be isolated from all the other bureaucratic, political, organisational and social factors that affect change. The implementation of research-based practice depends on an ability to achieve significant and planned behaviour change involving individuals, teams and organisations. This is borne out by experience gathered from multi-centre projects such as the Promoting Action on Clinical Effectiveness (PACE) programme (Dunning *et al.*, 1998; Dopson *et al.*, 1999) and the South Thames Evidence-Based Practice (STEP) project (McLaren & Ross, 2000). Both evaluations highlight the multi-faceted nature of getting research into practice. The PARIHS framework, presented in the following sections acknowledges this, and provides a conceptual map of the factors that influence the successful implementation of evidence into practice.

Promoting Action on Research Implementation in Health Services (PARIHS) framework

Analysis of practice development, quality improvement and research project work conducted throughout the last decade or so (e.g. RCN, 1990; Morrell *et al.*, 1995; Ward *et al.*, 1998; McCormack & Wright, 1999) indicates that a number of key factors appear to play a role in the successful implementation of research into practice (Kitson *et al.*, 1998; Rycroft-Malone *et al.*, 2002). The Promoting Action on Research Implementation in Health Services (PARIHS) framework (Table 6.1) represents the interplay and interdependence of the many factors influencing the uptake of evidence into practice.

The framework presents successful research implementation as a function of the relation between *evidence*, *context* and *facilitation*. The three elements: evidence, context and facilitation are each positioned on a 'high' to 'low' continuum. The proposition is that for implementation of evidence to be successful, there needs to be clarity about the nature of the evidence being used, the quality of context, and the type of facilitation needed to ensure a successful change process. Theoretical and retrospective analysis of four studies (Kitson *et al.*, 1998) led to a proposal that the most successful implementation seems to occur when evidence is scientifically robust and matches professional consensus and patients' preferences ('high' evidence), the context receptive to change with sympathetic cultures, strong leadership, and appropriate monitoring and feedback systems ('high' context), and, when there is appropriate facilitation of change, with input from skilled external and internal facilitators ('high' facilitation).

Since the framework's conception and publication in 1998 it has undergone some research and development work. Most notably this has included a concept analysis (after Morse *et al.*, 1996) of each of the dimensions: evidence, context and facilitation. This has

Table 6.1 Promoting Action on Research Implementation in Health Services (PARIHS) framework.

Elements		Sub-elements	
		Low	**High**
Evidence	Research	Poorly conceived, designed and/or executed research	Well conceived, designed and executed research, appropriate to the research question
		Seen as the only type of evidence	Seen as one part of a decision
		Not valued as evidence	Valued as evidence
		Seen as certain	Lack of certainty acknowledged
			Social construction acknowledged
			Judged as relevant
			Importance weighted
			Conclusions drawn
	Clinical experience	Anecdote, with no critical reflection and judgement	Clinical experience and expertise reflected upon, tested by individuals and groups
		Lack of consensus within similar groups	Consensus within similar groups
		Not valued as evidence	Valued as evidence
		Seen as the only type of evidence	Seen as one part of the decision
			Judged as relevant
			Importance weighted
			Conclusions drawn
	Patient experience	Not valued as evidence	Valued as evidence
		Patients not involved	Multiple biographies used
			Partnerships with healthcare professionals
		Seen as the only type of evidence	Seen as one part of a decision
			Judged as relevant
			Importance weighted
			Conclusions drawn
Context		Lack of clarity around boundaries	Physical, Social, Cultural, Structural, System boundaries clearly defined

Table 6.1 *Continued*

Elements	Sub-elements	
	Low	**High**
	Lack of appropriateness and transparency	Appropriate and transparent decision-making processes
	Lack of power and authority	Power and authority processes
	Lack of resources	Resources
	Lack of information and feedback	Information and feedback
	Not receptive to change	Receptiveness to change
Culture	Unclear values & beliefs	Able to define culture(s) in terms of prevailing values/beliefs
	Low regard for individuals	Values individual staff and clients
	Task driven organisation	Promotes learning organisation
	Lack of consistency	Consistency of individuals role/experience to value: • relationship with others • teamwork • power and authority • rewards/recognition
Leadership	Traditional, command and control leadership	Transformational leadership
	Lack of role clarity	Role clarity
	Lack of teamwork	Effective teamwork
	Poor organisational structures	Effective organisational structures
	Autocratic decision-making processes	Democratic inclusive decision-making processes
	Didactic approaches to learning/teaching/managing	Enabling/empowering approach to teaching/learning/managing
Evaluation	Absence of any form of feedback	Feedback on: • individual • team ⎫ Performance • system ⎭

123

Table 6.1 *Continued*

Elements		Sub-elements	
		Low	**High**
		Narrow use of performance information sources	Use of multiple sources of information on performance
		Evaluations rely on single rather than multiple methods	Use of multiple methods: • Clinical • Performance • Economic ⎫ Evaluations • Experience ⎭
		Inappropriate facilitation	Appropriate facilitation
Facilitation	Purpose	Task	Holistic
	Role	*Doing for others* • Episodic contact • Practical/ technical help • Didactic, traditional approach to teaching • External agents • Low intensity – extensive coverage	*Enabling others* • Sustained partnership • Developmental • Adult learning approach to teaching • Internal/external agents • High intensity – limited coverage
	Skills and attributes	*Task/doing for others* • Project management skills • Technical skills • Marketing skills • Subject/technical/ clinical credibility	*Holistic/enabling* • Co-counselling • Critical reflection • Giving meaning • Flexibility of role • Realness/authenticity

enabled some conceptual clarity to be gained about the constituent elements and as a result, a refinement of its content. The following sections outline the contents of the PARIHS framework following this concept analysis process. The intention is to provide readers with a theoretical perspective of why these factors appear to be important in implementing research into practice. In addition to this, examples from practice and research will be used to illustrate the points being made.

The nature and role of evidence

So far, this chapter has referred to getting *research* into practice. However, in reality a number of different sources of knowledge and information need to be combined and used in clinical decision-making with patients. More specifically, the PARIHS framework identifies these as research, clinical experience and patient experience (Fig. 6.1).

Evidence

Research Low   High

- Poorly conceived, designed and/or executed research
- Seen as only one type of evidence
- Not valued as evidence
- Seen as certain

- Well conceived, designed and executed research appropriate to the research question
- Seen as one part of a decision
- Lack of uncertainty acknowledged
- Social construction acknowledged
- Judged as relevant
- Importance weighted
- Conclusions drawn

Clinical Experience Low   High

- Anecdote, with no critical reflection and judgement
- Lack of consensus within similar groups
- Not valued as evidence
- Seen as only one type of evidence

- Clinical experience and expertise reflected upon, tested by individuals and groups
- Consensus within similar groups
- Valued as evidence
- Seen as one part of the decision
- Judged as relevant
- Importance weighted
- Conclusions drawn

Patient Experience Low   High

- Not valued as evidence
- Patients not involved
- Seen as the only type of evidence

- Valued as evidence
- Multiple biographies used
- Partnerships with healthcare professionals
- Seen as only one part of a decision
- Judged as relevant
- Importance weighted
- Conclusions drawn

Fig. 6.1 The meaning of evidence and its dimensions.

Research evidence

Research evidence often can only address one small part of the complex experiences surrounding healthcare. Therefore the implementation of research into practice should be viewed as part of the wider context of practice development and evidence-based practice. Arguably this is particularly the case for nursing practice and development where there are many issues that, as yet, do not have a sound research evidence base. Consider, for example, pressure ulcer risk assessment and prevention; there is good quality research evidence to suggest that if an individual is at risk of developing pressure ulcers they should be placed on an alternative surface to a standard mattress (Cullum *et al.*, 2000; RCN, 2000). However, to date, there is no definitive research evidence to indicate the type of surface this should be, or indeed how to accurately determine a patient's level of risk. In such cases, the experience of the clinical team, the preferences of the patient and the local contract with suppliers of mattresses all make up the jigsaw of decision-making.

Whilst research evidence is only one piece of the jigsaw, there are certain factors that should guide whether it should or should not be used in practice. Traditionally 'evidence' has been synonymous with research carried out using experimental designs (Sackett *et al.*, 1997), particularly research that emphasises effectiveness, for example, randomised controlled trials (RCTs). Cullum (1997), in a selective search of the literature on nursing interventions from Medline (1966–94) and a hand search of 11 nursing journals from their inception, found 522 papers reporting RCTs and 20 systematic reviews. As Close & Cheater (1999) point out, Cullum's work does identify some RCTs that evaluate aspects of nursing care but the numbers are small considering the scope of nursing practice. This means that there is insufficient *trial* evidence to inform many aspects of everyday practice, but about which nurses need to make decisions (e.g. Rycroft-Malone, 2001). In the absence of RCT evidence and in cases where this type of evidence is not warranted because it is not appropriate (i.e. when studying issues that are not about effectiveness), the use of best available evidence drawn from other designs and paradigms are more appropriate and is advocated. For example, if we wanted to know about the patient's experience of living with diabetes, conducting an exploratory interview study would be a more suitable approach than carrying out an RCT. Critically, PARIHS proposes that what is important in making a decision about whether research evidence should be considered for implementation is that it is well conceived (e.g. uses an appropriate design to address the particular research question), is well

126

designed and well conducted. This may, of course, draw on the findings of quantitative and/or qualitative research evidence and necessarily means that it has to be appraised in order to be judged credible.

Even having assessed the credibility of the research evidence there are still other factors that might influence its uptake in practice. Upshur (2000) points out that 'the production, interpretation, dissemination and implementation of evidence is a social process subject to the forces and vagaries of social life'. Further he draws our attention to the values and beliefs underscoring evidence pointing out that 'the evidence we seek is partly constituted by what we value and what we believe'. The notion of evidence having a social and historical value for individuals and groups has also emerged , for example, Ferlie *et al.* (1998, 1999) describe a two-stage case study investigating the progress of four clinical change issues across one healthcare region in England. They identified that the social and historical construction of evidence had been a significant influencing factor in its uptake into practice. More specifically they report that different individuals and groups had multiple perspectives and attached different meanings to the evidence being implemented. As a result the uptake of the research evidence into practice was patchy. Recent research conducted with nurses highlights the significant role that human sources of information play in making decisions about care (Thompson *et al.*, 2001a, b). If nurses turn, for example, to practice development nurses as their main source of 'knowledge', the practice development nurses' role and ability in particularising evidence for practitioners becomes crucial. In recognising the social aspects of evidence, the PARIHS framework indicates that individuals and teams need to agree on the results of the appraisal to reach a consensus about it so that it becomes valued as a valid source of evidence (or not). Moreover, this also points to the need for evidence to be particularised and translated into the context into which it is being implemented, requiring the assistance of skilled facilitators.

Evidence from clinical experience

The paradox about evidence-based practice, is that although research evidence is viewed as the 'gold standard', it is always tempered by clinical experience and expertise (Dickinson, 1998), whilst research evidence aids decision-making it does not dictate the process. The PARIHS framework acknowledges the interaction between research evidence and clinical expertise and considers clinical experience to be a second strand or form of 'evidence'.

Knowledge that practitioners develop over time from their practice and life experiences has been defined and conceptualised by Titchen (2000) as 'professional craft knowledge' or 'practical know-how'. A comprehensive account of professional craft knowledge is provided in Chapter 7 of this book. She defines it as the often tacit and sometimes intuitive knowledge that is embedded in practice. Expert practitioners, especially, may take this knowledge for granted, seeing it as so ordinary and everyday that it is not worth mentioning. Or they may not be able to express it in words. The relevance of this type of knowledge is that if the thoughts of an expert practitioner are made accessible to the less experienced, it helps them interpret their own experiences and acquire and develop their own knowledge (Titchen, 2000).

Titchen (2000) goes on to suggest that this professional craft knowledge can be made more widely available if it is 'articulated, critically reviewed, generated and validated, by individual practitioners and their peers, through critical reflection on practice'. Thus, there is the possibility for professional craft knowledge to be transformed to propositional knowledge and verified through critical reflection, critique and debate of clinical experience. This knowledge could then be disseminated out to other groups, who go through a similar process. In addition, as professional craft knowledge is used, there is the potential to develop and add to it. An individual's practical know-how can be tested against the professional craft knowledge of others, against research knowledge and against theoretical knowledge.

When knowledge from clinical experience is used as part of decision-making it is argued that it should be made explicit and verified through these processes. In a similar vein Upshur (1997) argues that clinical common sense needs to be evaluated to the same extent as trial evidence, otherwise no honing of clinical reasoning is possible. Combining these different forms of evidence in a systematic process involves testing them against each other, so that professional craft knowledge is tested against research knowledge and theoretical knowledge. These are complex processes which form part of the translation and particularisation of evidence into practice and as such require the skills of a facilitator to enable them to progress.

Evidence from those who use healthcare services

There is a great deal of rhetoric about patient or user involvement in decision-making and care. However, it is an issue that is complex and poorly understood. In recognising that patient experiences should be part of the decision-making process, patient narratives and experiences should also be seen as a valid source of evidence and is the third strand of evidence in the PARIHS framework. There are several different aspects to consider in relation to evidence from those with healthcare needs. Research evidence needs to be appropriately presented for informed decision-making, and lay perspectives are needed at all stages of the research process (Bastian, 1994; Oliver, 1997; Entwistle *et al.*, 1998).

Many qualitative findings will be firmly grounded in the experiences of individual patients. This, too, can be used as information to implement into practice. For example, *Ouch! Sort it Out: Children's Experiences of Pain* (RCN, 1999) provides an example of how patients', in this case children's, stories can be incorporated into the development of an evidence-linked guideline (the recognition and assessment of acute pain in children). Through techniques such as a drama workshop, video workshop, graffiti wall, sentence completion, play and interviews, children were given the opportunity to share their experiences of treatment and care, and what they would like to happen when they are in pain. This experience was then used as one of the evidence sources which fed into the development of a guideline that also incorporated research evidence and expert opinion evidence.

However, most use of information from patients may well be in the context of individual interactions with healthcare professionals. Knowing the world of the person has been described as necessary to 'find out exactly what is happening, to this person, at this particular time, and what sense and meaning they construct out of the experience' (Barker, 2000). The best way of generating and testing this evidence is in the early stages of development. Using stories from patients has been suggested as one way of understanding patient experiences. At the individual level it seems health professionals will need interpersonal skills, insight and an ability to combine both technical and humane decision-making within a partnership with service users. This process has been described as human based not data based (Barker, 2000). Whilst it is still unclear how best to combine patient's experiences in human-based rather than data-based decision-making, the value of participatory interactions are important.

Summary: the nature and role of evidence in research utilisation

So far, this chapter has highlighted that there are different forms of evidence that can inform nursing practice. The PARIHS framework places value on evidence from research, clinical and patient experience. The challenge remaining to practitioners and researchers,

Box 6.1 Questions for consideration about the nature of the evidence being implemented.

> - Is there any research evidence underpinning the initiative/topic?
> - Following critical appraisal is the research evidence judged to be well conceived, designed and conducted?
> - Are the findings from the research relevant to the initiative/topic of practice development?
> - What is clinician's experience and opinion about this topic?
> - Does the research match professionals' clinical experience about the initiative/topic (within and across the professions involved in the implementation)?
> - If it does not, why might this be so?
> - Do you need to try and seek consensus before trying to implement it?
> - What is the patient's experience/preference/story concerning the initiative/topic?
> - How does the research evidence and clinical experience relate to the patient's experience about the initiative/topic?
> - How can a partnership approach to implementation be developed?

however, is to understand how these are combined in clinical decision-making and how more effective care can be delivered by finding ways of using all the diverse aspects of this broader evidence base. Box 6.1 poses a number of questions derived from the PARIHS framework about evidence, which may require consideration when embarking on a project to get evidence into practice.

The context of implementation

Research has demonstrated that the factors in the setting in which evidence is to be used can have a significant impact (for example, managerial structures, staffing levels, the physical environment and so on; see Dunning *et al.*, 1998; Ferlie *et al.*, 1998, 1999; Wood *et al.*, 1998; Dopson *et al.*, 1999). As Wood *et al.* (1998) point out, in promoting innovation or a piece of research evidence we are not dealing merely with the uncomplicated dissemination of findings to a passive and receptive audience. Despite this growing acknowledgement, we are only just beginning to really understand the role that contextual factors can play in facilitating or inhibiting the research implementation process.

The context in which healthcare practice occurs can be seen as infinite as it takes place in a variety of settings, communities and cultures that are all influenced by (for example) economic, social, political, fiscal, historical and psychosocial factors. In the PARIHS framework, the term context is used to refer to the environment or setting in which people receive healthcare services, or in the context of getting research evidence into practice. In its most simplistic form, the term means the physical environment in which practice takes place. Such an environment has boundaries and structures that together shape the setting for practice. The context of practice with which individuals and teams interact is complex and always changing. This means that not only are there 'no magic bullets' for getting research into practice (Oxman, 1994), but there are also 'no magic targets' (Dopson *et al.*, 2002).

The following sections outline the contextual factors that the PARIHS framework promotes as key to the successful implementation of evidence into practice. These fall under the three broad themes of: culture, leadership, and evaluation (Fig. 6.2). The text for these sections has been primarily derived and summarised from a paper by McCormack *et al.* (2002). Readers are referred to this paper for a more in-depth analysis of the issues.

Culture

Culture is widely seen as central to both understanding and transforming organisations. For example, *A First Class Service* (DoH, 1998) explicitly states an intention to changing the organisational culture of the NHS through clinical governance, lifelong learning and self-regulation. As the linchpin to the UK government's quality improvement strategy, it sets out an expectation that clinical governance 'is about changing organisational culture in a systematic and demonstrable way'. Furthermore, *Learning from Bristol* (2001) dedicates a whole chapter to the need to change the culture of the NHS. The inquiry recommends the culture of the future to be one of safety and of quality, of openness and accountability in which collaborative teamwork is prized, one that is flexible and in which innovation can flourish in response to patients' needs. Whilst the goals are clear, what does this mean in terms of a culture that encourages the use of evidence in practice?

Manley (2000) after Drennan (1992) defines culture as the 'way things are done around here', and argues that culture is created at the level of the individual, team and organisation, such that it creates the context for practice (see Chapter 4). Following this line of argument, it could be proposed that if we want to make changes to the context of healthcare, changing the prevailing culture may enable this to happen.

131

Context

Low   High

- Lack of clarity around boundaries
- Lack of appropriateness and transparency
- Lack of power and authority
- Lack of resources
- Lack of information and feedback
- Not receptive to change

- Physical/social/cultural/structural/system – boundaries clearly defined
- Appropriateness and transparent decision-making processes
- Power and authority processes
- Information and feedback
- Receptiveness to change

Culture

Low   High

- Unclear values and beliefs
- Low regard for individuals
- Task driven organisation
- Lack of consistency

- Able to define culture(s) in terms of pre-vailing values/beliefs
- Values individual staff and clients
- Promotes learning organisation
- Consistency of individual role/experi-ence to value
- Relationship with others
- Teamwork
- Power and authority
- Rewards/recognition

Leadership

Low   High

- Traditional, command and control
- Lack of role clarity
- Lack of teamwork
- Poor organisational structures
- Autocratic decision-making processes
- Didactic approach to learning/teaching/managing

- Transformational leadership
- Role clarity
- Effective teamwork
- Effective organisational structures
- Democratic inclusive decision-making
- Enabling/empowering approach to learning/teaching/managing

Evaluation

Low   High

- Absence of any form of feedback
- Narrow use of performance infor-mation source
- Evaluations rely on single rather than multiple methods
- Lack of teamwork
- Poor organisational structures
- Autocratic decision-making processes
- Didactic approach to learning/teaching/managing

- Feedback on:
  - Individual
  - Team   } Performance
  - System
- Use of multiple sources of information on performance
- Use of multiple methods:
  - Clinical
  - Performance } Evaluations
  - Economic

Fig. 6.2   The meaning of context and its dimensions.

132

The concept of a learning organisation (Senge, 1990) is promoted by the PARIHS framework as the type of organisation that embraces the key characteristics to facilitate learning and the implementation of change. It is believed that these organisations value individual's contributions, are open, have decentralised decision-making, a shared vision and quality organisational systems. In turn these factors tend to build innovative, facilitative cultures. These are also the types of organisations which writers of policy documents deem to be critical to fulfilling the government's agenda on, for example, clinical governance (e.g. *A First Class Service*, DoH, 1998). To move towards these types of cultures requires the implementation of strategies and processes that value individual's self development, reduce the contextual factors that mediate self-fulfilment and develop ways of translating tacit knowledge into explicit knowledge without relying on traditional management procedures (McCormack *et al.*, 2002). Clearly the challenges inherent in this shift are considerable, complex and not to be underestimated.

Many diverse and conflicting cultures can operate within the organisational context with many different values, beliefs and assumptions embedded within it (Bate, 1994). Therefore the starting point is to gain an understanding of these as a prerequisite to introducing evidence into practice. This is supported by the practical experiences of others (e.g. Dopson *et al.*, 1999). For the PACE projects a contextual analysis identified the receptiveness of the context(s) to change. This information was not only important in terms of identifying potential barriers to change (individuals and structures) but also useful when planning strategies to overcome obstacles or engaging support.

Leadership

Leaders have a key role to play in transforming cultures and are therefore influential in shaping a context that is ready for change. Leadership is about knowing how to make visions become reality (Kitson, 2001). In the PARIHS framework leadership summarises the nature of human relationships in the practice context. In this sense, leadership has the potential to bring about clear roles, effective teamwork and effective organisational structures. The underpinning philosophy of the framework is the belief that everyone can be a leader of something. Accordingly, it is this leadership potential in individual practitioners that needs to be developed and released.

Transformational leaders, as opposed to those that command and control, have the ability to transform cultures to create contexts that are more conducive to the integration of evidence into practice (Schein, 1985). Furthermore it is argued that transformational leaders create a culture that recognises everybody as a leader of something. These types of leaders inspire staff to have a shared vision and do so in a stimulating, challenging and enabling way. Mintzberg (1975) suggests that the qualities and skills required by transformational leaders include: emotional intelligence, rationality, motivational skills, empathy and inspirational qualities and the intellectual qualities of strategic sensing, analytical skills and self confidence.

The significance to the successful implementation of evidence into practice is that effective, transformational leaders have the ability to bring the 'science' component of healthcare practice (the application of science and technology) together with the 'art' component (the translation of different forms of practice knowledge) into caring actions (Manley, 2000). Further research, however, is required to understand the cause and effect relationship between leadership and culture.

Evaluation

An additional component of the environment that seems to play a role in shaping its readiness for implementation is that of evaluation. Measurement generates evidence on which to base practice and is part of the evaluation or feedback process that demonstrates whether or not changes to practices are appropriate, effective and or efficient. Traditionally, in the health service there has been an emphasis on collecting 'hard' outcomes data about performance and effectiveness of practice. Indeed, the focus of recent reforms through, for example, clinical governance serve to reinforce and perpetuate hard outcome measurement. However, this approach has been criticised as being too narrowly focused and not reflective of the complexities involved in the delivery of healthcare (e.g. Nolan & Grant, 1993).

Guba and Lincoln (1989), Pawson and Tilley (1997) and Quinn-Patton (1997) argue that evaluation frameworks need to reflect the complexity of organisational systems and the multiple realities of stakeholders. A framework of evaluation such as this would be congruent with the current emphasis on user involvement, practitioner reflections and practice narratives (McCormack *et al.*, 2002). It is therefore argued through the PARIHS framework that contexts in which evaluation relies on broad and multiple sources of evidence of effectiveness, in addition to 'harder' outcomes, tend to be those that are more receptive to change. This is because such contexts not only accept and value different sources of feedback information but also create the conditions for practitioners to apply them into practice as a matter of course.

Summary of the context of implementation

The context of practice and thus of research evidence implementation is complex and dynamic. PARIHS proposes that a context's characteristics are key to ensuring a more conducive environment to get evidence into practice. More specifically it is proposed that a 'strong' context, where there is, for example, clarity of roles, decentralised decision-making, staff are valued, transformational leaders and a reliance on multiple sources of information on performance will make the chances of successful implementation more likely.

Box 6.2 poses a number of questions derived from the PARIHS framework about context, which may require consideration when embarking on a project to get evidence into practice.

The role of facilitation

It is proposed that a facilitator has a key role to play in not only affecting the context in which change is taking place but also in working with practitioners to make sense of the 'evidence' being implemented (Harvey *et al.*, 2002). Kitson *et al.* (1998) describe facilitation as 'a technique by which one person makes things easier for others' (p. 152). Facilitation has been applied in different fields and

Box 6.2   Questions for consideration about the context of implementation.

- Is the context of implementation receptive to change?
- What are the beliefs and values of the organisation, team and practice context?
- Does the context have features of a learning organisation? (e.g. decentralised and transparent decision-making, pay attention to individuals and group processes, utilise a facilitative management style)
- Is the leadership style 'transformational' rather than 'command and control'?
- Are individual and team boundaries clear?
- Is there effective team working (inter- and multidisciplinary)?
- Does evaluation of performance rely on broad and varied sources of information?
- Are there processes in place to ensure that this performance information is fed back to clinical contexts?

disciplines both within and outside of healthcare, including practice development, health promotion, clinical supervision, quality improvement, audit, action research, education, counselling, and management. In healthcare, there are also other strategies thought to be effective in terms of promoting individual and organisational change that include a mixture of change agent roles and change management techniques, such as academic detailing, educational outreach visits, audit and feedback, social influence and marketing approaches (see, for example, Lomas *et al.*, 1991 and Locock *et al.*, 2001). There is evidence to suggest that some of these approaches are effective in some situations and that the most effective implementation strategies are those that adopt a multi-faceted approach (Oxman 1994; Bero *et al.*, 1998; Halliday & Bero, 2000).

In the context of the PARIHS framework, facilitation refers to the process of enabling (making easier) the implementation of evidence into practice. Thus, facilitation is achieved by an individual carrying out a specific role (a facilitator), which aims to help others. This indicates that facilitators are individuals with the appropriate roles, skills and knowledge to help individuals, teams, and organisations apply evidence into practice. What is key, is that appropriate facilitation is instigated, where 'appropriate' may encompass a range of roles and interventions depending on the needs of the situation. The following sections outline the key facets of facilitation which enable the successful implementation of evidence into practice. These fall under the three broad themes of: purpose, role, and skills and attributes (Fig. 6.3). The text for these sections has been primarily derived and summarised from a paper by Harvey *et al.* (2002). Readers are referred to this paper for a more in-depth analysis of the issues.

The purpose of facilitation

The concept of facilitation emerged from the fields of counselling and student-centred learning, influenced largely by humanistic psychology and, in particular, Carl Rogers' work on therapeutic, client-centred approaches to counselling (1983). In Rogers' work and subsequent developments (see, for example, Reason & Rowan, 1981; Heron, 1989), facilitation refers to a process of enabling individuals and groups to understand the processes they have to go through to change aspects of their behaviour or attitudes to themselves, their work or other individuals. Hence, the focus is on facilitating experiential learning through critical reflection.

A similar understanding emerges from some approaches to practice based learning in healthcare (e.g. student centred learning,

Facilitation

Low	High
No mechanisms, or inappropriate methods of facilitation in place	Appropriate mechanisms for facilitation in place

⇩

Purpose, Role, Skills

Purpose Task — Holistic

Role Doing for others — Enabling others

• Episodic contact • Practical/technical help • Didactic, traditional approach to teaching • External agents • Low intensity-extensive coverage	• Sustained partnership • Developmental • Adult learning approach to teaching • Internal/external agents • High intensity-limited coverage

Skills and Attributes Task/doing for others — Holistic/enabling

• Project management skills • Technical skills • Marketing skills • Subject/technical/clinical credibility	• Co-counseling • Critical reflection • Giving meaning • Flexibility of role • Realness/authenticity

Fig. 6.3 The meaning of facilitation and its dimensions.

problem based and experiential learning) that have applied frameworks of reflective practice and clinical supervision (Johns & Butcher, 1993). The aim with this type of approach is to challenge existing practice and support the development of new ways of working. For example, in Titchen's model of facilitation described as critical companionship (Titchen, 2000) and seated within a practice development approach to developing person-centred care, clinical and facilitation expertise are developed through experiential learning. Here, the emphasis is on facilitating learning from practice and, co-creation of new knowledge through critical reflection, and dialogue between the practitioner (or learner) and an experienced facilitator (the critical companion). The role of the companion is to help individuals and groups of practitioners to use the new theoretical insights to transform self and social systems that hinder improvements in practice.

In contrast, in other fields, such as quality improvement and some health promotion activities, the purpose of facilitation appears to be on achieving specific tasks and goals. For example, in some models of health promotion (e.g. 'Oxford Model', Fullard, 1994), although the emphasis is on helping, it is more specifically focused on the achievement of tasks (e.g. putting health checks in place) than on exploring relationships at team and individual levels.

There are of course hybrid models of facilitation that would fall some way between the developmental and the task orientated role. For example, in the Dynamic Standard Setting System (DySSSy) (RCN, 1990) facilitation is identified as one of the key building blocks of a method that aims to promote the local implementation of standards and audit. Facilitation is consequently focused on two key aims, namely the achievement of specific goals (the implementation of standards and audit in practice) and the development of processes to enable effective teamwork (Morrell & Harvey, 1999). Additionally, in practice development and action research there is evidence that facilitation can encompass different modes, providing a range of technical, practical and emancipatory support during the change process (Jackson *et al.*, 1999; Titchen, 2000; Garbett & McCormack, 2002; Manley & McCormack, 2003).

The PARIHS framework acknowledges that the purpose of facilitation can vary from a focused process of providing help and support to achieve a specific task ('Task') (e.g. 'Oxford Model') to a more complex, holistic process of enabling teams and individuals to analyse, reflect and change their own attitudes, behaviours and ways of working ('Holistic') (e.g. 'Critical Companionship'). As the approach moves towards the holistic, facilitation is increasingly concerned with addressing the whole situation and the whole person(s). However, the key to 'appropriate' facilitation is matching the purpose, role and skills to the needs of the situation.

The facilitator role

Just as the purpose of facilitation appears to vary within the literature, there are also multiple interpretations of the facilitator role in practice. These range from a practical 'hands-on' role of assisting change to a more complex, multi-faceted role (Harvey *et al.*, 2002). In the models of health promotion which explicitly employ a facilitator, the emphasis is on external facilitators using an 'outreach' model to work with several primary healthcare practices, providing advice, networking and support to help them establish the required health promotion activities (Fullard *et al.*, 1984). In contrast, approaches to facilitation that are rooted in the fields of counselling and experiential learning are strongly influenced by underlying theories of humanistic psychology and human inquiry. Consequently, the facilitator's role is concerned with enabling the development of reflective learning by helping to identify learner needs, guide group processes, encourage critical thinking, and assess the achievement of learning goals. For example, in some of the reported practice development initiatives, the facilitator role is concerned with enabling cultural change in organisations, through facilitating individuals and teams to analyse and challenge current ways of working through methods of reflection using action learning and mentoring (Garbett & McCormack, 2002). This often involves models of external–internal facilitation, where facilitators from outside the change setting work with identified internal facilitators, using a range of support and supervisory methods to enable the development of the internal facilitator's own skills and knowledge in managing change (Binnie & Titchen, 1999; McCormack & Wright, 1999).

PARIHS proposes that the operationalisation of the facilitator role will depend on the underlying purpose and interpretation of the facilitation concept. A broad distinction can be made between a facilitator role that is concerned with 'doing for others' and a role whose primary emphasis is on 'enabling others' (Loftus-Hills & Harvey, 2000). The 'doing' role is likely to be practical and task-driven, with a focus on administrating, supporting and taking on specific tasks where necessary. In contrast an 'enabling' facilitator role is more likely to be developmental in nature, seeking to explore and release the inherent potential of individuals. In reality, many approaches contain elements of both these characteristics.

Skills and attributes of facilitators

In order to fulfil the potential demands of the role, facilitators will require a wide repertoire of skills and attributes. However, there appears to be little concrete evidence in the literature as to the mix and relative importance of the different skills needed for the successful performance of the facilitator role. Generally it seems that a mixture of personal attributes and personal, interpersonal and group management skills contribute to the development of effective facilitation. Table 6.2 outlines the different facilitation skills and attributes that have been identified from studies using facilitation in three different activity areas.

Whilst there are core skills, such as interpersonal and communication skills that are believed to be a prerequisite requirement of

Table 6.2 Skills and attributes required to be an effective facilitator.

'Oxford' or Health promotion	DySSSy	Practice development

Allsop (1990)
 • Supplying technical or clinical advice Networking
 • Offer suggestions
 • Formulate solutions
 • Help shift attitudes
 • Political skills
 • Vision
 • Energy
 	
 Fullard (1994)
 • Catalyst for change
 • Resource agent
 • Helping hand
 • Teambuilding
	Morrell et al. (1995)
	 • Empowering clinicians
	 • Recognition of other's skills and abilities
	 • Local credibility
	 • Highly developed communication skills
	
	 Harvey (1993)
	 • Knowledgeable and up-to-date
	 • Innovators
	 • Help with group dynamics
	 • Understanding the system
	 • Lateral thinking
	 • Sensitive
	 • Good communicator
	 • Allowing people to learn by their own processes
		Garbett and McCormack (2002)
		 • Being pragmatic
		 • Risk taker
		 • Belief in the worth and value of people
		 • Patience
		 • Commitment
		 • Having vision
		 • Being motivated
		 • Being empathetic
		 • Experiential
		
		 Titchen (2000)
		 • Attending to whole person through use of self
		 • Facilitating:
		   • cognition, meta-cognition, intuition and their interplay
		   • use of different kinds of evidence
		   • particularisation of research findings
		 • Ability to create an environment of high support and high challenge

any facilitator role, it appears that to be effective, facilitators require a tool kit of skills and personal attributes that they can use depending on the context and purpose. Arguably, the expertise is in having the flexibility to be able to recognise the requirements of an individual situation. This may mean drawing on a combination of skills and qualities in the course of any implementation and change process.

Summary – the role of facilitation

Facilitation and facilitators have key roles to play in the implementation of evidence into practice. Whilst there is still some

Box 6.3 Questions for consideration about facilitation.

- Consider the answers to the questions posed in Tables 6.1 and 6.2 – what work needs to be achieved in order to implement evidence into this particular practice context?
- What might be the appropriate method of facilitation required for the needs of the initiative/topic?
- What tasks or processes will require facilitation?
- Based on the tasks and processes that require facilitation – what approach(es) is going to be appropriate to adopt?
- What type of skills and attributes will the person(s) facilitating require to be effective in the role?
- Would it be appropriate to draw on the skills and knowledge of an external facilitator to work with internal facilitators?
- What role might the facilitator have in evaluating the outcomes of the project?

conceptual clarity to be gained about how it may differ from other change agent roles (see Harvey *et al.*, 2002 for a discussion of this), the PARIHS framework proposes that fundamentally, the facilitator role is one which supports practitioners to change their practice. This is likely to include the need to work with practitioners to particularise and translate different types of evidence into practice, as well as working with individuals and teams to affect changes to the context of implementation in order for it to be transformed into the type of practice environment that is conducive to change. Box 6.3 poses a number of questions derived from the PARIHS framework about facilitation which may require consideration when embarking on a project to get evidence into practice.

Summary and conclusions

Mounting pressure is being exerted to ensure that the delivery of care is evidence-based and clinically effective. Both health and nursing policy documentation consistently remind us of this message. Whilst the message is clear, the solution is less easily found. Getting research evidence into practice is a complex, demanding and often messy undertaking. Traditionally it has been assumed that giving practitioners pieces of evidence and developing their individual capacity to be able to appraise and understand them, would lead to an expectation that they would be automatically used in practice. This naïve assumption has predominated in both policy and practice literature.

The complexities and challenges posed by implementing research into practice demand more innovative and multi-faceted approaches. This chapter has presented the PARIHS framework which attempts to present a conceptualisation of the key ingredients involved in the implementation of evidence into practice. It represents successful implementation of evidence into practice as dependent upon the nature of the *evidence*, the quality of the *context*, and the type of *facilitation* used. These need to be considered as interdependent and operating simultaneously during implementation processes. It is proposed that implementation is more likely to be successful when:

- Research evidence is well conceived, designed and executed, clinical experience reflected on and tested out by individuals and groups, and patient experience valued and integrated into the implementation and development process.
- The context in which the evidence is being implemented is characterised by a clarity of roles, decentralised and transparent decision-making processes, transformational leadership, effective team work and a reliance on multiple sources of information on performance.
- Facilitation mechanisms appropriate to the needs of the situation, have been instigated.

There are still questions and issues that need to be better understood including the relationship(s) between evidence, context and facilitation, and the relative importance of them when implementing evidence-based practices. This research work continues in the quest to increase our understanding so that we can be better placed to help practitioners plan and implement effective change and development strategies. In the meantime, the framework as outlined here, provides a useful conceptual coat hanger, by raising key issues for consideration and action that are appropriate to the work of practice developers.

References

Allsop, J. (1990) *Changing Primary Care: The Role of Facilitators*. King's Fund, London.

Barker, P. (2000) Reflections on caring within an evidence-based culture, *International Journal of Nursing Studies*, **37**(4), 329–36.

Bastian, H. (1994) The power of sharing knowledge: consumer participation in the Cochrane Collaboration (1994) Retrieved August 2000 from http://www.update-software.com/ccweb/cochrane/powershr/htm

References

Bate, P. (1994) *Strategies for Cultural Change*. Butterworth-Heinemann, Oxford.

Bero, L., Grilli, R., Grimshaw, J.M., Harvey, E., Oxman, A.D. & Thomson, M.A. (1998) Closing the gap between research and practice: an overview of systematic reviews of interventions to promote the implementation of research findings. *British Medical Journal* **317**, 465–8.

Binnie, A. & Titchen, A. (1999) *Freedom to Practice: The Development of Patient-centred Nursing*. Butterworth-Heinemann, Oxford.

Briggs, A. (1972) *Report of the Committee on Nursing (Briggs Report)*, Cmnd 5115. HMSO, London.

Burrows, D.E. & McLeish, K. (1995) A model for research-based practice. *Journal of Clinical Nursing*, **4**(3), 243–7.

Closs, S.J. & Cheater, F.M. (1999) Evidence for nursing practice: clarifying some issues, *Journal of Advanced Nursing*, **30**(1), 10–17.

Cullum, N. (1997) Identification and analysis of randomised controlled trials in nursing: a preliminary study. *Quality in Health Care*, **6**(1), 2–6.

Cullum, N., Deeks, J., Sheldon, T.A., Song, F. & Fletcher, A.W. (2000). Beds, mattresses and cushions for preventing and treating pressure sores (Cochrane Review). In: *The Cochrane Library*, Issue 1, Oxford: Update Software.

Department of Health (DoH) (1997a) *The New NHS: Modern, Dependable*. Stationery Office, London.

Department of Health (DoH) (1997b) *Research and Development: Towards an Evidence-Based Health Service*. Stationery Office, London.

Department of Health (DoH) (1998) *A First Class Service*. Stationery Office, London.

Department of Health (DoH) (1999) *Making a Difference*, Stationery Office, London.

Department of Health (DoH) (2000) *Towards a Strategy for Nursing Research and Development*, Stationery Office, London.

Dickinson, H.D. (1998) Evidence based decision-making: an argumentative approach. *International Journal of Medical Informatics*, **51**(1), 71–81.

Dopson, S., FitzGerald, L., Ferlie, E., Gabbay, J. & Locock, L. (2002) No magic targets! Changing clinical practice to become more evidence based. *Healthcare Management Review*, **27**(3), 35–47.

Dopson, S., Gabbay, J., Locock, L. & Chambers, D. (1999) *Evaluation of the PACE Programme: Final Report*. Oxford Healthcare Management Institute & Wessex Institute for Health Services Management.

Drennan, D. (1992) *Transforming Company Culture*. McGraw-Hill, London.

Dunning, M., Abi-Aad, G., Gilbert, D., Gillam, S. & Livett, H. (1998) *Turning Evidence Into Everyday Practice*. King's Fund, London.

Entwistle, V.A., Sheldon, T.A., Sowden, A. & Watt, I.S. (1998) Evidence-informed patient choice: practical issues of involving patients in decisions about healthcare technologies. *International Journal of Technology Assessment in Healthcare.* **14**, 212–25.

Ferlie, E., Wood, M. & Fitzgerald, L. (1998) Assuring high quality and evidence-based healthcare: a case study from HIV/AIDS services. *Quality in Health Care*, **7**(suppl), s24–s29.

Ferlie, E., Wood, M. & Fitzgerald, L. (1999) Some limits to evidence-based medicine: a case study from elective orthopaedics. *Quality in Health Care*, **8**(1), 99–107.

Fullard, E.M. (1994) Facilitating professional change in primary care. *Annals of Community-Oriented Education*, **7**(1), 73–8.

Fullard, E., Fowler, G. & Gray, M. (1984) Facilitating prevention in primary care. *British Medical Journal*, **289**, 1585–7.

Funk, S., Champagne, M., Weise, R. & Tornquist, E. (1991) Barriers: the barriers to research utilisation scale. *Applied Nursing Research*, **4**(1), 39–45.

Garbett, R. & McCormack, B. (2002) A concept analysis of practice development, *Nursing Times Research*, **7**(2), 87–100.

Guba, E.G. & Lincoln, Y.G. (1989) *Fourth Generation Evaluation.* Sage, Thousand Oaks, CA.

Halliday, M. & Bero, L. (2000) Implementing evidence-based practice in healthcare. *Public Money and Management*, **20**(1), 43–50.

Harvey, G. (1993) *Nursing quality: an evaluation of key factors in the implementation process*, Unpublished PhD thesis. South Bank University, London.

Harvey, G., Loftus-Hills, A., Rycroft-Malone, J., *et al.* (2002) Getting evidence into practice: the role and function of facilitation. *Journal of Advanced Nursing*, **37**(6), 577–88.

Heron, J. (1989) *The Facilitator's Handbook.* Kogan Page, London.

Hunt, J. (1981) Indications for nursing practice: the use of research findings. *Journal of Advanced Nursing*, **6**, 189–94.

Hunt, J. (1996) Barriers to research utilization. *Journal of Advanced Nursing*, **23**(3), 423–5.

Jackson, A., Cutcliffe, J., Ward, M., Titchen, A. & Cannon, B. (1999) Practice development in mental health nursing: part 2. *Mental Health Practice*, **2**(5), 2–9.

Johns, C. & Butcher, K. (1993) Learning through supervision: a case study of respite care. *Journal of Clinical Nursing*, **2**(1), 89–93.

Kitson, A. (2001) Nursing leadership: bringing caring back to the future. *Quality in Healthcare*, **10**(Suppl II), ii79–ii84.

Kitson, A., Harvey, G. & McCormack, B. (1998) Enabling the implementation of evidence-based practice: a conceptual framework. *Quality in Health Care*, **7**(3), 149–58.

Learning from Bristol (2001). The Report of the Public Inquiry into Children's Heart Surgery at the Bristol Royal Infirmary 1984–1995. Stationery Office, London: www.bristol-inquiry.org.uk

Locock, L., Dopson, S., Chambers, D. & Gabbay, J. (2001) Understanding the role of opinion leaders in improving clinical effectiveness. *Social Science and Medicine*, **53**, 745–57.

Loftus-Hills, A. & Harvey, G. (2000) *A Review of the Role of Facilitators in Changing Professional Health Care Practice.* RCN Institute: Oxford.

Lomas, J., Enkin, M., Anderson, G.M., Hannah, W.J., Vayda, E. & Singer, J. (1991) Opinion leaders versus audit and feedback to implement practice guidelines. *Journal of the American Medical Association*, **265**, 2202–7.

McCaughan, D., Thompson, C., Cullum, N., Sheldon, T. & Thompson, D.R. (2002) Acute care nurses' perceptions of barriers to using research information in clinical decision-making. *Journal of Advanced Nursing*, **39**(1), 46–60.

McCormack, B., Kitson, A., Harvey, G., Rycroft-Malone, J., Seers, K. & Titchen, A. (2002) Getting evidence into practice: the meaning of 'context'. *Journal of Advanced Nursing*, **38**(1), 94–104.

McCormack, B. & Wright, J. (1999) Achieving dignified care for older people through practice development – a systematic approach. *Nursing Times Research*, **4**(5), 340–52.

McLaren, S.M.G. & Ross, F. (2000) Implementation of evidence in practice settings: some methodological issues arising from the South Thames Evidence Based Practice Project. *Clinical Effectiveness in Nursing*, **4**(1), 99–108.

Manley, K. (2000) Organisational culture and consultant nurse outcomes. Part 1: organisational culture. *Nursing Standard*, **14**(36), 34–8.

Manley, K. & McCormack, B. (2003) Practice development: purpose, methodology facilitation and evalution. *Nursing in Critical Care*, **8**(1), 21–9.

Mintzberg, H. (1975) The manager's job: folklore and fact. *Harvard Business Review*, July–August, 49–61.

Morrell, C. & Harvey, G. (1999) *Clinical Audit Handbook.* London: Ballière-Tindall.

Morrell, C., Harvey, G. & Kitson, A. (1995) *The Reality of Practitioner Based Quality Improvement: a Review of the Use of the Dynamic Standard Setting System in the NHS of the 1990s*, Report No. 14. National Institute for Nursing, Oxford.

Morse, J.M., Hupcey, J.E., Mitcham, C. *et al.* (1996) Concept analysis in nursing research: A critical appraisal. *Scholarly Inquiry for Nursing Practice: An International Journal*, **10**(3), 253–77.

Muir Gray, J.A. (1997) *Evidence Based Healthcare. How to Make Health Policy and Management Decisions.* Churchill Livingstone, London.

Nolan, M. & Grant, G. (1993) Service evaluation: time to open both eyes. *Journal of Advanced Nursing*, **18**, 1434–42.

Nolan, M., Morgan, L., Curran, M., Clayton, J., Gerrish, K. & Parker, K. (1998) Evidence-based care: can we overcome the barriers? *British Journal of Nursing*, **7**(20), 1273–8.

Oliver, S. (1997) Exploring lay perspectives on questions of effectiveness. In: Non-random Reflections on Health Services Research (eds A. Maynard & I. Chalmers). *British Medical Journal*, pp 22–291.

Oxman, A. (1994) *No Magic Bullets: A Systematic Review of 102 Trials of Interventions to Help Health Care Professionals Deliver Services More Effectively or Efficiently.* North East Thames Regional Health Authority, London.

Parahoo, K. (1999) A comparison of pre-Project 2000 and Project 2000 nurses' perceptions of their research training, research needs and their use of research in clinical areas. *Journal of Advanced Nursing*, **29**, 237–45.

Pawson, R. & Tilley, N. (1997) *Realistic Evaluation*. Sage, London.

Quinn-Patton, M. (1997) *Utilization-Focused Evaluation: The New Century Text* (3rd edn). Sage, London.

Reason, P. & Rowan, J. (eds) (1981) *Human Inquiry: A Sourcebook of New Paradigm Research*. John Wiley and Sons, Chichester.

Rogers, C.R. (1983) *Freedom to learn for the 80s*. Columbus, Ohio.

Rogers, S. (1994) An exploratory study of research utilization by nurses in general medical and surgical wards. *Journal of Advanced Nursing*, **20**, 904–11.

Rogers, S. (2000) The extent of nursing research utilization in general medical and surgical wards. *Journal of Advanced Nursing*, **32**(1), 182–93.

Royal College of Nursing (RCN) (1990) *Quality Patient Care: The Dynamic Standard Setting System*. Scutari, London.

Royal College of Nursing (RCN) (1999) *Ouch! Sort it Out. Children's Experiences of Pain*. RCN Publishing, London.

Royal College of Nursing (RCN) (2000) *Pressure Ulcer Risk Assessment and Prevention: a Clinical Guideline*. RCN publishing, London.

Rycroft-Malone, J. (2001) Formal consensus: the development of a national clinical guideline. *Quality in Health Care*, **10**, 238–44.

Rycroft-Malone, J., Kitson, A., Harvey, G., *et al.* (2002) Ingredients for change: revisiting a conceptual framework. *Quality and Safety in Health Care*, **11**, 174–80.

Sackett, D.L., Richardson, W.S., Rosenberg, W. & Haynes, B. (1997) *Evidence Based Medicine. How to Practice and Teach EBM*. Churchill Livingstone, Edinburgh.

Schein, E.H. (1985) *Organizational Culture and Leadership*. Jossey Bass, San Francisco, CA.

Senge, P.M. (1990) *The Fifth Discipline: The Art and Practice of the Learning Organisation*. Doubleday/Currency, New York.

Thompson, C., McCaughan, D., Cullum, N., Sheldon, T.A., Mulhall, A. & Thompson, D.R. (2001a) The accessibility of research-based knowledge for nurses in United Kingdom acute care settings. *Journal of Advanced Nursing*, **36**(1), 11–22.

Thompson, C., McCaughan, D., Cullum, N., Sheldon, T.A., Mulhall, A. & Thompson, D.R. (2001b) Research information in nurses' clinical decision-making: what is useful? *Journal of Advanced Nursing*, **36**(3), 376–88.

Titchen, A. (2000) *Professional Craft Knowledge in Patient-centred Nursing and the Facilitation of its Development*. University of Oxford DPhil thesis. Ashdale Press, Oxford.

Titler, M.G., Kleiber, C., Steelman, *et al.* (1994) Infusing research into practice to promote quality care. *Nursing Research*, **43**, 307–13.

Upshur, R. (1997) Certainty, probability and abduction: why we should look to C.S. Pierce rather than Godel for a theory of clinical reasoning. *Journal of Evaluation in Clinical Practice*, **3**(3), 201–6.

Upshur, R.E.G. (2000) Seven characteristics of medical evidence. *Journal of Evaluation in Clinical Practice*, **6**(1), 93–7.

References

Ward, M., Titchen, A., Morrell, C, McCormack, B. & Kitson, A. (1998) Using a supervisory framework to support and evaluate a multi-project practice development programme, *Journal of Clinical Nursing*, **7**, 29–36.

Wood, M., Ferlie E. & Fitzgerald L. (1998) Achieving clinical behaviour change: a case of becoming indeterminate. *Social Science and Medicine*, **47**(11). 1729–38.

7. *Helping Relationships for Practice Development*
Critical Companionship

Angie Titchen

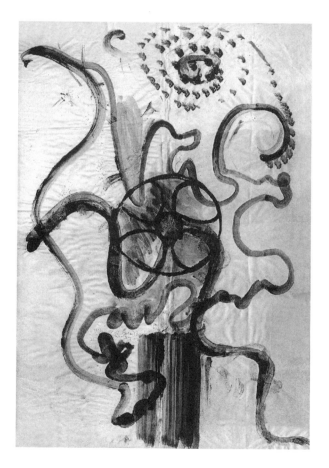

Fig. 7.1

Critical companionship is often highly intuitive, creative and magical, just as this phoenix arose quite by
itself with critical companionship at its heart.

(Angie Titchen, 2000)

Critical companionship is like eating a plate of
　spaghetti bolognaise
It has many ingredients, like spaghetti
　bolognaise
And it's difficult to tease out the individual
　strands of spaghetti
There are still many integral strands to unravel

Critical companionship is like thinking that you
　know
What is in the bolognaise but sometimes being
　surprised
When you discover a new ingredient

We learnt how to consume the spaghetti through
　the masterly companionship
Of a critical colleague and through observing and
　questioning
The strategies they use
And through critical conversations
About the different ways you could do it

Critical companionship has potential like bolog-
　naise sauce
To pervade everywhere

(Poem created by
Kim Manley, Kate Sanders,
Jennie Gill at
2002 RCN Institute Practice
Development School, Wales)

'Critical companionship' (Titchen, 2000) brings mind, heart, body, and creative imagination into helping relationships for practice development. It offers a metaphor and framework for an experienced facilitator (often, but not necessarily a colleague) who accompanies another on an experiential learning journey towards evidence-based, person-centred care. Creating trust and using 'high challenge' and 'high support',[1] critical companions enable individuals, teams and organisations to transform their roles, relationships, cultures and ways of thinking, being, doing and feeling. Companion and participants know that they will be together for the duration of this journey, with a mutual parting at the end. To establish, sustain and close the relationship, the critical companion uses the same practical know-how that they would use to make patient care person-centred. Thus the critical companion takes a person-centred approach to facilitating the practitioner's learning, becoming a role-model for using their true *self* (their personal qualities, as well as their professional behaviour and skills) in a helping relationship. As well as giving the practitioner direct experience of a person-centred approach, the critical companion also spells out the processes and strategies they use, to enhance the power of the role-modelling. This chapter explains this practical know-how of critical companionship and shows how people use it in their practice development work.

Although this critical companionship may seem simple, the work that Alison is doing here is very sophisticated (see box 7.1).

Box 7.1 Critical companionship expertise in action (all names except Angie Tichen and Alison Binnie are pseudonyms).

The Scene: Alison Binnie (AB), a senior sister and critical companion, and Dave (D), a staff nurse in his first year of qualified practice, are sitting in the staffroom of a busy medical ward. They are drinking tea while critiquing the care plan for Joe, Dave's patient. Alison and Dave have negotiated a critical companionship relationship with the purpose of helping Dave to acquire, in and from practice, the practical know-how of being person-centred. I am Alison's critical companion helping her to become a critical companion to the staff nurses (Binnie & Titchen, 1999). I observed and audio-taped this interaction.

AB: [Reading] 'Nursing action'. See here: 'Joe needs at present to feel that support is available, but just feels able to seek information for himself.' Now I just get bored reading sentences that long when I'm busy. I haven't got time. What I want to know is what you want me to do really. . . . If I look after him tomorrow, do you want me to do anything [pause] as regards these things?
D: Mm [long pause]. But not really no, because I'm the one he is talking to.
AB: So if I am looking after him tomorrow, it will be very helpful for me to know that.
D: Right.
AB: So, the most helpful thing for me is?
D: Don't talk to this man [laughs] that I am taking care [pause].
AB: 'I will manage information' – that's all really. So that I know it's being dealt with; it's planned, prescribed and I know it's you dealing with it. Just write what you want me to do, if he raises the subject and asks questions – and that's all.

Box 7.1 *Continued*

D: Say whatever you think is appropriate.
AB: So, 'I will take the major role in providing information. We have a strategy about his smoking or whatever'. That's it. That will do really! [All laugh].

Alison's intention in this dialogue was not just to focus on Dave's care plans, she was also thinking about the need to help him to focus his thinking because 'he is off in all directions all the time'.

Later, in critical dialogue with me:

AB: I think it is his difficulty in identifying saliency. . . . So it was easy to focus on that because you and I had agreed that I was going to help him to think about his style and thinking processes. So I wasn't just trying to work on his care planning, but also his thinking processes. . . . I was trying to ask him focusing questions. What comes over on the tape and which you pointed out at the time, it was a brilliant question – 'What do you want me to do tomorrow?' and there's a long pause [laughs] where he is *really* thinking now 'Gosh, well'. You can almost see his vision channelled down into a laser point [laughs] and that really put him on the spot! So that was a very good question. So coming in from a new angle.

(Titchen, 2000: 201)

It reveals how she:

- *knows what matters* in this situation, for Joe, for the nurse who will look after Joe tomorrow and for Dave in terms of helping him to become more focused;
- *knows* that Dave is not aware of what really matters here and that he will be comfortable with the supportive challenge that she is offering;
- *problematises* Dave's understanding of what needs to go on the care plan by looking at the plan from the angle of others in the team. Thus, she gently points out, without putting Dave down, that he is not being clear and succinct in his communication and that this could be problematic for the nurse tomorrow. She helps him to think deeply through the situation and come to a new insight himself;
- *role-models* the use of pithy, clear communication, free of extraneous detail, which is useful to other nurses caring for this particular patient – not only by the actual words, but in her delivery of them (synchronicity). Thus she is role-modelling the pace and

importance of focus in professional conversations that take place in hot action;

- *articulates her professional craft knowledge* (knowledge gained through professional experience) of writing person-centred care plans;
- *uses humour* to create a supportive space for challenge.

That Alison is able to do all this in a busy ward means she must *know the practitioner* (Dave), have awareness of her own qualities and of the environment and make *facilitative use of herself*.

Critical companionship is, first, about helping people to become more effective in delivering person-centred, evidence-based care and, second, about helping others to become critical companions. Becoming more effective requires the capacity to present evidence from our practice for critical review and evaluation by self and others. Such scrutiny leads, potentially, to both knowledge development and refinement to enhance our own practice and to contribute to the wider professional knowledge base. In order to critically review and develop new understandings about our practices, we have to understand the nature of our practice knowledge and how we use and create it in our everyday work (see Titchen, 2000). The evidence we review will come from many sources, from research and theory, from the knowledge that patients develop through their lives and experiences of illness and from the professional craft knowledge we develop from our practice and shape through our life experiences.

Developing a deep understanding of our practice knowledge, on our own, and/or articulating it fully to others is often difficult. This is because much of our professional craft knowledge is deeply embedded in our practices and our selves. So, it may either be very difficult to express in words, or, so taken for granted that we think it hardly worth mentioning. Critical companions help us to surface this knowledge and to become more aware, both of the way that we think, and of the way that intuitions and different types of knowledge inform our decision-making and practices. A critical companion helps us to check out the rigour and usefulness of all this evidence and to make sure that we are blending it appropriately, so that we can act effectively and imaginatively for each specific situation. In addition, critical companions help us to examine and challenge the often unconscious assumptions underpinning our actions and help us to free ourselves from the obstacles, either inner or outer, which get in the way of our development of evidence-based, person-centred care. Critical companionship is, therefore, a way of helping people to become reflective, person-centred practitioners, managers, clinical leaders, practice developers and practitioner-researchers.

In this chapter, I briefly describe the development and testing of the critical companionship framework. Then I present the framework and illustrate it and its impact with examples from RCN Institute practice development projects and practice development research. I end with messages for further journeys.

The creation of critical companionship

I created the term 'critical companionship' in 1998 and developed its theoretical perspectives and conceptual framework in my doctoral research, using action research and a phenomenological case study approach (see Titchen, 2000; 2001a, b). As mentioned above, I investigated how I, as a critical companion, helped Alison Binnie, a senior sister, to become an effective critical companion to the staff nurses who worked with her, in terms of helping them to become more patient-centred. The framework has since been tested and verified in other nursing settings (RCN, 2004; Wright & Dewing, 2003). It has also been used by other professions in educational and action research contexts (e.g. Higgs & Jones, 2000; Goodfellow *et al.*, 2001; Winter & Munn-Giddings, 2001).

The original critical companionship framework was influenced by four theoretical perspectives: (1) *critical social science* (e.g. Freire, 1985); (2) *humanistic existentialism* (e.g. Rogers, 1983); (3) *a spiritual perspective* based on a form of moderated love or graceful care (Campbell, 1984) which is most usually manifested in critical companionship as extraordinary generosity in terms of time, appropriate emotional engagement and caring; and (4) *a phenomenological perspective* concerned with the lived experience of practice, learning and researching. Since then, I have added a fifth perspective: (5) *nurturing the creative imagination* (see fig. 7.1) through creative arts (Seizing the Fire Collaborative, 2002). The framework is also complementary to the work of facilitation and reflection theorists, such as Mezirow (1981), Boud *et al.* (1985) and Heron (1989).

It is important to stress that, who the critical companion is, as a person, will shape the choice and emphasis of the theoretical perspectives used. For example, not all critical companions will want to use creative arts, so they could use other ways of helping people to express the hidden aspects of practice and of drawing out the creative imagination.

Whilst the framework itself is new, you may recognise some of the practical know-how, just like 'thinking that you know what is in the bolognaise'. This is not surprising, given that it has been developed by surfacing the professional craft knowledge of skilled facilitators. What the framework has done is put the know-how together in a new way. It also reveals the subtleties and nuances of embedded, everyday facilitation practice of which you may not be so aware. Maybe, you will be surprised if you 'discover new ingredients'.

The framework

The conceptual framework of critical companionship is laid out in a series of overlapping circles (see Fig. 7.2) which represent various practical know-how domains.[2]

1. The relationship between the critical companion and the practitioner, team or organisation.
2. *Relationship domain*, with four processes:

   * *Mutuality*: working with/partnership working
   * *Reciprocity*: reciprocal closeness, giving and receiving
   * *Particularity*: knowing the practitioner/team/organisation
   * *Graceful care*: using all aspects of self

   These processes stand in a 'prerequisite relationship' with each other, *working with* (mutuality) being the most dependent. For effective mutuality, then, all the other processes in the relationship domain must be used and well-developed by the critical companion.
3. *Rationality–intuitive domain*, with three processes:

   * *Intentionality*: acting intentionally or deliberately
   * *Saliency*: knowing what matters and acting on it
   * *Temporality*: attending to time, timeliness, anticipating, pacing

   These are practical tools to help use of the relationship and facilitation processes. They are, therefore, prerequisites for the relationship and facilitation processes. For example, to get to know the individual/team/organisation (*particularity*), we must use deliberate strategies (*intentionality*) to find out about them and the situation we're examining together. But they are not prerequisites for each other which is why they are set out in the same ring.
4. Strategies to put the relationship and rationality–intuitive processes into action.
5. *Facilitation domain*, with four processes:

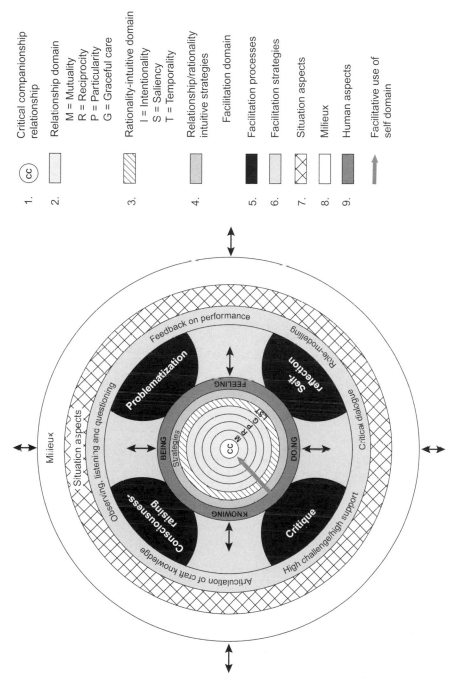

Fig. 7.2 Critical companionship: a conceptual framework for facilitating learning from experience.

- *Consciousness-raising*: bringing hidden or taken-for-granted knowledge to the surface
- *Problematisation*: raising awareness of problems in situations that are perceived as being problem-free
- *Self-reflection*: facilitating critical investigation of own self and practice
- *Critique*: developing new knowledge and critically reviewing it through debate.

These processes do not have prerequisite relationships with each other.

6. Strategies to put the facilitation processes into action.
7. The situation – the focus of the critical companionship or the broad aspects of the situation under examination (e.g. facilitating: learning in and from clinical practice; interdisciplinary team working; practitioner-research; or the articulation of knowledge embedded and taken-for-granted in expertise).
8. The milieux or the opportunities for reflection which can be seized or created by the critical companion (e.g. opportunistic and formal clinical supervision, action learning, 360° feedback sessions, work-based learning, practitioner-research, workshops and practice development strategy meetings). Little arrows indicate the *antennae* through which critical companions sense what is happening both internally and around them.
9. *Facilitative use of self domain* – the big arrow shows how critical companions take themselves as a person into their relationship with the individual/team/organisation, i.e. their own being, knowing, doing and feeling. The dotted lines around the arrow indicate how the companion 'picks up' the necessary bits of practical know-how in the relationship, rationality–intuitive and facilitation domains, and blends them together into a unique mix for working with each individual/team/organisation and situation. This domain is overarching: all the other domains and strategies interplay here, and are shaped by the personal qualities of the critical companion, the particular situation and the opportunities available to work together. There are any number of patterns and combinations, as the dotted lines show. This blending of know-how and bringing ourselves into our work as critical companions is part of professional artistry (see Titchen & Higgs, 2001; Titchen & McGinley, 2003).

Before going into the detail of the framework, I explain why I chose the particular examples to illustrate it.

The examples come from my original research and several RCN Institute projects, but primarily from the Expertise in Practice Project (EPP) (RCN, 2004; Titchen & McGinley, 2003) and the Gerontological Nursing Practice Development Programme (GNPDP) (Dewing & Wright, 2002; Wright & Dewing, 2003). These two projects represent different uses of critical companionship. In the EPP, critical companions helped nurses with expertise in a variety of nursing fields, to become practitioner-researchers, gathering evidence from their own patients and colleagues in order to develop a portfolio for accreditation by the RCN. The companions were mainly senior nurses who were already experienced facilitators or university educators. Even so, they needed support in their development of the critical companionship skills which was provided through action learning. The EPP is an example of critical companionship used over a one-off, intensive period. In contrast, the critical companions in the GNPDP are senior nurses (G to I grades) who have continuous responsibility for practice development within their organisational roles. They therefore work with many individuals and teams, but in the examples here, they are working with clinical leaders (F and G grades). These critical companions had no educational backgrounds and little or no previous experience of facilitation.

Finally, in the definitions of the critical companionship processes, I refer only to 'practitioner' for brevity, but equally, 'manager', 'clinical leader', 'practice developer', 'practitioner-researcher', 'nursing team', 'inter-professional team', or 'stakeholders' could be used.

Relationship domain

Mutuality

The critical companion and practitioner work together in a partnership that is carefully negotiated. Critical companions are alert to the practitioner's readiness to learn, making use of opportunities for shared experiences. They build on the practitioner's starting point and offer their knowledge and experience as a resource for the practitioner to draw on in solving problems and helping them learn from practice.

Strategies

- Creating equality in the relationship, especially in hierarchical organisations where a companion who is more senior or has specialist knowledge and expertise would be seen as the more powerful.

> A critical companion (CC) who is a Professor of Nursing Research took care to set up a contract with an expert practitioner (EN) in the EPP in which he explicitly valued the practitioner's expertise. The outcomes for EN were that she never sensed a huge gap between them and she experienced CC as always offering his own expertise with humility.

- Sharing responsibility with the practitioner for the structure, process and outcomes of the relationship.
- Helping the practitioner to understand the situation now and what is likely to happen.

> CC describes how she and EN have experienced difficulties developing their relationship. 'If the relationship is going to develop symbiotically then EN is going to have to reciprocate and provide the input that you would expect of the expert practitioner.' CC describes how EN perceives her as having expertise within their relationship and, therefore, as having the responsibility for it and for the project work. She realises that she should not take (all the) responsibility because the relationship needed to be more balanced. In order for the relationship to 'meet in the middle', CC felt she needed to step back.
>
> (EPP action learning set notes)

Creating a genuine partnership in which responsibility is shared is no easy task; however, it can be helped on the way by setting out a contract in which responsibilities and ways of working are made explicit, agreed and evaluated regularly. It is important to negotiate the strategies of critical companionship, for example, high challenge/high support and to talk about the kind of culture that you want within the relationship. Stepping back, whilst giving support, may be necessary to give people enough space to have a go at what may be a new activity.

Reciprocity

Reciprocity is the mutual, collaborative, educative and empowering exchange of feelings, thoughts, knowledge, interpretations and actions. Both companion and practitioner recognise that they receive gifts of care, concern, satisfaction and wisdom from each other.

Strategies

- Negotiating
- Receiving
- Learning

> CCs in the GNPDP valued the way that critical companionship skills had made them more effective in all aspects of their work, whilst many CCs in the EPP felt privileged and enriched by the wisdom and skilled know-how revealed to them by their ENs.
>
> Working with one of the ENs who participated in the EPP gave me insight into how to work collaboratively with a practitioner in using and developing new theoretical frameworks (Titchen & McGinley, 2003).

Particularity

Particularity is getting to know and understand the unique details and experience of the practitioner, within the context both of the specific learning situation and of people's lives (as far as they wish to disclose). Once the companion knows 'where the person is at', they take this as the starting point from which they can help people learn from their own experience. Each individual is seen as a unique, whole person, as well as a colleague, with individual needs that can be met in different ways. Organisations are also seen as unique with different needs.

Strategies

- Observing the practitioner's situation and responses, facilitating and listening to their stories and self-reflections, picking up on cues and clues
- Blending knowledge of the practitioner with the companion's self-knowledge, professional craft knowledge (know-how built up through professional practice) and facilitation theory and research, to design and evaluate unique learning experiences

If a critical companion is working with an organisation and stakeholders, it is important for the companion to meet as many key individuals and groups as possible. This enables the companion not only to get to know them and their ways of working, but also to get a sense of the kind of culture operating in the organisation that is expressed through their language and behaviour.

Graceful care

Graceful care is support given to the practitioner by the critical companion through their presence, touch and use of body language (including posture, speed of movement, tone of voice) to express both who they are as a person and their response to the practitioner, which makes them feel personally valued, and to promote emotional, psychological and intellectual growth.

Strategies

- being genuine and expressing self as a person
- being generous with self, knowledge and time
- giving undivided attention
- being physically and emotionally present with the practitioner in times of stress, disappointment and frustration, listening, engaging and giving reassurance
- maintaining a balance between absence and too much emotional closeness with the practitioner
- dealing with own negative or inappropriate emotions
- using humour to provide support
- valuing the practitioner as a person and their unique professional contribution

---

Graceful care has already been displayed above (see Box 7.1), in Alison's generosity in sharing her skills with Dave and in the way she did not put Dave down when she was giving him feedback on his care plan.

AB: When people are trying something new, if you knock them down early, it is hard to pick up. People are so fragile and sensitivity is important. They are very tentative, trying so hard and they need accurate feedback, in the sense that it is important to show them where they need to develop or improve. It needs to be done quite gently, so they are not just squashed. And if they feel that they have got half way there themselves, that just makes the rest of the criticism much more tolerable (Titchen, 2000: 137).

Staff Nurse: Alison gives you good feedback, always honest. It never puts you down, it's very clever . . . I justify what I did and she will say, 'Yes, that's fine, now I understand why you've done it', instead of saying, 'No, that's wrong'. She takes on board what you have to say (Titchen, 2000: 138).

EN in EPP: When I asked a question, CC never indicated that the question was silly, inappropriate or showed my lack of knowledge. He never let me down or made me feel that I was wasting his time. If he disagreed with something I said, he never said so, rather he asked why, listened to my response and then presented me with another option. He never cancelled a teleconference without giving me an alternative date to avoid my disappointment. This gave me a sense of being cared for, rather than feeling brushed aside for something more important to him.

Graceful care is also part of the 'stepping back' of mutuality because it often has an emotional component. For example, like Alison working with Dave, critical companions might see the way forward clearly, but they will slow down and help practitioners to work it out for themselves. Graceful care would mean being patient and not letting any signs of irritation or frustration show.

Rationality–intuitive domain

Intentionality

Intentionality is consciousness, self-awareness and thoughtfulness of critical companions as they deliberately use all the critical companionship strategies.

> *EN*: The EPP action learning set facilitator intentionally used reflection at the end of the set meeting, not only to conclude, but also to help us to see the critical companionship domains in action during the meeting and how they were helping us to become researchers of our own practice. She asked us to use a critical companionship matrix to identify which processes and strategies we had used, how and how well. She explained that we don't have to use all the boxes all the time, that there will be different emphases according to the uniqueness of each situation.

Saliency

Saliency is the ability to know, both consciously and intuitively, what is important, of concern and of significance, from both the critical companion's and the other's perspectives. Using significant cues and clues to plan learning strategies to address what matters.

Saliency is at work in Alison's session with Dave. She knew that Dave was having difficulty, generally, with knowing what was important to attend to in his care, 'he is off in all directions all the time'. Seizing this opportunity, she helped him to focus down on what really mattered for Joe's care tomorrow.

> CC sensed that EN was stuck in relation to using the reflective tool (Johns, 2001) in practice: 'I was reading about it, but was not translating it into practice. CC let me go on for so long with this reading and then he gave me a set of questions. These questions helped me to move from theory to practice. He knew just what I needed.'

Temporality

Temporality means time, timing and pacing. The critical companion should understand the need to attend to what's happened in the past and the present and could develop in future. They should make time for this work, and act (or hold back) in timely ways at the right pace for the practitioner, anticipating their needs.

Strategies

- Acknowledging past, present and future time
- Making focused time
- Timeliness
- Regulating speed of interaction or balance of conversation

> In the GNPDP, a CC made focused time for a clinical leader by setting up a reflective session to discuss a difficult issue. Giving undivided attention, she could see that his past experiences of respite care for this particular patient and her family were influencing his current response to them. However, due to his defensiveness, CC knew that this moment was not right to challenge him and she waited for a more appropriate time (Wright & Titchen, 2003). Timeliness is also apparent in the EPP example just above.

Facilitation domain

Consciousness-raising

Consciousness-raising is bringing into the practitioner's consciousness the knowledge embedded in daily practice, and a recognition of the nature of this knowledge. This includes a practitioner's intuitions and behaviour and the effect they have whilst practising as clinicians, practice developers, clinical leaders, practitioner-researchers, critical companions and so on.

> The RCN facilitator was role-modelling consciousness raising – getting CC to see how the conceptual labels of the CC model could be applied to what, on the surface, seemed to be an 'ordinary' meeting with her EN. The facilitator ran through the model to help CC to do this . . . CC said that it 'is difficult to describe what the meeting was' in terms of the processes and strategies. The facilitator then explained where she saw them in action in the CC's description of the ordinary meeting . . .
> *Facilitator*: So that's brilliant, there's lots of evidence there.
> CC: More than I thought! It's strange when you break up a conversation.
>
> CC went away with an action plan to be more aware of how she was using the critical companionship processes in her work not only with EN, but also with her ward staff.
>
> (EPP action learning set notes)

162

Problematisation

Problematisation is helping the practitioner to become aware of, and to critique, the tacit understandings that have grown up around repetitive, routinised practice, pointing out areas which might need attention but are not perceived by the practitioner as problems. Where practitioners do see a problem but can't find a solution, the critical companion helps them to see things from a different perspective. If practitioners are unaware of inconsistencies or contradictions in their practice, the companion gently points them out.

> When I arrived EN looked fed up and said that he had had a very traumatic day with a particular patient. We talked in general terms about the project and what could contribute to evidence, but he was still preoccupied with the events of the day. I asked him to tell me about the incident and his role within it. He said he felt the incident had not gone well, but as he was telling the story I was aware of the *relationship domains* of skilled companionship (Titchen, 2001b) (parallel with critical companionship domains) and that this demonstrated *particularity*. What he was describing was *graceful care* within his relationship with the patient and *intentionality* of his response to a difficult situation. He had used *informed intuition* and *rational thinking* to respond in a way that assessed therapeutic risk and preserved the therapeutic relationship for the future. . . . I reflected back to him that the story was, in fact, his evidence of expertise and that in itself would make a powerful narrative to capture the essence of his practice.
>
> (RCN, 2004)

Self-reflection

Self-reflection is a cyclical process in which practitioners critically reflect upon and evaluate their experiences, thinking and intuitions in a particular situation. The critical companion helps them to describe the important features of their actions, behaviours, what happened and their thoughts and feelings. The companion encourages a focus on positive feelings and dealing with negative ones. The companion also supports the analysis by making people aware of their thinking and reasoning processes. New knowledge is linked with what they already know. People are then helped to draw conclusions about these experiences, to use theory to deepen understanding, and then use their conclusions to inform action plans.

> *CC*: I was to facilitate a reflective session for the staff on a ward, based around a complaint they had received. I was aware that this was a very dispirited team (*particularity*), but also that I needed to challenge some practice in order to do the complainant justice (*saliency* and *intentionality*). I used *high challenge with high support*. I used *saliency* to focus on the causes of the problems, not the outcomes. I listened to their accounts and questioned at points where I considered *deeper reflection* might be useful. I asked the team to seek support when needed. We drew up an action plan.
>
> I enjoyed the process. I was able to challenge and received a good response from them – they accepted the challenge and rose to it. The feedback was that they came away feeling motivated. I have realised that a lot can be learned from reflection and negative emotions can be turned around.
>
> (GNPDP reflective account)

> *CC*: You say that reading Carper (1978) and Benner (1984) helped you to increase your awareness, but did they offer you anything else to help you to get to where you are now?
>
> *EN*: These people gave me a framework to interpret my practice . . . I realised that everybody has to start as a novice [and Benner's framework] gave me a goal towards developing expertise [in assessing people's pain and needs].
>
> (EPP portfolio)

Critique

Critique is a collaborative, critical reflection on an experience and the situation in which it took place. Personal and professional issues and meanings in the situation are uncovered, and the influence of cultural, social, historical and political factors/constraints explored. The companion and practitioner debate these in the light of their newly gained insights, understandings and interpretations of practice. Refined understandings are then used to develop new knowledge about how to change the situation within the practitioner's own sphere of work, within social, cultural, historical and political constraints.

The following example shows how critique builds on the three other facilitation processes.

The RCN Institute worked with NHS Trusts to help them to implement and evaluate clinical supervision for nurses. This work involved the development of learning cultures. At the beginning, we encountered 'them' (management) and 'us' (practitioners) cultures within which blame cultures existed. There was often a marked lack of trust and a fear of reprisals. For example, nurses were fearful about being supervised by their managers, stating that they would not expose weaknesses or mistakes in supervision, even though they knew that this would be the most effective use of it. To address this concern, we:

- *raised* practitioners' and managers' *consciousness* of the kind of culture that would support clinical supervision;
- helped practitioners and managers to see that their deeply-held, perhaps unconscious, attitudes, language and behaviours were getting in the way of changing the culture, even though everyone said that they wanted it to change (*problematisation*);
- enabled *self-reflection* on these attitudes, language and behaviours and helped people to explore the historical, cultural, social and political reasons why these cultures had developed. We felt reassured by research that shows how hard it is to change behaviours that are deeply socialised into our practices and use of language;
- together we *critiqued* their new self-understandings and insights into the old and new cultures to inform discussions on culture change. The practitioners came to see how they could take the strategic lead within the Trust to ensure that clinical supervision was sustained and built into the Trust's clinical governance and business plans. They formed themselves into a Trust-wide steering group.

Practitioners and managers reported shifts towards a learning culture. One steering group reported that the programme had enabled:

- Opportunities to develop practice, challenge poor practice, contribute to Clinical Governance;
- Use evidence-based practice and link it with PREP;
- A shift from a blame culture to improving skills and practice;
- Access to continuing professional development and personal growth;
- Empowerment to develop capacity to be reflective and thoughtful.

(Clinical Supervision Steering Group, 2002)

The four facilitation processes can be put into action by the following strategies.

Strategies

- *Role-modelling* evidence-based, person-centred skills and strategies, critical, creative and independent thinking processes and the use and blending of creative imagination and rigorous evidence/knowledge of all kinds.

- *Articulating craft knowledge* about these practices through, for example, telling stories, describing one's logic, rationale, intuitions, intentions, what one is trying to achieve and how.
- *Observing, listening and questioning* practitioners going about their everyday work and asking questions about the shared experience, such as 'What sense were you making of the situation?', 'What options were running through your head?', 'Why did you make the choice you did?', 'What was the consequence?' or 'Why did you say or do (a specific thing) at that point?' The simple 'why' question can be devastatingly powerful. The rewards for overcoming logistical barriers that sometimes make observation of practice difficult are immense, both in terms of the wisdom made available to others and in helping practitioners to value their taken-for-granted knowledge.
- *Feeding back* on these observations and conversations, providing detail and examples of what went well and what didn't.
- *High challenge/high support* means offering challenge in a supportive way, often achieved through the strategies of graceful care, just as we saw Alison challenging Dave's practice in a way that made the three of us laugh and in her words, 'it needs to be done quite gently'. High challenge does not mean confronting the practitioner in a blaming or threatening way. Rather, we make a judgement, for example, that a practitioner may have allowed her negative emotions to enter into her interaction with the community team. We do not share the judgement with the individual, but are prompted into action by it. For instance, we might *feedback on performance* to help the practitioner to see the important features of the situation, so that she could make her own evaluation. This is a supportive way of challenging because it never feels so bad when we have the opportunity to identify our own weaknesses and then have our critical companion say, 'Yes, I think you are right there.'
- *Drawing out creative imagination through creative arts media.*[3] Engaging practitioners in creative visualisations, collage-making, poetry writing, painting, clay modelling and movement can be used in a variety of practice development processes, for example, in creating a shared vision and common purpose for practice development and its evaluation, for gathering evidence of expertise or for 360° feedback. Such media can also be used to 'dig out' embedded knowledge and to disseminate, in powerful and memorable ways, the processes and outcomes of practice development projects.

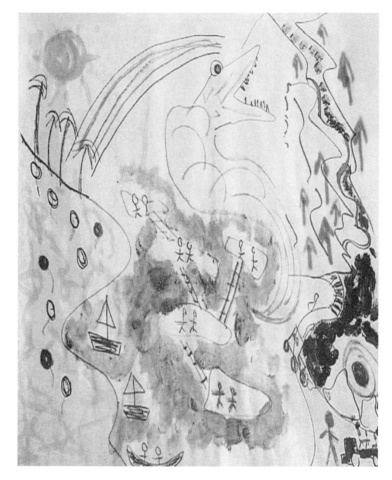

Fig. 7.3 A practice development journey.

The picture and story in Fig. 7.3 were created during a clinical supervision collaborative inquiry with senior practitioners and clinical leaders. Towards the end of our inquiry, I helped the group to imagine their individual experiences of the inquiry as a landscape and journey through it. They expressed their experience through painting and then told the story of their painting to each other. We used the paintings and stories to identify key themes and shared meanings which are shown in their composite journey (Fig. 7.4). A poster, with the paintings, the composite journey and evidence of outcomes for patients, staff and the organisation, was presented to key stakeholders and at a conference (Hill *et al.*, 2001). It was met with great interest at both events.

167

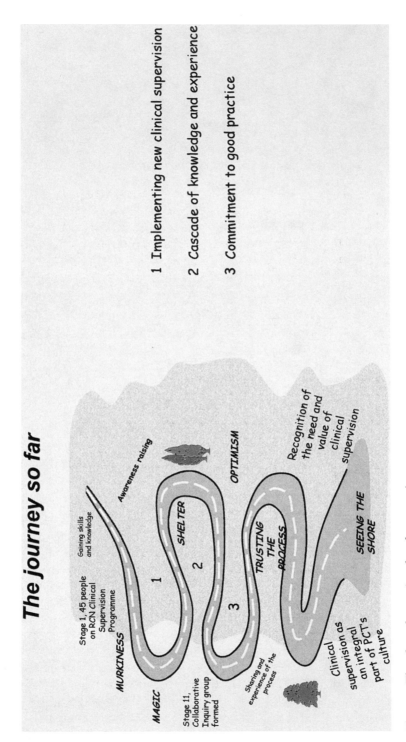

Fig. 7.4 The shared practice development journey.

168

- *Critical dialogue* to critically review, evaluate and debate the knowledge that has been surfaced through all or some of the above strategies.

A CC in the EPP helped the EN to reflect critically on how, in the past, she had been influenced by traditional ideas of teaching as transmitting information. They explored how these ideas were influencing her current practice of responding for requests for information or advice from her colleagues by just 'spoon-feeding' them, rather than helping them to think through the issue/problem for themselves. CC helped her to discover the potential of becoming a critical companion for her colleagues to enable them to make their care more evidence-based and person-centred. Subsequent use of a matrix (published in Titchen, 2003) to map the aspects of critical companionship that emerged in her work with her colleagues, enabled the CC to discover where she was strong and when she needed to do some work.

The impact of critical companionship

Having shown the effect of individual critical companionship strategies on practitioners and clinical leaders in the examples above, I now give a flavour of the overall impact on the participants in the EPP and GNPDP projects and on patients in my original work.

At the beginning of the EPP, many of the ENs were reluctant to consider themselves as having expertise. By the end, their portfolios showed that they now know that they have the expertise to change some patients' worlds. Moreover, whilst claiming their expertise in public, they did so in ways that showed their authenticity and humility. ENs felt empowered by having language to describe their expertise:

EN: Participating in this project has helped me develop as a practitioner. Analysing and reflecting on what I do, and how and why I do it, in a systematic way has helped me recognise my own skills and knowledge. Prior to this project, I did not recognise a lot of what I do, articulating them has made them visible to me. I feel this portfolio can make them visible to others. At the beginning of the project I found it difficult to pick out concise and specific evidence relating to expert practice, and immensely difficult to write down. I would sit at my computer for hours and produce what felt like a pathetically small amount of work. The writing flows now, and that feels like a gift to me (RCN, 2003).

> CC: The level of focus and exploration has afforded me greater insights into my own practice and my relationships with others. To understand and declare our own expertise is an empowering and powerful process (RCN, 2004).
>
> An EN and her CC both identified the experience as *'one of the best and most fulfilling experiences of my career'* (Brown & Scott, 2002).

In the GNPDP, critical companionship skills became integrated with other aspects of their work:

> (Being a critical companion) has helped me personally to maintain a clinical and practice development focus alongside my senior management role – beneficial in this time of reconfiguration and organisational change. It also helps me to consider and recognise that service developments should be first and foremost patient/person focused.
>
> (Wright & Titchen, 2003)

Critical companionship also makes a difference to patients, from their perspectives (Binnie & Titchen, 1999; Titchen, 2000; RCN, 2004; Titchen & McGinley, 2003) and from the nurses' own.

> The nurse gets to know your problems and you get to know her. I think it helps. You feel as though you know the person you are talking to and it helps you to relax. When you need something, you know she'll help you if she can.
>
> If it hadn't been for Rosemary, I think I wouldn't have calmed down so much. She's more like a friend I've known for years. She sits on the bed and has a little chat.
>
> They make me feel I have something to live for. It's the way they talk to me, the time they take to explain, being nice to me.
>
> (Binnie & Titchen, 1999: 186)

A reflective account, written by a participant in the GNPDP, detailed how a person with dementia had exhibited behaviour which staff and other patients found disturbing. The team worked hard at looking beyond the behavioural manifestations and assessing the person's emotional needs. Care was planned accordingly and the behaviour that had been causing the consternation diminished markedly. The nurse summarised the team's interventions:

> This lady's behaviour was often labelled 'challenging' and attributed to her dementia, but was obviously an expression of unmet emotional need/ill-being. When we stopped trying to control the behaviour . . . and began to understand the message behind the behaviour, we met the emotional need. (Wright & Titchen, 2003)

How can we develop effective critical companions?

Using the critical companionship framework starts as a challenge for many (see RCN, 2004; Titchen & McGinley, 2003). The imagery and phraseology will often only begin to make sense to beginning companions as they start to work alongside individual practitioners.

> Once the partnership began to unfold and flourish, the critical companions were more able to make sense of what was required of them by returning again and again to the theoretical underpinning of the model and were greatly encouraged by their enhanced understanding of what it was they were doing.
>
> (RCN, 2004)

Critical companionship, at least in the context of facilitating practitioner-research, is 'a very difficult and skilled thing to do'. We find that even those with supervision/facilitation experience, need support in developing critical companionship skills. This support will vary according to the individuals' starting points, but wherever they are, development needs to be offered by skilled facilitators (RCN, 2004). This is such a priority that explicit facilitation standards have developed and tested to enable RCN accreditation of one-to-one and group and work-based learning facilitation to increase the pool of skilled facilitators and critical companions in UK health care (see www.rcn.org.uk/pd for details).

Resting place

My purpose in this chapter has been to 'tease out the individual strands of spaghetti'; to unravel the complexity and nuances of critical companionship processes and strategies. Briefly describing its development, I spelt out the critical companionship framework, giving examples from my doctoral research and RCN Institute practice development research and projects. Now, rather than presenting a set of conclusions that imply a point of arrival, I offer three key messages for future journeys.

First, critical companionship came from, and was verified in, practice development research (Binnie & Titchen, 1999; Titchen, 2000; RCN, 2004). In this research and in the work of RCN practice development projects (e.g. Wright & Dewing, 2003), critical companionship has been shown to have a powerful effect on the development of individuals, teams and organisations to enable the delivery of evidence-based, person-centred care. It is effective in supporting experiential learning in and from practice, developing expertise and enabling practitioner-research. Yet, critical companionship is constantly developing and evolving and, as the spaghetti poem suggests, 'there are still many integral strands to unravel'. But we have made good headway. We have imagery and frameworks that are meaningful and helpful for people in the de-construction and re-construction of their practices, as they develop and refine them.

Second, critical companionship is a resource for all professionals, practice developers, educators and researchers who help others to learn in and from practice.

Third, critical companionship could ultimately benefit patients and their carers. This could occur through the creation of explicit knowledge about evidence-based, person-centred care, generated in and from expert practice, to be shared and tested by other practitioners, through further critique, in ever-widening ripples throughout the profession (see Titchen & Higgs, 2001).

Acknowledgements

My thanks go to the people who have helped us to develop and test critical companionship.

Notes

1 Term 'high challenge/high support' coined by Johns (1997).
2 A domain in this framework is a collection of different kinds of knowledge that have a conceptual connection in some way.
3 The picture and the poem at the beginning of this chapter provide examples.

References

Benner, P. (1984) *From Novice to Expert: Excellence and Power in Clinical Nursing Practice.* Addison-Wesley, London.
Binnie, A. & Titchen, A. (1999) *Freedom to Practice: The Development of Patient-Centred Nursing.* Butterworth-Heinemann, Oxford.

References

Boud, D., Keogh, R. & Walker, D. (1985) *Reflection: Turning Experience into Learning*. Kogan Page, London.

Brown, A. & Scott, G. (2002) Working with critical companionship. Seminar at RCN Congress. Harrogate, 23 April.

Campbell, A.V. (1984) *Moderated Love*. SPCK, London.

Carper, B.A. (1978) Fundamental patterns of knowing. *Advances in Nursing Science*, **1**(1), 13–23.

Clinical Supervision Steering Group (2002) *Our Journey: Getting Clinical Supervision on the Road*. Tower Hamlets NHS Primary Care Trust Clinical Supervision Steering Group, presented at RCN Congress, Harrogate.

Dewing, J. & Wright, J. (2002) *Practice Development for Nurses Working with Older People: The Story of Yesterday and Today*. Royal College of Nursing, London.

Freire, P. (1985) *The Politics of Education: Culture, Power, and Liberation*. MacMillan, Basingstoke.

Goodfellow, J., McAllister, L., Best, D., Webb, G. & Fredericks, D. (2001) Students and educators learning within relationships. In: *Professional Practice in Health, Education and the Creative Arts* (eds J. Higgs & A. Titchen), pp. 161–74. Blackwell Science, Oxford.

Heron, J. (1989) *The Facilitator's Handbook*. Kogan Page, London.

Higgs, J. & Jones, M. (2000) Will evidence-based practice take the reasoning out of practice? In: *Clinical Reasoning in the Health Professions* (eds J. Higgs & M. Jones), pp. 307–15. Butterworth-Heinemann, Oxford.

Hill, F., Hegarty, T., Richardson, R. *et al.* (2001) *Clinical Supervision Development*. Poster presented at Enhancing Practice Conference No. 1, University of Keele.

Johns, C. (1997) *Becoming An Effective Practitioner Through Guided Reflection*. Unpublished PhD thesis, University of Luton.

Johns, C. (2001) Reflective practice: revealing the art of caring. *International Journal of Nursing Practice*, **7**, 237–45.

Manley, K. & McCormack, B. (1997) *Exploring Expert Practice (NUM65U)*. MSc Nursing Distance Learning Module. Royal College of Nursing, London.

Mezirow, J. (1981) A critical theory of adult learning and education. *Adult Education*, **32**(1), 3–24.

Rogers, C. (1983) *Freedom to Learn for the 80s*. Charles E. Merrill, London.

Royal College of Nursing (RCN) (2004) *Expertise in Practice Project: Exploring Expertise*. Royal College of Nursing Institute, London.

Seizing the Fire Collaborative (2002) *Nurturing creativity in health and social care and education*. Unpublished presentation at the Nuffield Trust, London.

Titchen, A. (2000) *Professional Craft Knowledge in Patient-Centred Nursing and the Facilitation of its Development*. University of Oxford DPhil thesis. Ashdale Press, Oxford.

Titchen, A. (2001a) Critical companionship: a conceptual framework for developing expertise. In: *Practice Knowledge and Expertise in the Health*

Professions (eds J. Higgs & A. Titchen), pp. 80–90. Butterworth-Heinemann, Oxford.

Titchen, A. (2001b) Skilled companionship in professional practice. In: *Practice Knowledge and Expertise in the Health Professions* (eds J. Higgs & A. Titchen), pp. 69–79. Butterworth-Heinemann, Oxford.

Titchen, A. & Higgs, J. (2001) Towards professional artistry and creativity in practice. In: *Professional Practice in Health, Education and the Creative Arts* (eds J. Higgs & A. Titchen), pp. 273–90. Blackwell Science, Oxford.

Titchen, A. (2003) Critical companionship: part 1. *Nursing Standard*, **18**(9), 33–40.

Titchen, A. & McGinley, M. (2003) Facilitating practitioner-research through critical companionship. *Nursing Times Research*, **8**(2), 2–18.

Winter, R. & Munn-Giddings, C. (2001) *A Handbook for Action Research in Health and Social Care*. Routledge, London.

Wright, J. & Dewing, J. (2003) *Practice Development for Nurses Working with Older People in Community Hospitals*. Royal College of Nursing Institute, London.

Wright, J. & Titchen, A. (2003) Critical companionship. Part 2: Using the framework. *Nursing Standard*.

Part 2

8. Including the Older Person with a Dementia in Practice Development

Jan Dewing and Emma Pritchard

Introduction

Our ageing population means that practice development work in nursing and multi-agency care will almost inevitably involve older people, some of whom will have a dementia. There are deeply rooted power inequalities in relationships between the older person living with a dementia and others in society at personal and social levels. The exclusion of the old with mental health problems causes a number of challenges for practice developers. This chapter explores ways in which the older person with a dementia can be compassionately included in practice development. The chapter does not describe one project in detail but discusses some key methods to support practice development in dementia care.

The first section establishes why practice development is a necessity in dementia care by considering the experience of care from the perspective of the person with a dementia. The next section will explore why the person with a dementia should or could be involved in practice development work and why practice developers should avoid or discontinue the approach used in research and policy for so long of involving carers instead of the person with a dementia. The main section focuses on describing some of the methods practice developers can use to promote involvement. Throughout the chapter, examples from the authors' practice development work are used to illustrate the discussion.

Rationale for practice development in dementia care services

Services are usually shaped by professional agendas. Funding and work load divisions within and between health and social care and other local authority services (such as housing) lead to the 'guarding' of professional territory and have contributed to a seg-regated rather than integrated approach to care (Smyer, 2001). The current focus on service development or restructuring does not necessarily achieve long-term cultural change (modernisation) or change the person's day-to-day experience of care delivery. Chang-ing service structures and systems has little impact at the interface between those who provide and receive care.

Over the past decade the evidence base advocating person-centred values and social inclusion underpinning dementia care practice has grown (Dewing, 2000). The literature demonstrates advances such as person-centred assessment, support and educa-tion groups for people with a dementia and their supporters/carers, advances in dementia diagnosis disclosure, and growth in the use of counselling and a range of psychotherapeutic approaches, to name a few. How embedded these innovations are in day-to-day dementia practice across the UK is debatable. Clarke & Keady (2002) state that despite these encouraging therapeutic trends, there is little to suggest these advances have permeated practice. Every-day practice tends to focus on traditional approaches, for example, reliance on risk prevention, reality orientation and control and con-straint (Pritchard & Dewing, 2001). This distance between evidence and practice in dementia care mirrors a more general concern in nursing and healthcare for older people, about the quality of prac-tice and how evidence is (or is not) used to inform practice in reality (DoH, 2001a).

We need to explore both how evidence-based, and how compas-sionate or person-centred, dementia care is. These two areas under-pin practice development. The work of Kitwood (1997a), amongst others, in dementia care has been key to promoting person-centred care for older people in general. However, person-centred care is not yet the norm in many dementia care areas, or other healthcare areas, where many with a dementia find themselves. Many practi-tioners can 'talk' person-centred care, that, is they espouse a belief in it. Yet when it comes to expanding on this belief or illustrating it with compassionate evidence, they struggle. If we focus on the day-to-day experience of the older person with a dementia there is plen-tiful evidence that practice development is necessary. The extracts in Box 8.1 are taken from reflective diaries or evaluation data from a variety of practice development projects. They demonstrate attrib-utes of the traditional culture of dementia care (Kitwood, 1997a, b). For example, the person with a dementia feeling not wanted and misunderstood and being told and controlled by staff to the point

Box 8.1 Extracts from field notes in areas where older people with a dementia are cared for.

> *No-one here asks you anything about what . . . [pause] how anyone here might want it to be . . .*
>
> Said during a conversational interview by a woman attending a day centre. At the same time a member of staff came and asked the woman if she would like a drink. She said, *'coffee'*. The woman was given tea.
>
> *Would someone shut that bloody row up!*
>
> Said by resident to staff who were talking and laughing at the nursing station. The radio was also on, playing music.
>
> An exchange observed between a domestic worker and a patient:
> *Give me some sugar for me tea!*
> *I've put sugar in already.*
> *You haven't. It's not right. Give me the sugar here!*
> *I have. You're not getting any more.*
> *For Christ's sake I only want a bit of bloody sugar for me tea. What's this – a prison camp?*
> *You've got plenty of sugar. I'm not giving you any more.*
> The domestic worker starts to walk away with the tea trolley. The patient gets hold of the trolley and tries to help himself to sugar and spills his tea. The domestic worker reprimands him for spilling his tea. At this point a nurse intervenes, having responded to the raised voices. This exchange was witnessed several times in one afternoon as if a video was being re-run.
>
> During a baseline evaluation of care observation, two care assistants were heard to say:
> *You okay, Clarice? Breakfast's that way . . . no, you've forgotten, it's not sup-pertime, it's breakfast now.*
> Whilst in an intervention with this person, one care assistant said in a loud voice to the other, 'Has Mr S been toileted yet?'
>
> In an interview where staff were telling a story about their typical day at work, a care assistant said:
> *We get handover when we get in, then we go and get people up at 8 o'clock. The night staff will have got some done already, they tend to leave the heavies to us. Everyone has their own room and they can bring things to decorate their rooms. Their families do that sometimes.*
> *After breakfast it's the drug round. That takes about half an hour to go round everyone. Then we get people settled in the living room and put on some music. Sometimes in the afternoon we have a singer or entertainer.*

Box 8.1 *Continued*

> *We all go for our breaks then and most of the residents go to sleep – it's very hot here. We haven't had an activity organiser since I've been here, I'm not sure there's much the patients could do anyway, some of them have behaviour problems. The nurse does the dressings and other stuff and we sit in the living room with the residents. There are a few I really like talking to. The nurse is usually in the office . . . there's a lot of paperwork.*
>
> *Lunch is at 1 o'clock. We do the toileting before lunch for some people and after for others. Then there's another drug round. If there are any changes the nurse lets us know. They tell us what to do. Everyone has their own seat in the dining room and we all know who needs feeding.*
>
> *Visitors are allowed most of the time. It's good because sometimes you just can't do everything yourself. Supper is just a sandwich and soup now. Then it's the last drug round. If you're on a late you start getting everyone to bed around 7 o'clock. But it depends on who's on. It's quite confusing really. Some people spend a lot of time in bed, others are up all night, and some of them shouldn't be here really.*

that their reality is not believed. A reliance on routine is shown by the way things happen at pre-set times. The language the assistants used suggests a task-orientated culture where persons with a dementia are seen as workloads to be got through. Carers are seen as additional pairs of hands for the staff rather than friends or intimate associates of the person with a dementia. Psycho-social care seems ad hoc and reliant on whether the staff like the person or not and it probably relies too much on reality orientation which can undermine the person with a dementia.

A hierarchical culture with 'command and control' rather than transformational leadership style is evident, with the registered nursing focus being on paperwork and delegation. Staff are preoccupied with providing 'lounge-centred' care where the focus is on getting people out of bed and ready to sit in the lounge for the day. There is no sense that dementia care should focus on developing relationships between the carer and person with a dementia. The care assistants view the people with a dementia in terms of what they are unable to do, characteristic of a dementia care culture underpinned by a traditional biomedical model of dementia.

In the type of environment the last example in Box 8.1 the person with a dementia will become increasingly disempowered. In turn they may become withdrawn or behave in a way that others find difficult to deal with. If the person with a dementia is seen as less of a person because of their condition, this will pervade the engagement and interactions of healthcare professionals. It will then be difficult for professionals to see beyond the decline to other possibilities that dementia can often open up, such as new ways of thinking and feeling, and expression through art and music. Interestingly in our experience, staff in this sort of culture have much more in common in many ways with the people with a dementia than they may realise as they, too, experience devaluing and disempowerment.

Look out – here comes a person with dementia!

The emergence of the person with a dementia is a definite theme in much contemporary literature in gerontology. In the area of policy for example: the National Service Frameworks for Mental Health and Older People (DoH, 1999a; 2001a), *Forget Me Not* (Audit Commission, 2000; 2002) and *The Essence of Care Framework* (DoH, 2001b) all stress user involvement. Clinical Governance frameworks also set out the importance of involving users. Local and national organisations for older people have supported the principle of user involvement. For example the HOPe Group (Help the Aged, 2000) a group of fifteen older people, have created nine standards for health and social care. Whilst Joseph Rowntree have set out models of involvement for older people (Carter & Beresford, 2000) and the Alzheimer's Society (2000) aims to involve persons with a dementia in their research development programme.

In research there is a rapidly growing body of knowledge, mainly from social gerontology and social policy research, exploring ways and means of working with persons of all ages who have a dementia. The practice developer can certainly learn from this body of work. In the UK quite a lot of work has been done around service evaluation that has included the person with a dementia to some degree. See for example: in practice, Barnett (2000), Pritchard & Dewing (2001), Walker *et al.* (2001) and Allan (2002); in research, Cotrell & Schulz (1993), Keady & Gilliard (1999) and Pratt & Wilkinson (2001); and in research planning and prioritisation (Corner, 2002). The growing emphasis of involving users in health and social care continues to be a major impetus but it is a challenge for practice development when it comes to the older person with a dementia. The emergence of the person with a dementia is a slow process.

Perhaps this is because many practice developers do not yet have the skills or confidence needed to work with this group. Key issues such as consent and cognitive capacity tend to exclude those who are unable to give informed consent (Dewing, 2002). This is often seen where evaluation research is carried out as part of practice development. Research and ethics proposals will set out exclusion criteria for patients based around the inability to give informed consent. A major challenge for practice developers is to incorporate the principles of process consent methods into practice development work (Dewing, 2002). After all, process consent is a key part of action research methodology and methods; it simply needs to be adapted for persons with a dementia.

Persons with a dementia as stakeholders?

Before rushing in to involve the person with dementia, practice developers need to debate what exactly is meant by involvement-inclusion in the context of persons with a dementia. Terms such as consultation, involvement and participation are used more frequently. The ideas of involvement and inclusion can be conceptualised as a continuum ranging from minimal and passive involvement to active and total inclusion. The following assumptions associated with a traditional culture of care place the person with a dementia as a victim and less likely to be involved in practice development:

- persons with a dementia have poor self awareness and insight, and are unable to participate in reflective processes or communicate in the same ways as ourselves, and therefore do not experience as 'we' do;
- displacement of the older person with mental health problems from being the centre of care activity. Rather than being a person to be cared about, 'they' become something to be attended to (Reed & Clarke, 1999);
- depersonalising and stigmatising people with a dementia through placing them as apart and different from ourselves. Seeing people with a dementia as 'them' helps control our own fear of developing dementia;
- therapeutic pessimism, a concept described as contributing to low expectations in terms of response to therapy, so therefore what's the point in trying?

However, the person with dementia has the ability to feel and experience:

- Shame and embarrassment (Post, 1998)
- Pride and maintaining dignity (Post, 1998)
- Concern for the well-being of others (Sabat, 2001)
- Formulation of goals (Sabat, 2001)
- Using different forms of communication to compensate for linguistic impairment (Killick & Allan, 2001)
- Ability to communicate effectively with another's facilitation (Dewing, 2002)
- Manifest indicators of well-being (Kitwood, 1997b)
- Experience and work effectively to maintain self-esteem
- Manifest spiritual awareness and expression (McCurdy, 1998)

In a similar way to Wilkinson (2002) in relation to inclusion in research practice, practice developers need to ask and critically reflect on several key questions: should we involve–include persons with a dementia in practice development? This can be reworded to ask: do persons with a dementia want to be involved–included? Are we (as practice developers) in a position to do this? How can we (as practice developers) best facilitate involvement–inclusion? It is vital that involvement–inclusion does not take place just because it's considered to be the 'in thing' or practice developers feel they ought to. Involvement–inclusion must be based on authentic values and beliefs. In many projects involvement will be minimal if the culture has been one of traditional dementia care.

Who to involve: carer or person with a dementia?

As carers' needs have gained prominence, persons with a dementia have been seen as incidental subjects and passive recipients in the process of their dementia (Keady & Gilliard, 1999). This is unsurprising if traditionally held views of dementia described earlier are part of the culture of care, that is, that the person with a dementia is unable to act as an agent or contribute because of memory problems or cognitive changes. In such a culture, it may seem valid to involve carers rather than the person with a dementia. This may also be indicative of lack of communication skills or abilities with people with a dementia. It is possible that such a culture makes it easy for practitioners not to confront and address their own inadequacies in a developmental way.

Over the past two decades the visibility of carers of people with dementia has greatly increased. Generally, the work of organisations such as the Alzheimer's Society and Carers' National Association have highlighted carers' needs. We now have legislation and guidance for carers' needs, through the *Carers Act* (DoH, 1995) and *Caring about Carers* (DoH, 1999b). Also, the body of research dedicated to understanding the care-giving experience has grown substantially. This may partly explain why the trend in dementia care research has been to substitute a carer's or relative's views for those of the person with a dementia (Stalker *et al.*, 1999). This has resulted in being others, such as healthcare professionals, carers and researchers, being involved rather than the person with a dementia (Bamford & Bruce, 2000).

It is essential that the traditional approach of a carer speaking on behalf of the person with a dementia is questioned. According to Clarke & Keady (2002) it is no longer acceptable for the person with a dementia to be present only through the carer. In particular, exploration is needed if carers, when they claim to be advocating on behalf of the person with dementia, are really speaking on behalf of themselves and other carers. There is no reason why carers should be any more skilled at representing the person with a dementia than professionals have been. Carers have had intense caring experience and may have known the person with a dementia extremely well as they were. But they may not be best placed, because of the effects of caring on themselves, to know that person as they are now. Some carers can separate their own needs from the person with a dementia and speak either for themselves or the person with dementia but this is not an easy thing for anyone to achieve. However, it should be recognised that carers can offer valuable insight and perspectives as stakeholders in their own right (Pratt, 2002). Nonetheless, ignoring the person with a dementia and relying on carers and relatives denies the experience and perspective of the person with dementia and is problematic for the following reasons:

- The views of the person and carer may be different (Maguire *et al.*, 1996; McWilliams, 1998; Webb *et al.*, 1998). It should not automatically be assumed that the views or involvement of a carer can be used as a proxy (Epstein & Olson, 1999). A carer may approach a situation from their own perspective, coloured by their own values, experiences and knowledge, even though much of this may be part of a shared past and present with the person with a dementia.
- A carer may have some insight into the views and perspectives of the person with a dementia and these may be extremely useful, for example, in contributing to joint interviews or to forming an ethical framework to support each individual's participation.

However, accumulating evidence suggests carers have greater emphasis on the views the person with a dementia may have had in the past. The person's views, perspectives and abilities may have changed and carers may find it harder to see the validity in supporting these because of their own values and beliefs held about dementia, or because of the therapeutic pessimism of professionals.

- Views from relatives or carers may also be influenced by their own feelings, for example, the relationship may be strained, or they may feel protective about the person with a dementia and see their role as one where they speak for the person rather than facilitate their contribution. Carers may also feel that they cannot criticise or comment on services they are reliant upon (Cotrell & Schulz, 1993; Barnett, 2000).
- Family history and relationship dynamics may impact on the involvement of the carer as proxy, who may have difficulty balancing their needs with those of the person with a dementia (Stalker *et al.*, 1999). Bamford & Bruce (2000) found in their work on outcomes that carers had difficulty separating outcomes they wanted for themselves from those of relevance to the person with a dementia. What is appropriate for carers and what meets their needs is not necessarily the same for the person with a dementia.

How to involve the person with a dementia

If we accept we need to increase our understanding of the experience of dementia and the lived experience of persons with a dementia as service users and stakeholders we have to find ways of facilitating the views and perspectives of persons with dementia themselves. However, the legacy of the traditional culture of dementia care means that many persons with a dementia are extremely disempowered; some to the point where they seem unable to express themselves in words or action. Involvement–inclusion must be sensitive to the local culture of care. Wilkinson (2002) comments on the power inequalities inherent in many situations in research contexts and suggests these need to be recognised with care and time allowed for people with dementia to participate as fully (or not) as they wish. In many settings involvement may be minimal to begin with. However, practice developers should always be prepared to be surprised by what the older person with a dementia can offer with expert facilitation.

How can we develop our ways of facilitation?

General methods

Currently, there is growing interest in research methods known to enable the voice of the person with a dementia to be encouraged, heard and understood (Dewing, 2002; Wilkinson, 2002). General strategies Clarke & Keady (2002) advocate aim for a collaborative approach involving active and ongoing partnership with the person, rather than one-off consultations. This helps develop mutually trusting relationships and helps the person with a dementia contribute to and question their care. Lots of attention must be given to creating or using a 'safe' context. This means attending to location, duration of time spent, and the pacing of the communication in order to minimise anxiety and tiredness (which reduces competence). One of the best processes to learn is that of letting and enabling the person with a dementia both lead the way and set the pace. Multiple interviews or encounters may be necessary. This allows a relationship to develop and leads to increased depth of discussion (Pritchard & Dewing, 2001). Practice developers must be prepared to respond meaningfully and attentively to the experiences and expressions of the person with a dementia whatever they may be. This may mean listening and talking, or time out for either the person with a dementia or the practice developer.

In a review of methods to involve persons with dementia in the evaluation of services, Cheston *et al.* (2000) suggest five methods: questionnaires or structured interviews, semi-structured interviews or conversations, observation, advocacy and working in a group. They suggest advocacy could be considered as a general means to promote involvement of the person with a dementia, whatever method is used, providing this resource is available. This is something for practice developers to consider when working with practitioners on setting out their practice development strategies and action plans.

Questionnaires and structured interviews

Questionnaires or structured interviews may be useful to involve people with very mild impairment. Cheston *et al.* (2000) stress that the person using such methods should know the person well. There is also a danger that the issues covered in interviews or questionnaires may not be those that match the concerns of the person with a dementia (Murray, 1996). Within practice development these methods could be of use in specific situations where areas of

concern for development are already highlighted and priorities
need setting. However, this needs careful planning and facilitation
so as not to disempower the person with a dementia as it may challenge areas of function they already find difficult, such as writing
or reading questions, rather than capitalise on the person's remaining or new abilities.

Semi-structured interviews and guided conversation

Interviews are increasingly being used in research involving people
with dementia. How to carry out interviews effectively with people
with a dementia is a question only just beginning to be addressed
(Pratt, 2002). Conversational and semi-structured interviews can be
useful for persons with greater disability. They are more relaxed in
nature. More importantly they tend to use questions or prompts
that focus on what the person feels or sees rather than what they
think. The use of props and cues to prompt conversation (such as
objects and photos) can also be helpful and promote active involvement (Allan, 2001; Dewing, 2002). Where the person with a dementia is apprehensive or acts in a disempowered way the use of third
person questions can be a useful way in to talking together. For
example, 'what do others feel about . . . ?' followed by 'and what do
you feel?' Sometimes persons with dementia are able to increase
their involvement by being with others in a group. However, this
can sometimes go wrong when the group dynamics are not conducive. Discussions and interviews may need to be held within the
context to which they apply, as the person will draw on cues and
props around them to support their communication. Obviously
there are concerns and issues around confidentiality and privacy
included within this (see Box 8.2).

Observation

Observation is a widely used method in collecting evidence for
evaluation in practice development. Observational methods such as
Dementia Care Mapping (DCM) (Kitwood, 1997b) are widely used
in dementia care practice. However, DCM observations are complex
and time consuming and are usually done to the person with a
dementia, by trained mappers, rather than with them. Practice
developers can create opportunities to involve the person with a
dementia in less structured forms of observation, involving carrying out joint observations for example, or devising observational
criteria, or in giving feedback.

For example, members of a practice development group in a
nursing home for older people with mental health needs carried out

Box 8.2 Example of using semi-structured interviews and guided conversation.

The RCNI (1999) used semi-structured interviews informed by Ehernberger-Hamilton (1994) and Mills (1998) as frameworks for guided conversation. Time was spent in the group getting to know the clients and carers and becoming part of the group. The clients got to know the researcher who got to know individuals' contexts, behaviour, usual conversation, and usual activity pattern, levels of well-being and how these might be recognised. Also, importantly, the researcher learnt what may trigger ill-being in each client and how this may be recognised. Then individual interview approaches to each client were discussed with the care team and agreed. The clients ranged from having early to later stage dementia. The plan emerged to interview clients within general conversation; for example, one client within her context of being a 'group helper' and one client within the context of her husband (who also had dementia) having attended the group, and how she then viewed her own involvement with the service. A three-day time frame for interviews was allowed. Open questions were used such as: 'Can you tell me more about that?', 'What's it like?' and 'What matters?'. An open format helped the conversation to be as flexible as possible. Third-person questions were also used within conversation if an opportunity arose. The client's experience of the service, the individual's contexts, their life history and the wider context of the service itself were all taken into account when developing questions and cues to suit the person and their immediate context. Items and situations occurring in the immediate context were brought into the dialogue for discussion. The client led the discussion, to keep a sense of their own agency of autonomy with the researchers gently guiding them towards certain issues. This approach meant being prepared to take turns in asking and answering questions and to listen with the aim of increasing the client's confidence within the conversation. It also allowed statements that at times appeared to have just been 'thrown in' to the conversation to be capitalised on. Observations during the interviews were also incorporated into the data. The client's body language, tone of voice and other paralinguistic cues were attended to, as well as noting what was happening in the surrounding environment at the time.

a series of seeing, hearing and smelling observation exercises. They took place at three different times in the day and lasted for 15–30 minutes each time. The exercises were then carried out again but this time with a resident leading the way and saying what they saw, heard and smelt. The exercise was also carried out with carers and the local church visitor. The residents' responses were audio-taped during the observation and played back to the residents for validation or clarification. The perceptions of the different stakeholder groups were discussed and compared with each other.

Working in groups

Group work with people with a dementia has been, in theory, an established part of dementia care practice for some years. For example, groups in validation therapy, early stage support, memory training, reminiscence and art. Within practice development, group work can involve a range of groups such as workshops, focus groups, user forums and advisory or steering groups. Persons with dementia can be involved–included in the strategic and project management aspects of a project if this is their preferred way. Practice developers need to look at how they run meetings and groups so that they do not cognitively outpace the person with a dementia. We can also begin to explore more creative means of communication as we expand our evidence base that shows persons with dementia can often express themselves more readily through creativity (Killick & Allan, 2001).

Communication

Communication expertise is a core attribute in facilitating the involvement–inclusion of persons with dementia in practice development and is likely to be a two-way challenge for both the person with a dementia and the person facilitating. Keady & Gilliard (1999) note that the person's awareness of their dementia, how it is affecting their abilities and how they may be perceived by others, in turn can affect their willingness to be involved. Additionally, the person communicating with them may not have expertise in this area and may either purposefully or unknowingly put up barriers to effective communication leading to the concerns and issues of people with a dementia being ignored (Pritchard & Dewing, 2001). Evidence also suggests that people with a dementia are extremely receptive to others' communication (Kitwood, 1997a; Sabat, 2001) although they may not react immediately or in ways that others generally find easy to understand.

Older persons with dementia are not a homogenous group and communication needs to be developed according to need. One way has been to focus on technical and cognitive aspects, responding to what is externally verifiable or objectively 'true' in a person's conversation. Unless this is limited to reinforcing information that is immediately practically or emotionally beneficial, e.g. locating the toilets or talking about an event that brings the person pleasure (Crisp, 1995), it can become threatening and frightening for the person with a dementia as it emphasises the need to retain facts and recall specific information, two difficult areas for people with dementia. This can lead to the person perceiving themselves and being perceived by others as a 'failure'. Thus the person with a dementia states they are at their sister's house and 'the food here isn't much to speak of'. Because the setting was factually inaccurate, the experience is dismissed too.

Another way of communicating emphasises the affective areas of emotion and creativity and accepts what the person says and does as being right and a valid way of communicating (verbally and non-verbally) and a process that the practice developer communicating has to work at in order to understand the feeling behind the words or actions. It is this second way that facilitates positive communication in dementia. Sabat (2001) describes using a way of communicating called 'indirect repair'. This is underpinned by the assumption that the person with a dementia has something meaningful to say and is trying to say it. Indirect repair refers to:

> inquiring about the intention of the speaker, through the use of questions marked not by interrogatives but by intonation patterns, to the use of rephrasing what you think the speaker said and checking to see if you understood his or her meaning correctly. Thus the responsibility for effective communication between people lies with the listener as well as the speaker.
>
> (pp. 38–9)

Communication needs to take into account the immediate context of the communication, the person's own values system and personal life history. By context of the communication we mean:

- knowing the person and how they are on a day-to-day basis, for example, attending to how they use eye contact, facial expression, body language and their voice;
- knowing the combination of verbal communication, written information or pictures to which they respond best;
- taking into account what is going on in the person's life at the time of interaction; for example, have they recently experienced any difficult events or transitions?
- what is going on around the person; for example is there a lot of activity (or not) and how does the person feel and react to this, what clues they are giving?

- having some knowledge of the culture of care that surrounds the person; that is, 'the way things are done around here' (Drennan, 1992);
- the purpose of the conversational interaction as the person with a dementia might perceive it.

Hence we can see why repeated encounters rather than single encounters work best for persons with dementia. Any sort of face-to-face involvement will bring the central challenge of knowing how to talk with the person and how to understand what they say. It is not possible to address both concerns in this chapter. In most communications with people with a dementia, a higher than usual level of interpretation is needed, Walker *et al.* (2001) state that lengthy conversations with people who have a dementia may only yield small amounts of relevant data that relate directly to the area of interest or concern.

Interpreting what's said

These strategies are often used in communication by persons with dementia as they develop increasing disability (adapted from Killick & Allan, 2001 and Crisp, 1998):

- Moving to broader categories, for example the word 'tea' may be used to describe any type of drink. The broader category may have an emotional dimension, for example a relative may be mis-named (calling the son by a dead brother's name) but this does not necessarily mean there is no sense of a relationship existing.
- Describing an object by talking about its function. For example, what is this?

  that shape with the legs that has the means to chew – when I can because my teeth are missing . . . them there go and plonk by it in any fashion hithering and tittering.

  Answer: the dining table. The person here was talking about how her meals were organised and her feelings.
- Links of likeness for example, a red post box could be identified as a phone box.
- Links in common usage for example, 'hot' may be substituted for 'cold'.
- Word substitution. For example: 'one, one hours' means two o'clock.
- Pronouns may be used in a different way.
- Pacing may be altered (very slow or very fast).

- Use of humour in a witty way, use of one liner or news head-lines, for example: 'Shock news of the day – it's time for lunch!' (lunch was being served as the national news was on the television).
- Use of singing.
- Use of metaphors (Sutton & Cheston, 1997).

Look again at the person who states that they are at their sister's house and 'the food here isn't much to speak of'. What we can inter-pret is that there is something about the atmosphere or the envi-ronment that is similar to her sister's house. Bamford & Bruce (2000) describe how they moved beyond their feeling that discussions in a focus group appeared superficial and tangential to extract really useful data.

It is important to work on the positive principle of ruling in, not the negative one of ruling out (Crisp, 1995). This means attending to all of what the person says to try to make sense of the commu-nication, rather than automatically discarding words or sentences that initially don't seem relevant. Focusing on achievement so that communication leaves a positive feeling for the person with a dementia is important, that is, that they have been listened to and responded to at an appropriate level that enhances their well-being (Dewing, 2000).

There are benefits for practice developers in learning to commu-nicate effectively with persons who have dementia. Learning about others is likely to educate us and enrich our own experience. It con-nects us to each other, closing the 'them and us' gap, allowing us to get in touch with our own fears of ageing and dementia. It chal-lenges our thinking as we need to be responsive and flexible in the methods we use to encourage involvement. Although it is demand-ing work, we learn more about the experience of dementia and what being a person means through enabling persons with a dementia to share their expertise with others. It is also the foundation work for any sort of involvement of persons with dementia in practice development.

Summary

Traditionally persons with dementia have been excluded from being stakeholders in their care and services. This has been based on a whole range of values and beliefs and basic assumptions that can now be constructively challenged and reframed. In order to involve–include persons with a dementia practice developers need to develop methods that enable persons with dementia to become involved–included in meaningful ways that move beyond tokenism. The purpose of practice development may be multiple, around person-centeredness and evidence-based care, but should also focus on putting compassion into dementia care.

Involving the person with a dementia is necessary for practice to develop in a responsive way to the needs of people with a dementia. Meaningful involvement is more likely to result in practice development projects being focused on the most relevant areas, as concerns and issues important to the person with a dementia and carers can be identified and worked with. This recognises people with dementia as being social and political equals and persons with agency with the ability to refute negative views and stereotypes of dementia.

If people with a dementia are excluded from practice development then there are a number of implications. A significant group of the population will not be heard and the resulting risk is that decisions taken will lead to practice development work that is inappropriate and ineffective. Assumptions that persons with dementia cannot participate, do not have views and cannot share them reinforces negative stereotypes and fails to put into action some of the fundamental principles underpinning emancipatory practice development. However, involvement–inclusion does bring with it a set of challenges that practice developers need to address through a spirit of collaborative inquiry with persons who have dementia and their carers or advocates. Finally, we will leave you with the words of a person who has dementia:

> Compassion means understanding and overcoming the tendency to blame or ignore the victim and refusing to worship a false god who abets this. It means healing interventions on a personal and societal level, and when nothing concrete can be done, to be in solidarity with the afflicted person and help him/her bear his/her burden.
>
> Friedell (2002)

References

Allan, K. (2001) *Communication and Consultation: Exploring Ways for Staff to Involve People with Dementia in Developing Services*. Joseph Rowntree Foundation, Bristol.

Allan, K. (2002) A sense of possibility. *Mental Health Today*, **April**, 18–21.

Alzheimer's Society (2000) Quality Research in Dementia needs you! *National Newsletter of the Alzheimer's Society*. February, 4–5.

Audit Commission (2000) *Forget Me Not.* Audit Commission, London.
Audit Commission (2002) *Forget Me Not (2002).* Audit Commission, London.
Bamford, C. & Bruce, E. (2000) Defining the outcomes of community care: the perspectives of older people with dementia and their carers. *Ageing and Society*, **20**, 543–70.
Barnett, E. (2000) *Including the Person with Dementia in Designing and Delivering Care: 'I Need to Be Me'.* Jessica Kingsley, London.
Carter, T. & Beresford, P. (2000) *Age and Change: Models of Involvement for Older People.* Joseph Rowntree Foundation, York.
Cheston, R., Bender, M. & Byatt, S. (2000) Involving people who have dementia in the evaluation of services: a review. *Journal of Mental Health*, **9**(5), 471–9.
Clarke, C. & Keady, J. (2002) Getting down to brass tacks: a discussion of data collection with people with dementia. In: *The Perspectives of People with Dementia: Research Methods and Motivations* (ed. H. Wilkinson). Jessica Kingsley, London.
Corner, L. (2002) Including people with dementia: advisory networks and user panels. In: *The Perspectives of People with Dementia Research Methods and Motivations* (ed. H. Wilkinson). Jessica Kingsley, London.
Cotrell, V. & Schulz, R. (1993) The perspective of the patient with Alzheimer's Disease: a neglected dimension of dementia research. *The Gerontologist*, **33**(2), 205–11.
Crisp, J. (1995) Making sense of the stories that people with Alzheimer's tell: a journey with my mother. *Nursing Inquiry*, **2**, 133–40.
Crisp, J. (1998) Towards a partnership in maintaining personhood. In: *Dementia Care Developing Partnerships in Practice* (eds T. Adams & C. Clarke). Bailliere Tindall, London.
Department of Health (DoH) (1995) *Carers (Recognition and Services) Act.* HMSO, London.
Department of Health (DoH) (1999a) *National Service Framework for Mental Health.* HMSO, London.
Department of Health (DoH) (1999b) *Caring about Carers: A National Strategy for Carers.* HMSO, London.
Department of Health (DoH) (2001a) *National Service Framework for Older People.* HMSO, London.
Department of Health (DoH) (2001b) *Essence of Care: Patient-focused Benchmarking for Healthcare Practitioners.* HMSO, London.
Dewing, J. (2000) Promoting well-being in older people with cognitive impairment. *Elderly Care*, **12**(4), 19–24.
Dewing, J. (2002) From ritual to relationship: a person-centred approach to consent in qualitative research with older people who have a dementia. *Dementia: The International Journal of Social Research and Practice*, **1**(2), 156–71.
Drennan, D. (1992) *Transforming Company Culture.* McGraw-Hill, London.
Ehernberger-Hamilton, H. (1994) *Conversations with an Alzheimer's Patient: an Interactional Sociolinguistic Study.* Cambridge University Press, Cambridge.

References

Epstein, M. & Olson, A. (1999) An Introduction to Consumer Politics. In: *Advanced Practice in Mental Health Nursing* (eds M. Clinton & S. Nelson). Blackwell Science, Oxford.

Friedell, M. (2002) Awareness: a personal memoir on the declining quality of life in Alzheimer's. *Dementia: The International Journal of Social Research and Practice*, **1**(3), 359–66.

Help the Aged (2000) *Health and Older People. Our Future Health: Older People's Priorities for Health and Social Care*. Help the Aged, London.

Keady, J. & Gilliard, J. (1999) The early experience of Alzheimer's disease: implications for partnership and practice. In: *Dementia Care Developing Partnerships in Practice* (eds T. Adams & C. Clarke). Bailliere Tindall, London.

Killick, J. & Allan, K. (2001) *Communication and the Care of People with Dementia*. Open University Press, Buckingham.

Kitwood, T. (1997a) *Dementia Reconsidered: The Person Comes First*. Open University Press, Buckingham.

Kitwood, T. (1997b) *Evaluating Dementia Care: The DCM Method*, 7th edn. Bradford Dementia Group, Bradford.

McCurdy, D.B. (1998) Personhood, spirituality, and hope in the care of human beings with dementia. *Journal of Clinical Ethics*, **9**, 81–91.

McWilliams, E. (1998) The process of giving and receiving of a diagnosis of dementia: an in-depth study of sufferers', carers' and consultants' Experiences. *PSIGE Newsletter*, **64**, 18–25.

Maguire, C.P., Kirby, M., Coen, R., Coakley, D., Lawlor, B.A. & O'Neill, D. (1996) Family members' attitudes toward telling the patient with Alzheimer's Disease their diagnosis. *British Medical Journal*, **313**, 529–30.

Mills, M.A. (1998) *Narrative Identity and Dementia: a Study of Autobiographical Memories and Emotions*. Ashgate, Aldershot.

Murray, A. (1996) Listening to people with dementia. *Signpost*, **1**, 13–14.

Post, S.G. (1998) The fear of forgetfulness: a grassroots approach to an ethics of Alzheimer's disease. *Journal of Clinical Ethics*, **9**, 71–80.

Pratt, R. (2002) 'Nobody's ever asked how I felt'. In: *The Perspectives of People with Dementia: Research Methods and Motivations* (ed. H. Wilkinson). Jessica Kingsley, London.

Pratt, R. & Wilkinson, H. (2001) *The effect of being told the diagnosis of dementia from the perspectives of the person with dementia*. Final Report. Mental Health Foundation, London.

Pritchard, E. & Dewing, J. (2001) A multi-method evaluation of an independent dementia care service and its approach. *Aging and Mental Health*, **5**(1), 63–72.

Reed, J. & Clarke, C. (1999) Older people with mental health problems: maintaining a dialogue. In: *Advanced Practice in Mental Health Nursing* (eds M. Clinton & S. Nelson). Blackwell Science, Oxford.

Royal College of Nursing Institute (RCNI) (1999) *An evaluation of SPECAL: a multi-method evaluation of the SPECAL service for people with dementia*. Report No 19. Oxford, RCNI.

Sabat, S.R. (2001) *The Experience of Alzheimer's Disease: Life Through a Tangled Veil*. Blackwell Publishing, Oxford.

Smyer, M.A. (2001) Russian dolls and Chinese Boxes: the ecology of Alzheimer's disease research. *Aging and Mental Health*, Supplement **5**(1), S149–S152.

Stalker, K., Gilliard, J. & Downs, M. (1999) Eliciting user perspectives on what works. *International Journal of Geriatric Psychiatry*, **14**, 120–34.

Sutton, L. & Cheston, R. (1997) Rewriting the story of dementia: a narrative approach to psychotherapy with people with dementia. In: *State of the Art in Dementia Care* (ed. M. Marshall). Centre for Policy on Ageing, London.

Walker, E., Dewar, B., Dewing, J. & Pritchard, E. (2001) *An Evaluation of Day Care Services for People with Dementia from the Perspectives of Major Stakeholders*. Queen Margaret University College, Edinburgh.

Webb, S., Moriarty, J. & Levin, E. (1998) *Social Work and Community Care and Community Care Arrangements for Older People with Dementia*. National Institute for Social Work, London.

Wilkinson, H. (2002) Including people with dementia in research: methods and motivations. In: *The Perspectives of People with Dementia: Research Methods and Motivations* (ed. H. Wilkinson). Jessica Kingsley, London.

Commentary

Charlotte L. Clarke

The development of healthcare practice has one fundamental purpose – it is important to meet the health needs of service users. This is obvious isn't it?

However, it is easy to forget this purpose. It is challenging to achieve. It is frequently obscured by the consuming fog that is generated by many organisational changes.

This chapter by Jan Dewing and Emma Pritchard strikes to the heart of some of these issues, considering why and how we might engage with people with dementia to develop healthcare practice. These are complex issues that are worthy of considerable exploration for any group of service users. The presence of a dementia serves to magnify the challenges but does not alter them. In other words, we must not be complacent in our thinking and assume that service user engagement is straightforward when there is no cognitive impairment present.

Let us start by considering some of the key issues. First, let us explode the notion of service user for we all are service users, all stakeholders. We use healthcare services not only to provide us with healthcare but sometimes to provide us with employment, to contribute to the national economy, to provide political ammunition and so on. We all have vested interests in healthcare services, those interests being wide-ranging and not necessarily concerned directly with 'soothing the fevered brow'. The service that we use is a dynamic organisation that needs to be nurtured and tended. Sometimes to the extent that it is hard to distinguish between the drive to meet the needs of the organisation itself and the imperative to meet the needs of those who require healthcare. So we must have absolute clarity about what we mean by service user. And we must consider at every step in whose best interests we are acting lest we merge in our minds the needs of the patients, the care givers and the organisation.

197

Second, let us explore this notion of health. If we are truly talking about health then we are not talking about healthcare services since they are at best a very partial component of the sum of measures that promote and harm the health status of the population. Indeed, perhaps it is the ill-health service – or as one person described it to me, as the disease-ridden service! If we are talking about health, then we must talk about housing, transport, environment, education and so on. The maintenance and management of health is woven into the fabric of our society and the way we play out our day-to-day lives. But so often we fail to see this large tapestry and applaud ourselves perhaps for being so daring as to encourage healthcare services to talk to social care services. Interagency working may be today's agenda (at least once we have modernised the NHS) but let us hope that tomorrow's agenda will cease to talk about services and start to adopt a more public and community health orientated perspective.

Third, let us ponder on the notion of development, and remember that 'to do differently' does not necessarily equate to development. For development to occur we must witness a closure in the gap between need and provision. Doing differently may well not achieve this for all that there has been change. Similarly, focusing on 'doing' may be less important than focusing on 'thinking'. Let us aspire to think differently and the subsequent doing differently will be effortless and will achieve development.

And this is where the points that Jan Dewing and Emma Pritchard discuss are so critical because what they lay out is a process that can lead us to think differently. They take us on a journey that helps us to listen. What we hear are the oppressed and silenced voices of people receiving healthcare services.

There are of course some challenges along the way – but we must all own those challenges for they lie not with the person with dementia alone. As a first step, that little matter of power inequalities needs to be addressed!

If service users are to be expected to work alongside practitioners to develop care, then we must acknowledge and respect the expertise that they bring with them, and we are required to develop ways of working that place the control with the service user rather than with practitioners. This requires considerable planning and challenges all parties to shift the balance of power in this relationship. There is then a considerable degree of preparation required to ensure that people with dementia are adequately supported, for example, through advocacy workers, and that staff are well facilitated to allow them to be open to hearing the views of the service user.

Commentary

A wave of health and public policy is promoting service user involvement at the moment – there is no barrier to achieving this other than our readiness to accept the challenge. Part of this readiness, however, includes finding ways of working effectively with people with dementia and their families. This chapter maps out a range of methods and considers how we could best interpret and act on what we hear. I do not underestimate the magnitude of this challenge, but the rewards for everyone make this a critical journey and, mirroring the authors' conclusion, let me emphasise the need to have solidarity with people with dementia that they may allow us to glimpse their world and enrich us all in our capability to practice.

9. Practice Development in Child Health Nursing

a Personal Perspective

Christine Caldwell

Introduction

This chapter reflects on practice development activities with which I have been associated, in order to examine one approach to promoting practice development within child health nursing. The chapter focuses on developments that took place within child health at the RCN Institute from the mid 1990s onwards and more recently in partnership with South Bank University, London. On the face of it these developments were primarily educational courses and one might therefore challenge why they should be the focus of a chapter on practice development. This challenge will be examined within the chapter. In doing so, it will also draw upon the practice development activities undertaken by me and other RCN Institute colleagues who have held joint posts within children's nursing education and practice.

The discussion within this chapter is centred upon a philosophical approach which is underpinned by three key beliefs:

- A commitment to the value of emancipatory approaches in the facilitation of learning and development;
- That effective leadership is crucial to sustaining positive change;
- That children and young people should be considered equal citizens in the process of developing a healthcare system which is centred around the needs of the patient and his/her family.

Background

Whilst the education arm of the RCN Institute, formerly the RCN Institute of Advanced Nursing Education (IANE), has a long history of providing education courses for nurses and midwives, prior to the early 1990s there was nothing on offer for children's nurses wishing to further their education to degree level and beyond, despite constant internal lobbying. This was not unusual and reflected the provision across the UK at this time.

The appointment of, first, Gosia Brykczynska and then Sue Mullaney was to change this situation. Whilst neither was appointed to facilitate educational programmes in children's nursing or child health, both are committed children's nurses and had a mission to develop children's nurses and child healthcare. With support from Sue Burr, the paediatric adviser, they quickly succeeded in establishing, first, one module/short course and then soon after, the first ever undergraduate degree in Child Health for UK children's nurses. Over the next few years three further programmes were developed and launched. The original BSc was revised to become the BSc (Hons) Child Health Nursing, a UK-wide Distance Learning degree in Child Health Nursing was successfully developed and an MSc programme in Child Health Nursing became established (Caldwell, 1995).

Arguably these developments have had an impact on the process of creating a culture for effectiveness in practice development in child health nursing across many healthcare settings, but particularly within acute settings. This is because these developments were underpinned by the philosophy and methods of practice development.

The curricula were developed through a collaborative and iterative process where practice expertise and knowledge relating to the facilitation of practice knowledge and skills development were engaged, whilst also taking on board strategic policy objectives through the involvement of those at the forefront of health policy for children's healthcare. Also central to this process was the fact that key individuals, including the author and colleagues, Anne Lindsay Waters and Kathryn Jones, were simultaneously engaged in practice development activities within clinical practice whilst facilitating practice-based learning and development within the classroom.

Knowledge and ideas generated in practice were incorporated into the education programmes, and ideas from the educational programmes were incorporated into practice development activities in a range of healthcare organisations, both at a clinical and strategic level. This process enabled a spiral of continual work-based learning and development for all those involved. Furthermore, the close relationship between the RCN Institute and the

RCN's membership groups, including the involvement of RCN Policy staff, including Anne Casey and Sue Burr, in the delivery of educational programmes, meant that there was a mutually beneficial relationship between education, policy and practice for the advancement of practice and policy in child health.

Practice development: purpose, intention and approach

The RCN Practice Development team (2002) state that their corporate objectives for practice development are as follows:

> Working with healthcare providers and users to develop systematic strategies relevant to everyday practice to enhance care to users.

This is achieved through:

- Facilitation
- Leadership
- Developing a patient/person-centred culture
- Using and developing evidence
- Evaluating effectiveness
- Influencing and shaping policy

Although the level at which one operates might vary, it can be argued that these objectives should underpin the work of any practitioner wishing to enable practice development, including those working within child healthcare.

The overall aim of our activities over the years has been to influence the creation of a culture of effectiveness in children's nursing for the provision of quality patient-centred services for children and their families. This has been achieved through working with individual nurses, both on a one-to-one and group basis as well as with whole services and organisations, both at a local and national level.

Garbett & McCormack (2002), suggest that the purpose of practice development is increased effectiveness in person-centred care. This is achieved through:

- Enabling nurses or healthcare teams to transform the culture and context of care
- Skilled facilitation
- Systematic, rigorous and continuous process of emancipatory change; and
- Developing knowledge and skill

(see Chapter 3)

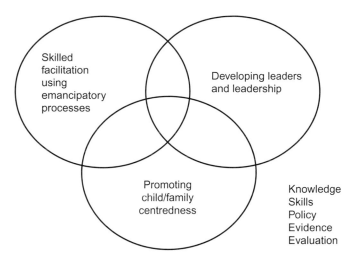

Fig. 9.1 Enabling a culture of effectiveness in child healthcare through practice development.

Manley & McCormack (2003) identify two related but different worldviews of practice development: technical and emancipatory. The activities described in this chapter can be located in an emancipatory approach, where the development and empowerment of practitioners is a deliberate and intentional purpose. The approach is summarised in Fig. 9.1.

The intentions of our work reflect Manley's characterisation of the elements of a transformational culture which she has demonstrated are essential for effectiveness in practice development (Manley, 2002, see Chapter 4) and how some of this has been achieved will be illustrated throughout the chapter.

Skilled facilitation using emancipatory processes

The educational programmes we have developed are clearly underpinned by the theories and methodology of critical social science. Critical social science is concerned with enabling a process of enlightenment, empowerment and emancipation (Fay, 1987). Davis (1998) provides a simple but helpful interpretation of Fay's ideas. She suggests:

Enlightenment – to understand who I am
Empowerment – to have the courage to change who I am
Emancipation – to liberate myself to become who I need to be

(p. 208)

The discussion here will focus on the first two elements of this process, enlightenment and empowerment, which ultimately enable us to take action – to become emancipated.

Enlightenment – to understand who I am

We have placed a huge emphasis upon challenging practitioners to look with fresh eyes on the things that they take for granted in their practice and in the environment in which they work and live. For those working with children, this is not just about understanding 'who I am' but also, and equally important, 'who you are' – the 'you' in question being each individual child for whom we care. It is easy to think that we know about children either because we once were children, because we have children of our own or because we have worked with children and young people for many years.

How adults view children and how children view

Traditionally most research about children's health has described the perspectives of mothers or of professionals working with children and this approach has underpinned the development of health policy and practice for children. Whilst this is now slowly changing, it reflects a longstanding assumption that children's interests are at one with their parents and that children are not capable of representing themselves. As Young (1997) argues:

> We wouldn't tell black people they aren't capable of making decisions about the things that affect their lives: or women that, bless them, they really don't know what is good for them. Nor would we suggest to disabled people that we understand more about their experience than they do. So why does it seem so easy to organize children's lives without consulting them?
>
> (p. 3)

Current debates about patient involvement as part of the NHS Plan's mission to ensure that the NHS more effectively meets the needs of its users, frequently bemoan the challenges of enabling the patient's voice to be heard and listened to in both policy development and implementation. The task of enabling patient/user involvement when the patient or user is a child is clearly a formidable task. One of the core aims of our work has been to challenge practitioners' beliefs in order to get them to recognise that children's views are not always the same as those of their parents or those caring for them and that children can eloquently represent themselves given appropriate opportunities. We also aim to inspire them to take action.

Secker (1997) outlines some of the reasons why the value of taking children's views into account should be promoted:

- As a counterbalance to the dominance of professional views about health and illness;
- Because we have recognised that people's own ideas about health and ill health must be understood if health professionals are to be able to find ways of helping to make sense of people's actual lives – children are no different in this respect and we must pay attention to their specific views;
- Because children must be recognised as people in their own right with their own views and feelings and not just as adults in the making;
- Because mental and emotional problems in childhood are far more common than has previously been recognised and may be on the increase – we need to understand how we can ensure that children can enjoy as happy and secure a childhood and adolescence as possible.

Listening to children, enabling their views to be heard and advocating for their rights requires a particular and overtly political stance underpinned by a set of values which also underpin our programmes of work:

- That children are able to communicate their own concerns
- That we have a professional responsibility to listen, to understand and to take seriously what children are saying to us
- That children and young people are not homogenous in their outlooks and views

(Brotchie *et al.*, 1998)

This stance reflects the so-called 'new sociology of childhood' which is underpinned by concerns about children's rights (James *et al.*, 1998). This standpoint suggests that history is not marked by an absence of interest in children but by their silence. Key features include the following, that:

- Childhood is understood as a social construction and (as distinct from biological immaturity) is neither a natural nor universal feature of human groups.
- Childhood is a variable of social analysis which can never be entirely divorced from other variables (such as class, gender and ethnicity) and comparative analysis over time and cultures reveals a variety of childhoods rather than a single and universal phenomenon.

- Children's social relationships are worthy of study in their own right, independent of the perspective of adults.
- Children must be seen as active, rather than passive, in the construction and determination of their social lives and the societies in which they live.

The recognition of children as a social group in their own right and one that should be given a voice is explicitly aligned with the claims of other oppressed groups (e.g. Roberts, 1983; Brotchie *et al.*, 1998) and is something that we debate within our programmes with regards to its implications for nurses influencing change.

It has proved a tremendous challenge, emotionally and intellectually, to our postgraduate students, who often have years of experience and great expertise in clinical practice or the education of children's nurses, to undertake practical activities listening to children and reading the words of young people explaining what it really is like to be a child growing up in contemporary Britain. By analysing these accounts and reflecting in a structured manner upon the impact, meaning and implications both for the students' personal practice and for professional practice within the services for which they have responsibility, these students have been able to consider changes which could be made in order to improve care for children and young people.

One student, a nurse teacher, undertook an analysis of one disabled teenager's written account of her experience of her parents' marriage breakdown and her father's subsequent new relationship (Atkinson & Dunbar, 1998). One of the outcomes of this exercise was that it led the student to reflect upon the extent to which children and young people were involved in the development of curricula for the education and preparation of children's nurses. Her conclusion was that, whilst in theory there was a commitment to involve users and their families, in reality this rarely happened to any significant extent. Furthermore, if users were involved, these tended to be either parents or children with chronic conditions or sick children with life-limiting conditions, because they have more contact with the health services, making it easier to solicit their views.

This student is currently undertaking a research dissertation which will use the 'draw and write' technique (Pridmore & Bendelow, 1995) to examine one group of children's perceptions of children's nurses. It is intended that this process will both provide data which can be fed into curriculum development and highlight other ways in which this tool might be used to access the user perspective in the curriculum development process to ensure that we are preparing children's nurses with the knowledge skills and attitudes required to care effectively for the client group.

Another student chose to adapt Johns' model of structured reflection (Johns, 1993) to first structure and then reflect upon a young child's emotional response to a life-threatening episode in the trajectory of his long-standing illness. This student is an expert practitioner and clinical nurse leader in an area of specialist paediatrics that has traditionally been nurse-led. Whilst the student had cared for many children in similar situations, the exercise enabled her to try and see the experience from the child's point of view by using Johns' prompt questions within her observations and conversations with the child and in examining his drawings. She then used structured reflection a second time to reflect upon what the experience meant for her professional practice, both personally and for the service which she leads. As well as achieving deep personal learning, she was able to develop and test a new practice theory and consequently influence future practice within a multi-professional context.

Equally challenging has been the process of facilitating children's nurses at all levels of experience to examine the degree of congruence between their beliefs and their actions. This is a central component of the leadership development activities which are fundamental to all the programmes, reflecting Argyris & Schon's (1978) work on theories of action. Action learning (Revans, 1982) is used in combination with structured reflection (Johns, 1993) as a core learning process to provide an opportunity for both undergraduate and postgraduate students to analyse how they act within their practice with children and young people (their theories in-use) and how they believe they should or do act (their espoused theories), in the light of what they are learning about effective clinical and strategic leadership. Once they are enlightened, this active learning process also supports the empowerment of participants to try out new leadership actions and reflect upon them within an environment of high support and high challenge so that they can become emancipated.

The process of enlightenment has also led those participating in our programmes to examine and look afresh at some of the espoused theories, core 'philosophies' and entrenched attitudes of children's nursing and child healthcare through such techniques as concept analysis (Whiting, 1997; 2001; Hutchfield, 1999) and primary research into the experience of parent participation and family-centred care (e.g. Gillhespie, 2002).

Empowerment – to have the courage to change who I am

Manley (1997) describes empowerment as the motivating and enabling force to act, arising from both the recognition of how we respond in certain circumstances and the need to take action or change what we do. It is a complex process which has been examined at length both from a theoretical and research perspective, both in nursing and elsewhere (e.g. Kalnins *et al.*, 1992; Gibson, 1995). Yet the idea of individuals and groups becoming 'empowered' is a very popular idea which is currently being promoted widely in Government policy. This may be, as Keiffler (1984) pointed out, because it is an intuitively appealing idea because of its psychological, ethical and political connotations. It also appears to fit well with current political ideology and, indeed, the empowerment of staff and patients is central to contemporary ideas about leadership in the NHS (DoH, 2001).

The empowerment of children and their families is also portrayed as a crucial element of contemporary child health nursing with the suggestion that in order to empower others children's nurses must themselves be empowered (Fradd, 1994). Empowering processes are central to our programmes and we seek to work with participants to address the associated challenges, some of which have been debated in a previous publication (Caldwell & Lee, 1998, see Box 9.1).

History, politics and policy in child health and the implications for nursing leadership

An increasing number of initiatives in recent years have provided potential opportunities for children's nurses to influence the health policy context in order to develop practice and improve healthcare for children and young people. Arguably, however, there has been little progress made and there is little evidence of significant nursing influence. The reasons for this may include:

- Lip service to issues concerning children in order to appear responsive to the requests of lobbying groups in order to avoid a loss of political support when there was little intention to act;
- Other competing priorities with child health issues not seen as enough of a priority and so receiving little time or financial resources;
- Children and those representing them were unable to find a strong enough voice to ensure that they were heard amongst more dominant groups nor had these groups sufficient power to be able to take action for themselves to ensure change.

Box 9.1   The challenges of promoting empowerment.

---

1. *Within healthcare generally:*

a) Those who are empowered must accept the burden of responsibility for their situation and its accompanying frustrations along with the benefits of the knowledge, confidence and competence they gain and the right to be heard by those who traditionally hold the power.

b) Healthcare professionals must feel confident in sharing their own knowledge and skills and be able to value others' expertise, in order to establish partnerships of mutual respect, open communication, active participation and sharing of power (this demands an organisational culture in which traditional power structures are flattened and healthcare professionals are themselves supported and empowered).

c) All parties in the empowerment process must work as part of a team, with the same agenda and a commitment to a common goal because empowerment is a continuous cyclical process; those who are empowered must be protected from 'responsibility overload' (Gibson, 1995) and it must be recognised that they will need support from a range of sources, particularly in 'new' situations or during crises.

2. *Within child healthcare:*

a) We must accept that children's own views and needs are valid even if they are different from adults' views.

b) We must strive to understand health and illness as children see them.

c) We must recognise that children are competent and are able to be full partners in healthcare planning and decision-making at both a strategic level and individually.

d) We must acknowledge the ability of children of all ages to identify their problems for themselves, to exercise choice and make decisions about action.

e) We must prepare children for these actions through appropriate education (e.g. life skills training) to enable them to take responsibility for their choices.

(from Caldwell & Lee, 1998)

In 1997, for example, the first ever House of Commons Select Committee on Children's Health published its wide sweeping recommendations in a series of reports (e.g. Health Committee, 1997). As part of their conclusion, the Committee stated that within child health services at the time there was poor communication and a lack of co-ordination, that services were often based upon custom and practice and professional self-interest rather than the needs of children and their families. The report stressed the importance of integration of health services for children and a requirement for multi-professional teams to function within a culture of mutual support and respect, valuing skills rather than qualifications and job titles (Casey *et al.*, 1997).

In mid-2001, the report of the public inquiry into excess mortality and morbidity amongst children undergoing cardiac surgery at Bristol Royal Infirmary (BRI) was published (Kennedy, 2001). Its many conclusions and recommendations, both generally and specifically in relation to children's health, closely resemble those of the Health Committee, as do those of the enquiry report following the child abuse case resulting in the death of Victoria Climbié (DoH, 2003). One way in which we can work to ensure that these reports have more impact in producing sustained and positive improvements to healthcare is through enabling a transformational culture within healthcare through practice development (RCN, 2001b; Manley, 2002).

There has been much debate regarding why nursing in general has failed to produce sufficient numbers of effective leaders both at clinical and strategic levels (e.g. Rafferty, 1993; Girvin, 1998), or alternatively why nurses consistently fail to take responsibility to exercise their capability for leadership, but rather wait for others to take the lead (Caldwell & Place, 2000). Potential reasons cited include the historical position of nursing within British society as a female vocational occupation requiring limited educational ability and dominated by medicine. This may have resulted in few individuals with the right kinds of leadership ability being attracted to nursing in the first place. Additionally, others argue that the education and socialisation of nurses and the way in which nursing has been treated by successive management changes within the NHS has further limited the development of its leadership potential.

Roberts (1983) discusses the characteristics and behaviours of oppressed groups such as African slaves in early America and relates this to nursing leadership. Nursing has been criticised for limiting its potential influence and increasing its powerlessness as a result of in-fighting and divisive arguments, dividing into factions to challenge and destroy those who attempt to lead change to benefit patients or failing to act to protect those who seek to harm through uniting in a powerful collective voice. Girvin (1998) believes that this in-fighting has held the profession back, and that it is also an easy weapon for others to exploit at the expense of nursing and the groups and individuals for whom nurses advocate.

210

It is interesting to consider this analogy to oppressed groups in the context of the historical development of children's nursing. Divisions were set up from the beginning and arguments continue in relation to, for example, educational preparation, and the need for separate registration, the care of 'sick' children versus the care of 'healthy' children, and battles between primary, secondary and tertiary care, leading to poor communication and professional isolation – all with consequent knock-on effects for those on the receiving end: children and their families.

Added to this, successive management restructuring within the NHS, and specifically in the organisation of children's services, has had a significant impact upon nursing leadership within children's nursing (RCN, 2001a). Inconsistent practices regarding the establishment or appointment of an appropriately qualified and experienced lead children's nurse is leaving some local communities without an effective nursing voice advocating and exerting strategic influence for children requiring healthcare in hospital. This situation is further complicated by limited career development opportunities and opportunities for succession planning, and, until recently, limited opportunities to pursue further educational development, which may lead potentially effective nurse leaders to leave children's healthcare in order to pursue better career development opportunities.

If this historical context is accepted, it could be argued that child health nursing does exhibit some of the characteristics of an oppressed group. Roberts (1993) identifies three steps that nursing can take to break free from exhibiting these behaviours:

1. Recognise the situation and expose the reality of the dominant/subordinate relationships that exist in the health service;
2. Develop leadership amongst the grass roots through dialogue and a shift to focus on the interests of the bulk of nurses, rather than those of an elitist group;
3. Rediscover nursing's cultural heritage and the values that underpin it (such as caring and its patient focus) through the development and dissemination of new and existing knowledge for practice.

Developing leaders and promoting leadership in child health nursing

Based upon the work of the RCN Leadership Programme, which has carried out research and designed development programmes for nurse leaders at all levels of healthcare organisations, Antrobus (2001) has identified what she believes to be the skill set required of the twenty-first century nurse leader. She suggests that nurse leaders must be able to transform the culture of an organisation through:

- Strategic change
- Continual learning
- Whole systems thinking and partnership working
- Managing conflict and facilitating teams
- Managing self

This work also supports the RCN's position regarding the centrality of effective leadership in facilitating and enabling practice development.

Furthermore, the key to effective leadership according to Rafferty (1993) and Antrobus & Kitson (1999) is the need for nurse leaders to become 'bilingual' operators so that they can communicate with the dominant culture, introduce the language of nursing to that dominant culture and thus interpret and translate it to bridge the gap between nursing practice and the policy context. Within child health nursing there is the added requirement of clinical nurse leaders to be able to communicate effectively with the users of the service – children and young people and their families, ensuring that they have a voice and are listened to in relation to clinical, strategic and policy agendas. There is little to be gained, as perhaps we have seen to date, in inviting contributions from child health nurses in the development of policy for children and in including them in implementation teams if they do not have the necessary leadership ability to make an effective contribution in advocating for children and their families.

Over a number of years of working as a practice developer both in child healthcare and more broadly, it has become increasingly evident that one of the keys to success is good leadership (Caldwell & McPherson, 2000; Caldwell *et al.*, 2000). This conclusion is also supported by colleagues (e.g. Kitson *et al.*, 1998; Antrobus & Kitson, 1999; Rycroft-Malone *et al.*, 2002). Good leadership is required at all levels of the organisation in which practice development is to take place. This leadership needs to be enabling and supportive of change and the development of all those who wish to take part in the change process, regardless of the level of seniority or experience (Caldwell *et al.*, 2000).

From her in-depth research into the development of a culture of effectiveness for practice development, Manley (1997) concludes that a specific kind of leadership is required – transformational leadership (Kouzes & Posner, 1987). Transformational leadership is also being promoted by the UK Departments of Health as being fundamental to the current task of modernising healthcare (NHS Confederation, 1999; National Nursing Leadership Project, 2003). Any programme of activity aimed at practice development needs to incorporate a strategy for ensuring that there is good transformational leadership in place. This has therefore been a central component of our activities.

The combined activities of our educational programmes, including specific leadership development modules, have sought to enable students to acquire the skill set of a twenty-first century nurse leader. Whilst much in the undergraduate programmes focuses on the uniqueness of the role of the child health nurse, the programmes are not isolationist or exclusive. They are open to all nurses whose primary role is in the healthcare of children and young people and we emphasise learning from a wide range of sources across the whole spectrum of nursing and beyond. We have developed leadership programmes that see nursing as a united profession with a common vision, yet enable nurses to identify and develop the unique knowledge and skills they require to succeed in their specific roles.

In addition, within the distance learning degree programme we have taken on board the specific issues related to leadership in child health nursing (RCN, 2001a) and are seeking to ensure that clinical leaders are prepared not only to influence and shape policy and practice locally but are also able to think and act strategically. Rather than ending their degree with a traditional thesis, we have incorporated a module entitled 'The child health nurse as strategist'. The aim being to maximise the impact of their new knowledge and skills in child healthcare practice. This module has been used by one NHS Trust, facilitated with a group of senior nurses, in order to help support and prepare them to be proactive in the face of major organisational change.

We have helped students to question whether the poor contexts described in recent reports are similar in some respects to those in which they work. The next step in this challenging process is to empower them through providing knowledge and support to have the courage to change themselves. Through this process they develop the confidence to take action to free themselves from taken for granted aspects of their own practice and from constraints in their environment, and through this emancipatory process may help their colleagues too.

A number of those participating in our programmes are nurses who began their health service careers as nursing auxiliaries or enrolled nurses, or were registered nurses with little confidence in their ability to undertake degree studies. Others, when they commenced their studies, had been employed in the same post or role for many years, where there had been little change in their own practice or patient care during that time. There have been many different motivators for participants to join the programmes, sometimes personally derived and sometimes linked to service developments encouraging them to join. The emancipatory nature of the programmes has been most evident in these groups, with hugely beneficial consequences for the development of child health practice.

Past participants included one nurse who through the degree programme realised the extent of her skills, expertise and influence in an aspect of chronic healthcare. Helped by her learning on the programme, she was able to recognise that the context in which she was practising was not enabling her to progress as she wished in order to develop the services for children which they and their families were requesting. As a result she moved organisations and has now set up and leads a thriving service which is nationally recognised and has gone on to become an RCN accredited Expert Practitioner in her field.

Our joint roles in education and practice have enabled us to encourage colleagues to take the first step in their studies through our practice development work in clinical practice. For example, from an early stage, we were able to validate a professional development programme for E and F grade children's nurses at Guy's & St Thomas' Hospitals NHS Trust as an elective module of the BSc (Hons) Child Health Nursing programme, giving it academic credit and providing a non-threatening work-based taster of degree studies and a stepping-stone onto a degree programme.

Increasingly participants on the programmes who have come from or moved into areas of child health practice are breaking the traditional mould. A number of students have developed ambulatory and primary care based services enabling children to access healthcare without unnecessary disruption to their family and school lives. The skills and knowledge gained from our programmes have assisted them in acquiring the confidence to challenge the systems and cross traditional boundaries, harnessing the support of colleagues in other areas of healthcare as well as education and social care services, enabling them to progress.

But is it practice development?

Some readers might challenge whether indeed some of the activities which are referred to within this chapter can be rightly included under the heading of practice development. Page (2002) concludes that practice development has the following key characteristics which are broadly congruent with the work of Manley (2002) and Garbett & McCormack (2002):

- It focuses upon the improvement of patient care
- It incorporates a range of approaches
- It takes place in real practice settings
- It is underpinned by the development and active engagement of practitioners
- It is collaborative and interprofessional
- It is evolutionary
- It is transferable rather than generalisable

It is therefore worth briefly examining such a challenge using this framework.

Focus upon the improvement of patient care

Page states that the patient is the focus of practice development rather than the practitioner, profession or department. This is clearly the case for some of our work. One could argue, however, that when a student embarks on an educational programme, their personal development is the main focus. However, the programmes which we have developed for children's nurses within the RCN Institute and in the workplace have been developed in line with our own and the organisations' philosophies and missions, which demonstrate a clear commitment to continually improving care for children and their families central to any development activity. In order to be successful in the programmes individual participants have to demonstrate their commitment to improving patient care through the assessment process.

Furthermore, organisations that have contracted with us to place their staff on the programme have done so precisely because of the focus on improving care for children and their family. This was certainly the case for the Children's Unit at Chelsea and Westminster Hospital NHS Trust, where a Lecturer Practitioner type role was introduced, in collaboration with the RCN Institute, to work across both organisations, but specifically to facilitate the integration of new learning into practice through enabling an effective culture for practice development.

Incorporating a range of approaches

Page states that practice development draws on and synthesises theory and activity from a number of fields with the end result being more than the sum of its parts. An excellent example of this is Anne Lindsay Waters' work at Great Ormond Street Hospital NHS Trust and the RCN Institute. Anne has been able to develop her work on clinical supervision in the workplace and integrate this into both face-to-face and distance learning education programmes for children's nurses, and through working collaboratively with clinical colleagues, incorporate real life clinical supervision exemplars to facilitate the development of theoretical knowledge and skills in clinical supervision in subsequent participants on these programmes.

Conversely, Anne has capitalised upon her involvement in the development and delivery of the curriculum and learning resources for the BSc (Hons) Child Health Nursing by introducing and facilitating the use of some of the modules of this programme within the Trust to enable clinical and strategic leadership skills and research awareness as part of the Trust's strategy for developing a culture for child and family-centred practice development.

Taking place in real practice settings

Many of the ideas within the education programmes have evolved from practice development activities undertaken as part of our joint roles such as the clinical supervision and leadership development work as already mentioned. In addition, the learning approaches which we use require that students test out their learning and skills within the real practice setting as part of the learning and assessment process. For many of the participants, however, authorising time away from their 'real practice setting' in a comfortable and safe environment has been a catalyst for the processes of enlightenment and empowerment which precede emancipatory change. Added to this, participants have had the opportunity to network with colleagues from other areas of practice and other organisations across the country, and some have found this to be one of the most beneficial and enlightening elements of the programme.

Underpinned by the development and active engagement of practitioners

Page (2002) suggests that because of the patient focus practice development can only succeed when patients become engaged in the process. He cites Clarke & Proctor (1999) who assert that practitioners need to integrate technical and theoretical evidence with the values and context of their practice environment. I believe that

216

this has been demonstrated through the emancipatory processes adopted within our work.

Collaborative and interprofessional

Whilst our direct work has been confined to nurses, the focus of our work especially around leadership clearly demonstrates a vision which is collaborative and interprofessional.

Evolutionary

Practice development is undertaken within multiple complex and ever-changing contexts (Bell & Proctor, 1998) and requires creative, individualised and eclectic interventions which evolve over time (Manley, 1997). This can be seen in the evolutionary nature of our programme development described at the beginning of the chapter.

Transferable rather than generalisable

We have sought to integrate generic ideas from practice development with the specific issues facing nurses working in child healthcare. We have then, in turn, worked with practitioners to interpret and adapt these ideas to their specific practice setting in order to generate unique solutions to the challenges in the services which they are seeking to provide.

Towards the future . . .

This chapter has suggested that there is some congruence between the values and aims of practice development and the Government's vision of a modern health service. For example, this vision includes the provision of:

• Fast and convenient care
• Delivered to a high standard
• Services provided when people require them
• Tailored to their individual needs

Through:

• Seeing things through the patient's eyes
• Looking at the whole picture
• Respecting and giving front line staff the time and tools to tackle the problems

(Modernisation Agency, 2002)

The modernisation of child health services is planned through the implementation of a National Service Framework (Ainsley–Green,

217

2001). The first part of the NSF, relating to acute healthcare, is currently awaited.

Potentially the NSF may revolutionise health services for children. The mission and philosophy of the Children's Taskforce reflect many of the approaches incorporated within our work. For example, the group believes that the focus should be on child life rather than child health and that children must be considered as people now rather than adults in the making (Ainsley-Green, 2001). Their mission is to 'improve the lives and health of children and young people through the delivery of an appropriate, integrated, effective and needs-led service'. To achieve this, they believe that there is a need for a period of prolonged action and cultural change at both macro- and micro- levels across health, education, social care and environment sectors.

As discussed already in this chapter, unless sufficient attention is paid to the development and preparation of those who will deliver the service to enable them to fully contribute, through the kind of work which we have sought to undertake, this opportunity might be lost in the same way that past opportunities have been lost.

References

Ainsley-Green, A. (2001) *The Children's Taskforce and NSF: Exploiting the opportunity for change.* Paper presented at Paediatrics, 2001, Commonwealth Centre, London.

Antrobus, S. (2001) *Nursing Leadership, Study Guide, MSc Nursing.* RCN, London.

Antrobus, S. & Kitson, A. (1999) Nursing leadership: Influencing and shaping health policy and nursing practice. *Journal of Advanced Nursing,* **29**(3), 746–53.

Argyris, C. & Schon, D.A. (1978) *Organisational Learning.* Addison Wesley, Reading, MA.

Atkinson, R. & Dunbar, J. (1998) *I Like Being Horrid, Me and My Electric,* pp. 24–42, Mammoth, London.

Bell, M. & Proctor, S. (1998) Developing nurse practitioners to develop practice: the experiences of nurses working in a nursing development unit. *Journal of Nursing Management,* **6**(2), 61–9.

Brotchie, J., Allan, H., Caldwell, C. & Mullaney, S. (1998) *The Socio-political Context of Care, Study Guide, BSc (Hons) Child Health Nursing.* RCN, London.

Caldwell, C. (1995) Mastering child health. *Paediatric Nursing,* **7**(5), 7.

Caldwell, C. & Lee, K. (1998) Nursing's contribution to the healthcare of children and adolescents: some principles for practice. In: *Nursing Practice and Healthcare* (eds S. Hinchliff, S. Normon & J. Schobes), 3rd edn, London: Arnold.

References

Caldwell, C., Lynch, F. & Komaromy, D. (2000) Working together to improve record-keeping: towards action-centred clinical leadership. *Nursing Standard*, **14**(47), 37–41.

Caldwell, C. & MacPherson, W. (2000) Leadership skills for ward sisters and charge nurses. *Nursing Times*, **96**(43), 37–8.

Caldwell, C. & Place, B. (2000) *Nursing Leadership, Study Guide, BSc (Hons) Child Health Nursing*. RCN, London.

Casey A., Young, L. & Rote, S. (1997) Integrating services for children. *Paediatric Nursing*, **9**, 5 and 8.

Children's Health Committee (1997) The Specific Health Needs of Children and Young People. HMSO, London.

Clarke, C. & Proctor, S. (1999) Practice development: ambiguity in research and practice. *Journal of Advanced Nursing*, **30**(4), 975–82.

Davis, M. (1998) The rocky road to reflection. In: Transforming Nursing Through Reflective Practice (eds C. Johns & D. Freshwater). Blackwell Science, Oxford.

Department of Health (DoH) (2001) *Shifting the Balance of Power Within the NHS: Securing Delivery*. Stationery Office, London.

Department of Health (DoH) (2003) *The Victoria Climbié Inquiry (Chaired by Lord Laming)*. The Stationery Office, London.

Fay, B. (1987) The basic schema of critical social science. In: *Critical Social Science: Liberation and its Limits* (ed. B. Fay) pp. 27–41 and 219–20, Polity Press, London.

Fradd, E. (1994) Power to the people. *Paediatric Nursing*, **6**(3), 11–14.

Garbett, R. & McCormack, B. (2002) A concept analysis of practice development. *Nursing Times Research*, **7**(2), 87–100.

Gibson, C.H. (1995) The process of empowerment in mothers of chronically ill children. *Journal of Advanced Nursing*, **21**(6), 1201–10.

Gillhespie, K. (2002) *A study using a series of qualitative interviews examining nurses' experiences of how they carry out participation in care on the paediatric unit*. Unpublished MSc thesis. Royal College of Nursing/University of Manchester.

Girvin, J. (1998) *Leadership and Nursing*, pp. 1201–10. Macmillan, Basingstoke.

Habermas, J. (1972) *Knowledge and Human Interests*, trans J.J. Shapiro. Heinemann, London.

Health Committee (1997) *Hospital services for children and young people*. Fifth report of the House of Commons Health Select Committee (Session 1996–7). HMSO, London.

Hutchfield, K. (1999) Family-centred care: a concept analysis. *Journal of Advanced Nursing*, **29**(5), 1178–87.

James, A., Jenks, C. & Prout, A. (1998) *Theorizing Children*. Polity Press, Cambridge.

Johns, C.C. (1993) Professional supervision. *Journal of Nursing Management*, **1**(1), 9–18.

Kalnins, I., McQueen, N.D.V., Backett, K.C., Curtice, L. & Currie, C.E. (1992) Children's empowerment and health promotion: some new directions in research and practice. *Health Promotion International*, **7**(1), 53–8.

Keiffler, C. (1984) Citizen empowerment: a developmental perspective. *Prevention in Human Sciences*, **3**(2/3), 9–36.

Kennedy, I. (2001) *The Bristol Royal Infirmary Inquiry Report*. HMSO, London.

Kitson, A., Harvey, G. & McCormack, B. (1998) Enabling the implementation of evidence based practice: a conceptual framework. *Quality in Healthcare*, **7**(3), 149–58.

Kouzes, J.M. & Posner, B.Z. (1987) *The Leadership Challenge: How to Get Extraordinary Things Done in Organizations*. Jossey Bass, San Francisco, CA.

McFadyen, H.A. (1999) *A phenomenological study of the experience of in-patient minor surgery for children*. Unpublished MSc thesis. Royal College of Nursing/University of Manchester.

Manley, K. (1997) Practice development: a growing and significant movement. *Nursing in Critical Care*, **2**(1), 5.

Manley, K. (2002) *The Components of a Transformational Culture and Related Cultural Indicators*. RCN, London.

Manley, K. & McCormack, B. (2003) Practice development: its purpose and methodology. *Nursing in Critical Care*, **8**(1), 22–9.

Modernisation Agency (2002) *Improvement in the NHS*. HMSO, London.

National Nursing Leadership Project (2003) www.nursingleadership.co.uk

The NHS Confederation (1999) *Consultation: the modern values of leadership and management in the NHS*. The NHS Confederation and the Nuffield Trust.

Page, S. (2002) The role of practice development in modernising the NHS. *Nursing Times*, **98**(11), 34–5.

Pridmore, B. & Bendelow, G. (1995) Images of health: exploring beliefs of children using the 'draw and write' technique. *Health Education Journal*, **54**(4), 473–88.

Rafferty, A.M. (1993) *Leading questions: a discussion paper on nursing leadership*. King's Fund, London.

Revans, R. (1982) *The Origin and Growth of Action Learning*. Chartwell Bratt, Bromley.

Roberts, S.J. (1983) Oppressed group behaviours: implications for nursing. *Advances in Nursing Science*, **5**(4), 21–30.

Royal College of Nursing (RCN) (2001a) *Children's services: acute healthcare provision – a report of the follow-up UK survey upon children's' nursing leadership*. RCN, London.

Royal College of Nursing (RCN) (2001b) *RCN Response to the BRI Inquiry*. RCN, London.

Royal College of Nursing Practice Development team (2002) www.rcn.org.uk/practice_development/practice_processes1.html

Rycroft-Malone, J., Kitson, A., Harvey, G. *et al.* (2002) Ingredients for change: revisiting a conceptual framework. *Quality in Healthcare*, **11**(1), 174–80.

References

Secker, J. (1997) Giving young people a voice. In: *How we feel: an insight into the emotional world of teenagers*, (eds J. Gordon & G. Grant), pp. 126–36. Jessica Kingsley, London.

Whiting, L. (1997) Health promotion: the role of the children's nurse, *Paediatric Nursing*, **9**(5), 6–7.

Whiting, L. (2001) Health promotion: the views of children's nurses, *Paediatric Nursing*, **13**(3), 27–31.

Young, R. (1997) Kids can hack it. *The Guardian*, 5 November, 3.

Commentary

Patric Devitt

Caldwell thoroughly explores the nature of practice development in paediatric nursing. However, there are three areas that, while she addresses them, require some further exploration. The three areas are: the unique nature of paediatric nursing, the environment of paediatric nursing, and the challenge of turning education into learning and ultimately into practice development.

The unique nature of paediatric nursing

This applies only to the client group and not, I hasten to add, to paediatric nurses themselves. No other area of nursing has a client group that is so diverse; from newborn babies to adolescents on the cusp of adulthood. The developing nature of children makes user involvement in practice development problematic. Multiple methods taking into accounts the attributes of children from pre-school through adolescence need to be developed. Also recognition needs to be given to those children who face challenges in communication, although they may be regular users of health services. Some steps are already being made towards this; for example, Noyes (2000). She has used approaches such as show and draw play techniques to ascertain the views of children with no verbal communication. Morris *et al*. (2002) have drawn on techniques such as 'circle time', familiar to children as they are used as a learning method in education, to ascertain their views. However, such measures need to be used on a larger scale and tested for reliability and validity.

The focus of paediatric nursing is also unique. It is only in considering the child within the parameters of their family that their healthcare needs can really be assessed. All care and developments must be planned taking this into account. The many and varied forms that the family can take must also be considered to maximise user involvement.

222

The environment of paediatric nursing

Whilst relatively few children are being cared for in hospital, it is still here that the majority of paediatric nurses are based. Those working in children's hospitals can expect to find child (and family) friendly policies and environments in place. This should make practice development easier. Those working on children's areas within District General Hospitals can often find themselves arguing about matters concerned with children as a group distinct from adults, rather than about practice development. A third group can often find their position even more difficult. These are nurses working in predominantly adult areas but charged with caring for children. These areas include accident and emergency departments, specialist surgery e.g. ear, nose and throat, or ophthalmology, and general outpatient departments. These nurses may not even have a paediatric qualification. They are nevertheless expected to champion the rights of children and families in the face of an overwhelmingly adult centred view of the world. If practice development is truly to have an impact upon the care of the child and family in hospital, methods of engaging with nurses in isolated areas must be developed. Perhaps local inclusive networks of interested individuals may be one way of generating support for the nurses who feel that in caring for children in an adult area they are swimming against the tide.

Developing learning into practice development

This chapter suggests that the basis of practice development can be further education, particularly to first or indeed master's degree level. The challenge is how to translate this theoretical education into learning and this learning into practice development and how to ensure it continues once the course of study is complete, i.e. develops into life-long learning. There is also the challenge of trying to translate experience into knowledge. Reflection on action is often suggested as a way of meeting both these challenges. However, there is relatively little empirical evidence to show what the impact of standard forms of reflection is on practice and its development. Brockbank *et al.* (2002) suggest that all reflective cycles such as those advocated by Kolb can provide an increase in competence and confidence, i.e. learning for improvement. What, they suggest, is really required is double-loop learning, where an individual is challenged both by other knowledge of the problem and a wider knowledge of the context in which it occurs. This extra stimulus provided by this additional knowledge is difficult to generate in solitary reflection. It is only within a group that sufficient levels of both challenge and support can be generated to allow the individual to develop a new understanding – so called double loop learning. This new understanding can then be used to inform radical practice development.

Whilst clinical supervision may provide the environment conducive to double loop learning it may well not. There is already a high level of confusion about the nature and purpose of clinical supervision with patchy uptake. The introduction of another goal for clinical supervision is unlikely to lessen either of these problems. Perhaps the local networks mentioned above could provide the framework that would allow double loop learning to be applied to all environments where children are nursed.

Conclusions

It is clear that whilst there is much happening in relation to practice development in child health nursing there is also much more to do. It appears that paediatric nursing is often isolated. This may be on a local level, where nurses caring for children do not communicate as they work for different parts of an organisation, or because the paediatric unit does not communicate with the rest of the Trust. Alternatively it may be on a more area or national basis, i.e. paediatric units or hospitals not communicating with other paediatric units or hospitals. The first can be addressed through local networks, but the latter is perhaps a larger problem. There are, however, networks that paediatric nurses interested in practice development should consider joining. These include the Foundation for Nursing Studies developing practice network, the Association of British Paediatric Nurses (ABPN) and the Royal College of Nursing's Research in Child Health (RiCH) network. It is by sharing and moving forward together that we can really make a difference.

References

Brockbank, A., McGill, I. & Beech, N. (2002) *Reflective Learning in Practice.* Gower, Aldershot.

Morris, K., McCabe, A., Mason, P., *et al.* (2002) *The National Children's Fund Evaluation: A Feasibility Study.* Children's and Young People's Unit, London.

Noyes, J. (2000) Enabling young 'ventilator dependent' people to express their views and experiences of their care in hospital. *Journal of Advanced Nursing*, **31**(5), 1206–15.

10. *Acute Mental Healthcare:*
Transforming Cultures, a Practice Development Approach

Mary Golden and Steve Tee

Introduction

> I spent about five months as a patient in six mental hospitals. The experience totally demoralised me. I had never thought of myself as a particularly strong person, but after hospitalisation, I was convinced of my own worthlessness.
>
> (Chamberlin, 1988: 5)

Experiences such as those described above are not uncommon and will no doubt strike a chord with many individuals involved in mental healthcare, be they service users, carers or providers. Acknowledgement that such situations still exist, and a desire to find ways to bring about change, were the two main drivers for the practice development work described in this chapter.

In introducing this work it is necessary to reflect on the formative context which extends back almost two decades to the publication of a report by the Camden Consortium (1987). *The Good Practice in Mental Health* report into psychiatric hospitals concluded that admission to hospital was unsafe, unhelpful and untherapeutic. Over a decade later similar concerns to those reflected in the above quote, are still being raised about the quality of care for those admitted to acute in-patient services (Sainsbury Centre for Mental Health, 1998; SNMAC, 1999; MIND, 2000; Ford, 2002).

Despite these concerns and lack of supporting evidence regarding effectiveness, acute care continues to be used, often because there are few alternatives. Whilst the *National Service Framework for Mental Health* (Department of Health, 1999) supports the development of alternatives, such as crisis teams, assertive outreach and home treatment services, these are not yet in place and so pressure on in-patient beds is unrelenting. Even with such alternatives in place it is difficult to foresee a time when admission to some form of acute in-patient facility will no longer be needed.

The problem of providing high quality acute care is further compounded by difficulties recruiting and retaining staff (Sainsbury Centre for Mental Health, 2000; Department of Health, 2001). The poor perceptions of the role of acute in-patient nurses, compared to community colleagues, have led to shortages in skilled staff and over reliance on temporary staff. Acute in-patient nurses often report feeling less valued than their counterparts in the community and cite the examples of difficulty undertaking professional development and further training, and lack of available time to engage in activities, such as clinical supervision, as evidence for this.

Such problems inevitably have a pervasive effect on the culture of acute care services, which are reflected in the attitudes and behaviours of staff. As Morgan (1998) points out, where there is a perception of feeling under-valued and powerless then rule-following and adherence to the prevailing norms will continue. Achieving cultural change in such circumstances requires significant opportunities for change that promote a newly desired culture. This is clearly difficult when there is little time available for staff to undertake valued practice roles such as spending meaningful time with service users. The majority of nurses see this as a central component of their work and experience frustration and dissatisfaction at not being able to achieve it. Such issues have been identified as key reasons for the decision to leave the mental health nursing profession (Tingle, 2001).

In an attempt to begin to address these issues, the Department of Health (2002) published the *Mental Health Implementation Guide*. Although published after the commencement of the project described in this chapter, the guide's focus on the needs of acute in-patient services has been extremely useful in helping to develop our thinking further and enabling the project group to map activity against the key target areas presented (Box 10.1).

Understanding the socio-political context in which acute residential mental healthcare is provided was part of a process that began to identify key drivers for us and potential resisters to change. This was essential to appreciating the pressures staff were

226

Box 10.1 Key target areas.

> - To define the purpose and place of adult in-patient care in the context of the National Mental Health Policy whole systems approach
> - To establish effective means of service co-ordination of acute services to provide a safe structured and therapeutic in-patient experience
> - To develop effective service-user centred decision-making processes and ward arrangements
> - To address the need to enhance the role, status, training, support and career development of in-patient staff
> - To direct clinical leadership and management attention and expertise on the organisation and management of in-patient services
> - To ensure adequate clinical and support inputs to in-patient wards and to maximise the time spent by staff therapeutically engaged with service users
> - To promote ways in which future provision can project a more positive and socially inclusive view of mental health
>
> (Adapted from Department of Health, 2002)

facing and the possible reactions to this project, which would ultimately determine the level of ownership at a local service level.

Background to the project

The local picture

The members of practice teams who agreed to participate in this work were based in the acute in-patient units which, at the commencement of the work (October 2001) were all part of Portsmouth Healthcare NHS Trust. These services were provided in three units on two different sites, some 15 miles apart. All of these were 30-bedded units with integral intensive care facilities. Two were situated in the grounds of what was formerly the large local psychiatric hospital, whilst the third, a relatively new facility, was built in the grounds of an old learning disability hospital.

As a result of the reorganisations that took place in April 2002 these services are now managed separately. One of the units on the psychiatric hospital site is now attached to the local Primary Care Trust, whilst the other two are part of a Specialist Mental Health and Learning Disability Trust. All three have strong links with their Local Implementation Teams. Despite the changes, close contact is still maintained, especially as the pressure on beds sometimes means that patients are admitted to units not within their own geographical locality. This places considerable emphasis on the importance of maintaining, and continuing to develop, good relationships across all components of the organisations.

Establishing the project group

The issues ultimately addressed through the project had formed the basis of many discussions for several months before the plan to develop this work was formalised. Clinicians and service managers had become increasingly concerned about the anxieties being voiced by service users and carers, and ward-based staff were expressing dissatisfaction at what they saw as their inability to provide good quality care. As a result of this, the project group was almost self-selecting as those contributing to the discussions were asked to participate in the initial workshops. Many of these people chose to stay involved with the work that grew out of this. One of the local university mental health teams which has already established user-led and user-focused approaches to teaching and learning agreed to participate with a view to supporting any further educational developments that may emerge. No terms of reference or formal agreements were established regarding the work to be done as it was felt these should be generated by the wider group and reflect the priorities described by the participants, and not by the service providers.

Approaches to practice development

Having set up the group it was necessary to achieve a consensus as to the purpose of the project. However, the nursing literature reveals a lack of agreement as to the definition of practice development. This lack of clarity, whilst potentially inhibiting, was overcome by the use of Garbett and McCormack's (2002) definition. Their description of a facilitative process that created cultural transformation, leading to belief and behavioural change, reflected clearly our aspirations.

From a philosophical perspective our approach could also be described as postmodernist, which subscribes to the view that science and technology will never provide the answers to the complex interpersonal challenges of providing person-centred acute mental healthcare. In constructing the framework of the project, the team drew heavily on the principles of human inquiry, which advocates, from the outset, that the people who use the service should be full participants in any change (Reason, 1994). To achieve this it was important to create valid, non-tokenistic systems for collaborating as it is argued that through such dialogue institutions can learn to adapt.

Structuring the project

Whilst acknowledging that the local picture broadly reflected the national one, in considering how best to approach the sustained development of practice, it was helpful to adopt a framework that would apply some order and logic to the process. The scale of the task could have been overwhelming, however, structuring the process allowed us to set some parameters, prioritise and clearly articulate the purpose of and rationale for the work undertaken. Conceptualising the process as a clinical improvement project allowed questions to be asked in a relatively schematic way and provided sequential opportunities for reflection and modification. Langley *et al.* (1996) have identified several questions summarised in Box 10.2.

What are we trying to achieve?

To achieve the level of partnership and collaboration required to make a success of the project it was helpful to refer to the King's Fund report *Collaboration for Change* (Smith, 1988). This report highlights the importance of changing existing patterns of delivery from working 'on' people, to working 'with' people. Working 'on' people essentially requires the recipients to adopt a passive position, accepting and accommodating what is delivered to them, whilst the central focus of working 'with' people is ensuring that full participation and active contributions from all, is achieved.

In relation to the work of Langley *et al.* (1996) defining what we were trying to achieve would clearly only be possible if the 'we' involved service users and carers throughout the whole life of the project. Ascertaining the concerns of service users and carers about their experience of acute residential services would then provide the basis on which practice development activity would be planned.

Box 10.2 Summary of questions to help structure the process.

1. What are we trying to achieve?
2. How can we find out what needs improving?
3. What changes can we make that will result in improvement?
4. How will we know that a change is an improvement?

How can we find out what needs improving?

In recognition of the fact that those of us working within the services had already had time to discuss and consider some of the issues we felt were important, it was agreed that the initial group work, undertaken in October 2001, would focus on the service users' and carers' experiences. The first half-day was thus set aside for an external facilitator and one of the local facilitators, to meet with the users and carers who had agreed to participate. The first part of this session was used to provide background information to the work and ensure time was available for all present to seek clarification and gain an understanding of what we hoped to achieve. Following on from this we asked the group to identify the things that caused them most concern. The following statements give a flavour of the concerns that were commonly expressed:

> Nurses are often not available or have gone off duty before they have spent time with you.
>
> Staff are in the office but not with patients.
>
> They say they have just come on duty and do not have time.

This behaviour was interpreted as creating a therapeutic distance between the staff and patients:

> There is a lack of warmth between nurses and patients.
>
> Nurses don't come over as caring.
>
> Nurses are there as minders rather than carers.

Consequently the service users felt this behaviour was at the root of a great many problems such as poor communication with their relatives and carers, adding:

> What do we need a registered nurse for? . . . We value the unqualified staff more as we get more from them.

They suggested that there were some simple and achievable solutions:

> The nurse should speak to each patient at least once per day.
>
> They need support, supervision and reflection without fear of recrimination. They need to rediscover the caring attitude.
>
> They need to change the culture of blaming the family and carers for what is happening.

What became evident, as the session progressed was that, whilst both users and carers were prepared to be very clear and direct in describing the things they saw as problems and failings, they all expressed considerable concern and understanding for the nursing staff. Those present felt that nursing staff were, generally, very committed to their work and were trying to offer the best quality service, often under difficult circumstances. However, despite this acceptance all were clear that what presently existed was not acceptable and needed to change.

Drawing from the issues identified by the service users the project group set some broad aims, which would provide direction for the work:

- Shifting the balance of power from professionals to people that use services
- Identify the most appropriate and effective ways of developing user-led services, based on participation and shared ownership of all stakeholders
- Transforming acute mental healthcare environments and cultures so that they cater for the needs of individual patients
- Provide opportunities for all to be involved in shared learning that will lead to the development of the necessary knowledge, clinical skill and decision-making ability, to work effectively in an acute residential care environment

Learning from each other

The first workshop was helpful in identifying the service users' concerns but would be of little value if it was processed and reinterpreted by professionals. It was important that those people involved in providing the service had an opportunity to appreciate the meaning of the service users' and carers' experience. However, in sharing such information we also had to be sensitive to the fact that many of the comments were critical of staff. We wanted to avoid early antagonism as this could create defensive responses. Our aim was to promote an atmosphere of shared learning.

A second workshop was held the day after the service users' workshop. This involved the same service users and carers and other key stakeholders including nurses, educators and service managers. This workshop presented additional challenges as it brought people together who had not worked in such a way before. It created opportunities for participants to question traditional power relationships, to set the agenda, influence decisions and plan action. Consequently there were some initial anxieties about how to behave and what could be said to whom. However, skilled group facilitation enabled people to feel comfortable enough for the work to proceed.

The aim of the first part of this workshop was to encourage the service providers to be as open and honest about the problems and challenges they face, i.e., providing service providers with a similar opportunity to that of service users. What emerged could be organised into three distinct themes:

Theme 1: The status of acute services and the developmental needs of staff
- Residential care being seen as second class
- The need for specialist status
- The training needs of staff to focus on reflective practice and individualised care
- Poor staffing levels and recruitment/retention difficulties
- Trained staff caught up in housekeeping and environmental issues

Theme 2: The culture of the environment
- Practice perceived as stuck in time 'it is the way things are done around here'
- Little collaboration of good practice between service providers
- New staff made to 'fit in'
- Students do not feel able to question practice
- Lack of effective clinical role models

Theme 3: Communication
- Poor communication between professional service users and the community agencies
- Staff withholding information from carers
- The need to adopt more collaborative approaches which treat people as equals

The process of recording these themes on paper does not adequately reflect the level of critical self-reflection and frankness that was evident during the workshop. Whilst at times emotionally and perhaps professionally painful for the clinical staff present, they remained willing to engage with the process. However, it was essential for the success of the project that there was honesty and ownership of the problems. The emerging themes were then compared with those identified by the service users and carers and common issues agreed.

- Communication and information delivery
- Lack of or loss of skills amongst staff
- Acknowledgement of each other's skills (staff and service users)
- Lack of time with service users and too much time spent on housekeeping

- Experienced staff having insufficient contact with service users and carers
- Basic attitudes of caring and user involvement in clinical decisions
- The low profile of acute services and lack of staff resources

This was a significant step as it represented common agreement, and therefore ownership, of the main problems that would provide the focus of any practice development. What was also affirming was the remarkable similarity between this list and the key target areas identified earlier in the *Mental Health Implementation Guide*. However, identifying a common list of problems, whilst important, did not inspire or encourage individuals to think outside the box about what might be possible. To address this issue the participants were taken on a journey that would allow them to think more creatively about the sort of service they wanted to ideally provide or receive. The participants were then formed into small groups to envision the future, explore challenges to be overcome and identify critical issues to be addressed in the process. This culminated in four groups developing a collective vision and practical concerns that would need to be addressed in the action plan. This was done using a three-step process, involving identifying a 'collective dream', indicating issues that would need to be addressed to make the dream a reality (the realist) and finally identifying the barriers to the change happening (the critic).

Collective dream

The collective dream attempted to identify a utopian concept of the provision of acute residential care. Many of the ideas focused on the redistribution of power and reduced professionalism. There was an emphasis on greater equality, collaboration and clearer leadership from all levels of the organisation, which included extra resources. There was also a belief that people would feel valued in whatever role they were in and boundaries between users, providers and professionals would no longer exist. Staff would have a positive attitude and be highly skilled with developmental opportunities to fulfil their role. They would engage early with people and have time to provide high-quality, evidence-based care with services being truly person-centred. The service would become a centre of excellence with recruitment no longer being an issue. New staff would be recruited jointly by service users and the Health Trust.

233

The realist

The second stage of the process required participants to adopt a realistic approach to the vision and determine what could be achieved given the existing service constraints. Interestingly, many present felt that the vision would be achievable given the commitment from staff. Other suggestions were that a positive structure needed to be present that brought people together, created opportunities for service users to influence all levels of the organisation, provided a forum for staff and service users to learn together and would enhance the humanistic skills which the staff required to do the job.

The critic

The third stage required participants to critique the vision and proposals suggested in order to identify the current barriers to achieving these changes. These were written as action-oriented statements listed below, which would then form the basis for planning specific outcomes in the final stage of the process.

- Everyone across the organisation must own the vision
- The culture of the organisation needs to be more inclusive at all levels
- Staff resistance must be overcome
- More resources for acute residential care need to be identified
- Negative attitudes must be challenged
- Staff and service users must be more involved in organisational change
- The blaming approach to staff needs to be replaced with one of mutual learning
- Support mechanisms need to be found for people who may become ill and are unable to make progress
- Services must be safe and supportive for both users and staff
- Revisit the role of the mental health nurse so that they can do the job they are trained to do
- Champions of change need to be supported
- Joint approaches involving service users and staff should be employed for recruiting staff

What changes can we make that will result in improvement?

This list identified key drivers and resisters that allowed for identification of specific practical actions that could be planned, moni-tored and reviewed as the work progressed. The actions essentially fell into one of three areas. Those that related to the whole organisation and its culture, those that identified strategies for greater user involvement and those that focused on staff development.

Organisational

- Communication of the collective vision across the organisation
- Senior management representative will take the lead on this work to ensure there is ownership at the most senior level of the organisation

User involvement

- Service users will be invited to be on the organisation's Executive Board
- Care Programme Reviews will routinely involve carers and relatives as appropriate
- Fora will be created that provide opportunities for service users, staff and student nurses to come together for mutual learning and support
- The Trust and University will develop recruitment processes that involve service users

Staff development

- The profile of acute residential care nursing will be raised
- New and specific career pathways will be identified for acute residential staff
- Through appraisal processes, staff will review existing nursing roles and identify their development needs
- Peer supervision arrangements will be implemented

In identifying these actions we attempted to achieve a balance between our long-term ambitions to achieve a significant cultural shift and short-term more immediate results that would motivate those involved. As these actions represented a work that was both complex and time consuming, it was agreed to establish three action-oriented groups to take responsibility for the implementation of the work into day-to-day practice.

These three groups were identified according to the main focus of their work:

- Learning and teaching together
- Raising the profile of residential care
- Collaborative working with users and carers

The 'learning and teaching together' group

This group aimed to meet once each month on each of the three acute residential units. Its purpose was for service users, both current and recently discharged, to meet together with staff and students, to discuss issues common to all and learn from each other's experiences. It is facilitated by someone outside the staff team and is usually of one hour's duration. There is no pre-determined agenda, allowing issues for discussion to be determined by the group members. The discussion is often wide-ranging but tends to focus on those problems important to the service users at the time, including medication and side-effects, treatment and therapies, the experience of mental health problems, preparation for discharge and the management of symptoms at home.

Raising the profile of residential care

The initial aim of this group was to retain a broad focus, and membership, that would enable staff, service users and carers from all three units, to continue working together. Unfortunately the practicalities of this, in terms of finding a suitable venue, ensuring transport was available and transport costs met where necessary, and agreeing on the best times to meet, proved more challenging than the groups had envisaged. This became more complicated following reconfiguration as the two organisations, whilst generally being committed to this work, had different service agendas and time scales. However, work done in identifying the main problems and possible actions to overcome these, has been communicated to the groups now working to establish Acute Care Fora, as described in the *Mental Health Implementation Guide* (Department of Health, 2002).

Collaborative working with users and carers

Strong user and carer groups exist within the three geographical locations covered by this project. Service user and carer support and project workers are in place and users and carers are permanent members of Local Implementation Teams (established by the English Department of Health's 'Modernisation Agency' to help develop healthcare systems locally) and participate in a wide range of working groups and fora. The participants in the project used their existing networks to pass on information about this work and collect comments, feedback and suggestions as to how things could best progress. Quality of communication between service providers, users and carers was a common theme as was the lack of good, clear information. Individual experiences of hospital settings and perceptions of attitudes of staff varied considerably although where problems had been experienced issues such as poor communication were found to be central features. Again, the logistics of keeping one large group together proved problematic and so it was agreed that work would continue separately in each area.

Two further project group workshops have taken place, one after six months and the second at the end of the first year, and these have provided opportunities for progress between groups and across areas, to be discussed. Other work done to support this project has included the production of a formal report which was sent, with a covering letter, to Trust Board members and senior managers, and attendance, by the local facilitator, at a range of meetings in order to describe this work. Trust representatives have also been invited to attend the next workshop as some participants remain unconvinced that there is real commitment at this level, to support this work.

The challenges: how will we know that a change is an improvement?

It is important to maintain the credibility of the project, that thorough evaluation is undertaken to assess the value and effectiveness of what we are trying to achieve. Through the process of evaluation the project group can learn from their actions and determine changes that need to be made. The process would also enhance the partnership by ensuring that the outcomes clearly reflected improvement in the experiences of those using mental health services. The values compass (Kashkouski & Neuhauser, 1998: see Fig. 10.1) was helpful in identifying the relevant dimensions of improvement.

Evaluation of the impact of the project at different points on the values compass requires a range of methods and tools. As this project is fundamentally concerned with improving the functional health and quality of life outcomes for service users admitted to acute residential care, a design was chosen that involved an adaptation of the Carers' and Users' experience of Services (CUES) tool (Lelliott *et al.*, 2001). This involved developing benchmark statements relating to the experience of acute in-patient care. The tool is a self-reported questionnaire that asks the individual to rate their experience against each statement. The experience of service users is also being evaluated through interviews with service users who have had recent experience of acute residential care and questionnaires have been distributed through the 'teaching and learning together' group.

Measuring changes in the clinical outcome dimension present particular challenges. Whilst length of hospital stay could be

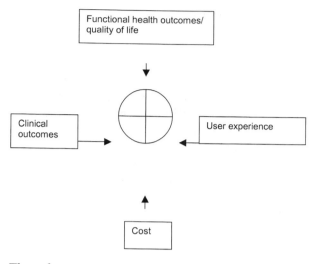

Fig. 10.1 The values compass.

calculated it would be difficult to determine a causal link to this project in view of the many other factors that impact on admission rates. However, it could be possible to suggest a relationship between improvements in the care experience of service users and reduced symptoms and increased confidence and self-esteem.

The project is also being evaluated from the perspective of the staff who work in each of the acute residential units to assess the impact on their practice. Methods used will include observations of care and interviews. One other important source of data are the evaluations of student nurses who receive training in the units. Our colleagues in the University are collating this data.

Successes: initial evaluations of each development

The evaluation data, collected through direct observation, interview and questionnaire suggests a high level of satisfaction with the teaching and learning together group. The level of attendance, often in excess of 20 people, and degree of participation, indicate that it serves a useful purpose in creating a forum where concerns and frustrations can be aired in a safe and supportive environment. The staff are quick to respond positively to issues to improve the quality of the person's experience of care. There is also an atmosphere of democracy and power sharing which appears to be impacting on the service user's perceptions of the staff's behaviour.

The solutions generated within the discussions relating directly to the problems raised are also identified as an important part of the recovery process for the service users and are greatly valued. At a very fundamental level the group brings people together who have similar problems.

Such data represents only the beginning of an iterative process of action and evaluation that extends over a significant period of time. In addition to the evaluation of each of the groups the workshop held at the end of the first year provided an opportunity for all of the participants to review progress made and clarify the on-going challenges. This was very useful as it provided some very positive feedback about the changes apparent to those who have been recently in receipt of services:

> I have only just been in hospital and had a very good experience. I attended the teaching and learning together group and found it helped me to share with others how I was feeling.
>
> (Service user)

> As a member of staff I have certainly noticed a positive difference in the way that staff are working with people.
>
> (Staff member)

Reflections and lessons learnt

This ongoing project, whilst stimulating and enjoyable, has presented significant challenges for all participants. The willingness of those involved to stay committed to this work is impressive, despite the speed of progress which (with any work requiring significant culture change) is slow.

Although our aim was to develop a collaborative project, it has been necessary at various points, to provide leadership. In many ways this has required a transformational style using such skills as inspiration, intellectual stimulation and individual support. It was important to ensure that this was offered in a way that enabled others to take charge where needed and did not suggest that any central or service provider 'control' was being imposed. However, more than this, it has required great sensitivity to the feelings of all involved by constantly attending to the potential for anxiety and conflict and carefully monitoring the atmosphere in order to create a more harmonious environment in which people can work together.

Unfortunately the organisational restructuring during the course of this work resulted in different acute services on the same site being managed by different organisations. This created considerable uncertainty for staff regarding future roles and responsibilities resulting in some initiatives being delayed, which meant extra effort at maintaining staff's commitment to the process over a long period of time.

The process of organisational change and the fight against the existing culture and institutional processes remains an ongoing battle. Achieving the right balance between valuing staff through support whilst also challenging and motivating them toward achievement of the vision requires determination and resilience. Key to such cultural change has been achieving acknowledgement, acceptance and support of the project from senior managers in each of the provider organisations.

What has been perhaps the most energising experience of all is the tolerance, encouragement and enthusiasm of the service users and carers. They have been both supportive and willing to accommodate the service's problems as the organisation embarks on what is likely to be a long journey toward truly person-centred services. This process of collaboration has perhaps been the most rewarding and enlightening aspect as it reveals the day-to-day struggle that people encounter when they use services. It has also required sensitivity to the dynamics between users and caregivers who are likely to use services again.

Our engagement in the process has at times been a very intense experience characterised by highs when service users report improvements and lows when efforts are frustrated by the institution. Perhaps one over-riding achievement has been the raised profile of acute care and those people that use it or work within it. We have experienced relationships where traditional boundaries have been broken down and people have been able to work together toward mutually valued goals. It would have been very easy to jump on the accusatory bandwagon and blame nurses for the inadequacies of acute services. However, throughout this work we have encountered enormous enthusiasm and commitment to making change. It has felt in many respects like pushing at an open door despite the fact that fatigued staff are often carrying huge responsibility. In progressing such a project we were struck by the significance of Barker's (2001) suggestion that: 'the kind of care that nurses need to deliver, . . . given the context of care and the often limited resources available, can represent acts of extraordinary courage and compassion.' (p. 238).

It is through reporting such practice development work that the skill of acute mental health nursing can be acknowledged and celebrated for what it is.

References

Barker, P. (2001) The tidal model: Developing an empowering, person-centred approach to recovery within psychiatric and mental health nursing. *Journal of Psychiatric and Mental Health Nursing*, **8**, 233–40.

Camden Consortium (1987) *Good Practices in Mental Health. Treated Well? A Code of Practice for Psychiatric Hospitals*. Camden Consortium, London.

Chamberlin, J. (1988) *On our Own*. MIND, London.

Department of Health (1999) *National Service Framework for Mental Health*. HMSO, London.

Department of Health (2001) *National Service Framework for Mental Health, Workforce Planning, Education and Training*. The final report of the Workforce Action Team. HMSO, London.

Department of Health (2002) *Mental Health Implementation Guide: Adult Acute In-patient Care Provision*. HMSO, London.

Ford, R. (2002) Acute care. *Mental Health Practice*, **5**(9), 26.

Garbett, R. & McCormack, B. (2002) A concept analysis of practice development. *Nursing Times Research*, **7**(2), 87–100.

Kashkouski, S. & Neuhauser, D. (1998) *Personal Continuous Quality Improvement Workbook*. Case Western University, US.

Langley, G.J., Nolan, K.M., Nolan, T.W., Norman, C.L. & Provost, L.P. (1996) *A Practical Approach to Enhancing Organisational Performance*. Jossey Bass, San Francisco, CA.

Lelliot, P., Beevor, A., Hogman, G., Hyslop, J., Lathlean, J. & Ward, M. (2001) Carers' and users' expectations of services – user version (CUES – U): A new instrument to measure the experience of users of mental health services. *British Journal of Psychiatry*, **179**, 67–72.

MIND (2000) *Environmentally Friendly? Patients' Views of Conditions on Psychiatric Wards*. MIND publications, London.

Morgan, G. (1998) *Images of Organisations*. Sage, London.

Reason P. (1994) *Participation in Human Inquiry*. Sage, London.

Sainsbury Centre for Mental Health (1998) *Acute Problems: A Survey of the Quality of Care in Acute Psychiatric Wards*. Sainsbury Centre for Mental Health, London.

Sainsbury Centre for Mental Health (2000) Finding and Keeping. *Review of Recruitment and Retention in the Mental Health Workforce*. Sainsbury Centre for Mental Health, London.

Smith, H. (1988) *Collaboration for Change: Partnership Between Service Users, Planners and Managers of Mental Health Services*. King's Fund, London.

Standing Nursing and Midwifery Advisory Committee (1999) *Addressing Acute Concerns*. SNMAC, London.

Tingle, A. (2001) Mental health nurse: do they care? *Mental Health Practice*, **4**(9), 12–15.

Commentary

Ann Jackson

The current focus on acute in-patient mental healthcare (Department of Health, 2002) could be described as a double-edge sword. On one edge of the sword, there is the unprecedented opportunity supported by national policy to change the way in which traditional care has been given and services have been developed and delivered. There has been an overwhelming, but arguably, necessary critique of services and care from the professions, managers, politicians and, importantly, service users and carers. Most powerfully, this critique has centered on the experiences of people who have used the services and would define themselves as *survivors* of a system that is oppressive and often abusive.

On the other edge of the sword, the level of critique over the last ten years, culminating in the English Department of Health's policy response last year, has done little to improve the image and morale of psychiatric and mental health nursing in these areas. Unfortunately, much of the critique has focused on the quality of nursing care at a time when we have a national problem with recruitment and retention, and services are desperate to encourage staff to work in acute services. Scant attention has been paid, in terms of policy, to other professions within this area of care, and yet the criticisms of service users often implicate the structure and cultures of traditional (medical model) psychiatric practice.

However, it is important that the psychiatric and mental health nursing profession make the most of the opportunity radically to improve what we have now, but more importantly, influence the development of future services in line with the growing demand for 'alternative solutions'. This demand for alternatives to admission is two-fold. First, the *National Service Framework* (Department of Health, 1999) is directing the development of services that are provided in the community such as crisis teams, intensive home treatment(s) and assertive outreach. Second, there is growing appreciation of more radical survivor-led service models that are effective and *desirable* in providing non-institutionalised care (Faulkner *et al.*, 2002). We must heed the warning not to do 'the same but better' by developing services and practices within modernist constructions of 'mental illness' and previously ordained roles of professionals and those receiving care (Peck, 2000).

At the same time, psychiatric and mental health nurses are being implored to value and practice the skills which users of the service find the most helpful. These skills and attributes are well documented and have been for some considerable time (Rogers *et al.*, 1993), and are constantly being flagged up in psychiatric and mental health nursing conferences and academic debate (personal observation). These attributes and skills are often referred to as the humanistic qualities; and is well illustrated within this practice development project with a direct quote from a service user, 'They need to rediscover the caring attitude'. It has been argued (and contested) that this has been lost along the journey towards 'evidence-based' practice.

However relevant or not this debate is, in itself it is not enough. We currently need to be able to offer services which provide timely and skilled interventions for people requiring a broad range of psychiatric and mental healthcare. Such needs might range from the often underestimated need for asylum or sanctuary (Nolan, 2003 personal communication) to those requiring skills of assessment and interventions based on current 'best practices' and best available evidence(s) from the range of sources, but particularly from people who use services. There is an urgent need for a more inclusive taxonomy of 'evidence' that gives equal status to non-academic knowledge(s) and experiences of people who use services (Rose, 2001). It is the systemic inclusion of service users and carers in all levels of representation and decision-making which might provide the basis for a radical shift in power-relations within existing culture(s) and structures of care provision. This might then pave the way for 'a dynamic partnership between agencies, service users, carers, academics, professionals and managers' (Department of Health, 2001).

We currently have a situation where the language of 'involvement' 'collaboration' and 'partnership' is evident in all policy documents relating to the mental healthcare modernisation agenda. Whilst this is to be welcomed, there are varying degrees to which service providers, professionals and service users are: a) able to engage in a shared *language* of participation; b) able to engage with a *political* agenda of 'participation'; and c) able to influence the way in which the development of alternative services can be resourced,

243

particularly through the voluntary sector (Bates, 2002; Beresford, 2002).

In order to be truly 'participative' or 'collaborative' there is a considerable amount of attitude change and the reinstatement or discovery of a value base that provides an enlightened context for sustained change. This practice development work as described by the authors is a good illustration of the purpose and processes involved in the development of services which respond to the explicit claims, concerns and issues (Guba & Lincoln, 1989) of participant stakeholders. The level of 'collaborative' *intent* is evident in the detailing of workshop identification of issues and the development of action-planning and implementation. The evaluation evidence suggests that a range of mechanisms have been constructed across the organisation and with the Local Implementation Teams systemically to involve 'staff,' service users and carers and managers in implementation of their 'collective vision', although explicit examples of collaborative decision-making will be an important addition to the richness of the work. The authors draw our attention to the importance of Trust Executive level commitment and the ongoing need for this to be demonstrated in order to engage and motivate all stakeholders in the pursuit of philosophical and cultural change.

The work describes the beginning of the *journey* towards person-centred service-development. It is an ambitious attempt to overhaul the way in which care is provided within a framework of collaboration and shared vision. Importantly, there are a range of evaluation methods that will provide the detailed evidence to support the genuine hopes and aspirations of their collective development. The work is important in that it illustrates the complexity of developing acute services to be more helpful places to receive care and better place to work in.

References

Bates, P. (2002) (ed.) *Working for Inclusion*, London, Sainsbury Centre for Mental Health.

Beresford, P. (2002) Thinking about 'mental health': towards a social model (Editorial). *Journal of Mental Health*, **11**(6), 581–4.

Department of Health (1999) *National Service Framework for Mental Health: Modern Standards and Service Models*. HMSO, London.

Department of Health (2001) *The National Institute for Mental Health in England: Role and Function*. Department of Health Publications, London.

Department of Health (2002) *Mental Health Policy Implementation Guide: Adult Acute In-patient Care Provision*. HMSO, London.

Faulkner, A., Petit-Zeman, S., Sherlock, J. & Wallcraft, J. (2002) A home away from home. *Mental Health Today* March, 18–21.

Guba, E.G. & Lincoln, Y.S. (1989) *Fourth Generation Evaluation.* Sage, USA.

Nolan Peter (2003) Personal communication.

Peck, E. (2000) Modernising mental health services in a post-modern world (Editorial). *Journal of Mental Health*, **9**(4), 347–50.

Resisters (2002) *Women Speak Out: Women's Experiences of Using Mental Health Services and Proposals for Change.* Resisters, Leeds.

Rogers, A., Pilgrim, D. & Lacey, R. (1993) *Experiencing Psychiatry – Users' Views of Services.* Macmillan Press Ltd, Hong Kong.

Rose, D. (2001) *Users' Voices.* The Sainsbury Centre for Mental Health, London.

11. *Developing a Corporate Strategy to Develop Effective and Patient-centred Care*

Jane Stokes

The purpose of this chapter is to provide an insight into the practice development journey undertaken in a large acute NHS Trust at a strategic and corporate level. It explores the steps taken over two years to develop strategies for both practice development and its evaluation. The context in which the journey began will be outlined and the challenges and opportunities presented to all the people engaged with the strategy will be described. At a corporate level practice development is defined as 'Working with healthcare providers and users, to develop systematic strategies relevant to everyday practice to enhance care for service users' (RCNI, 2002). How this is being achieved will be explored in the chapter by describing the variety of processes that have been established, throughout the organisation, to ensure that the vision for practice development becomes the reality for the patients at the centre of healthcare provision. It is an account of work in progress and so captures the practicalities of applying principles and processes developed within the practice development field to a large organisation.

The world of practice development is evolving, dynamic and complex. It is 'messy' and fast moving with the constant feeling of striving to 'keep all the plates spinning'. I would argue that the principles and processes collectively known as practice development provide a kind of 'recipe for practice development'. The ingredients that can contribute to its success are outlined in Box 11.1. However, like many recipes you may have tried, the ingredients and instructions look straightforward enough to begin with. But once you are cooking they may become quite complex; a key ingredient may have been missed out, and the outcome is vastly different from what

Box 11.1 A recipe for organisational practice development.

Recipe

To create a culture of effectiveness which is patient-centred and evidence-based (be warned it may take three years to see noticeable change in some aspects of the culture and 15 years to see sustainable change).

Ingredients

You will need:

Staff – nurses, doctors, allied health professionals and support staff
Practice development facilitators (PDF) (from within the organisation and from outside organisations too, if you can get them)
An understanding of the key concepts and theories underpinning practice development
A fully equipped practice development toolkit
Full commitment and support within the organisation
Energy, commitment, enthusiasm and luck!

Know how: key concepts and theories underpinning practice development

Practice Development – processes and outcomes (Manley, 2001; Garbett & McCormack, 2002)
Organisational Culture (Manley, 2000a)
Supportive helping relationships, for example, critical companionship (Titchen, 2000)
Reflective Practice (for example, Johns, 1994)
Learning from practice (for example, action learning, McGill & Beaty, 2001)
Creative approaches to evaluation (for example, Guba & Lincoln, 1989)
Understanding government agendas
Leadership (for example, transformational leadership (Kouzes & Posner, 1987))

Tools: A PD toolkit

Patient forum
A cultural assessment tool
Action learning sets
Clinical supervision
Facilitation standards
360° evaluation
Practice development workshops

Box 11.1 *Continued*

Essence of Care benchmarks
Patient and staff stories
Observation of care
Adverse incidents/clinical risk indicators database
Access to the Internet
Good communication (for example, an intranet site if possible)

was hoped for. Like a well-run, efficient and effective kitchen, practice development is about having the courage and support to take risks, to agree ways of working together, and to constantly review and revise the direction your journey is taking. Many recipes that work well have been developed in this way. As a consumer you will be presented with the finished product, which strives to meet with your approval, give you satisfaction, and an experience that you even enjoyed! This should be the patient's experience, and like a customer in a restaurant, they may not want to know, or be interested in, what goes on behind the scenes to achieve that result. What is important to them is their own experience.

Healthcare settings are being opened up to the consumer/the service user for their scrutiny, and their active participation and consultation is sought now at every level. The recipe for practice development is evolving and needs to be adapted and altered to meet the needs and challenges presented by each healthcare setting.

The context

Barts and the London (BLT) NHS Trust provides general hospital services to Tower Hamlets and the City of London and specialist services to the whole of London and beyond. It has over 1,100 beds spread over three sites. Each site has its own long and separate history. The Trust employs over 5,500 staff including 1,000 doctors and dentists and 1,600 nurses. It provides care to a population composed of diverse ethnic and cultural communities. The largest ethnic minority groups in east London are Bengali, Somali, Irish, Afro-Caribbean, Turkish, Chinese, Vietnamese and Jewish.

From April 2001 to April 2002 480,738 outpatients were seen at BLT; 98,457 patients were treated in the accident and emergency department and 85,633 patients were admitted. There were 24,699 theatre cases (18,738 scheduled cases and 5,961 emergency cases (source: www.bartsandthelondon.org.uk)). Nursing shared governance is well established in the Trust. Within the shared governance structure there are four teams composed of clinical practice, education, management and quality. The teams consist of self-nominated nurses from across the range of grades, roles and responsibilities. The teams report to a Trust-wide nursing policy board. The structure provides a framework where encouragement and support is given to all individuals to take responsibility for quality.

The practice development structure

There are presently 19 practice development nurses/facilitators across the nine directorates in the Trust. These practitioners are the co-researchers in this study. Other practitioners also contribute to initiatives intermittently but all activities are co-ordinated by the practice development team, which is guided by its own strategy. Participation from other disciplines is actively and constantly sought. The quality of care provided to patients and users does not rest with one discipline but requires effective teamwork, a characteristic of learning organisations (Manley, 2001).

There has also been a move away from using the term practice development nurse, replacing it with the title practice development facilitator. This was done to encourage colleagues from other professions and departments to get involved. Feedback from other disciplines suggested that there was 'nothing for them' on the practice development intranet site. On exploring this further it became clear that they had a valid concern, all the notes, resources and reports were nurse-focused although this had not been the intention. Changing the terms used is straightforward, using the terms 'practice developer' or practice development facilitator gives out a more inclusive message to others who might want to get involved. A further strategy to encourage the involvement of other disciplines was to re-visit the membership of the project steering group, it represented the key stakeholders identified at the beginning of the project. As the project evolved to involve the whole organisation the emerging questions and strategic objectives were relevant to all practitioners within the Trust. We have learnt that if the vision for practice development is to be realised in practice then the inclusion of all who have an impact on the patient's journey needed to be aware of the strategy and be given the opportunity to engage with the activity.

The process

The aim of the project is reflected in its two research questions: first, how do we (the practice development team) individually and collectively facilitate the achievement of the Trust-wide practice development strategy and vision? And, second, how do we individually and collectively evaluate progress towards the vision and achievement of the Trust's practice development strategy? The anticipated outcomes of practice development include patient-centred and evidence-based healthcare as well as a culture of effectiveness – termed a 'transformational culture' (Manley, 2001). These are associated with three characteristics: staff empowerment; practice development focused around the needs of patients; and specific workplace characteristics. Cultural indicators have been developed around these characteristics and measurable outcomes identified from a number of practice development and related organisational studies (Manley, 2001). These include:

- Patients having a range of opportunities to be more involved in their care
- Improved patient experiences
- Improved patient outcomes as indicated by reduction in clinical risk/adverse events
- Developing workplace cultures where all staff understand their responsibility to provide high quality and effective care
- Dynamic teams contributing to organisational development
- Empowered staff
- Improved staff recruitment and retention
- Leadership potential developed at all levels

Once completed, this study will further add to understanding about the practice development processes necessary to achieve a culture of effectiveness, one that is patient-centred and evidence-based. The study will also add to our understanding about how such outcomes can be demonstrated in day-to-day work.

Developing the strategy: agreeing the vision

Our plan in the first phase was to identify stakeholders in the overall project and undertake a values clarification exercise (Manley, 1992: see Box 11.2) with them in order to arrive at a shared vision for the work. The result of this work was presented to the Trust's Nursing Policy Board and to the executive board. A steering group was set up and strategies for practice development and the evaluation of its impact were developed in partnership with stakeholders. The project design was submitted to the local ethics committee. Securing the support of the Trust board was seen as an essential ingredient. As has been identified in previous practice development work, managerial support can provide support and ease the progress of project work (Manley, 2000 a, b).

Box 11.2   Values clarification exercise (adapted from Manley, 1992).

I believe our purpose in this unit/ward/Trust is . . .
I believe we can achieve this purpose by . . .
I believe an effective healthcare team is . . .
I believe individuals within a team feel valued by . . .
I believe I can be helped to become more effective by . . .
I believe I can help others to become more effective by . . .
Other values and beliefs I hold about patient care are . . .

It was agreed during the project planning stage that the strategy would involve the development of the following characteristics:

- A shared vision
- A learning culture
- Valuing leadership at all levels
- Valuing all stakeholders
- To be appropriate for the strategic direction of the Trust
- Flexible and adaptable to changes on the horizon

Practice development approaches can achieve these purposes through a number of key interrelated processes which guide the work of the practice developer:

- Skills which foster structured reflection and critique and the use of values clarification to enable espoused values to become a reality
- Fostering leadership potential in others
- Developing a patient/person-centred culture
- Developing a learning culture
- Focusing on the using and development of evidence
- Evaluating effectiveness
- Influencing, shaping and implementing policy

During phase 1 of the project the practice development workshop time was spent achieving a number of goals, one of which was to undertake a values clarification exercise and agreeing a shared vision. This was based on the same strategy used in the negotiation and planning in the initial stages on the direction the Trust was taking. Raising awareness of the proposal, and engaging the practice developers already working locally within the directorates, was essential. The members of the Nursing Policy Board and the four nursing teams, within the shared governance structure, had laid the foundations for the direction. Now it was the team of practice development facilitators who needed to be involved with writing the practice development strategy and identifying the evaluation questions and the strategic objectives. A shared vision is only the vision of those involved, each group of stakeholders needs the opportunity of owning the vision. The values clarification exercise (Manley, 1992) proved to be a useful starting point in achieving this goal.

Giving participants a voice: gathering claims, concerns and issues

One strategy that we used at the start of each workshop was to identify the participant's claims, concerns and issues about the strategy. This proved helpful in guiding the direction of the workshops and giving people an appropriate forum to share these important areas. The idea of claims, concerns and issues is drawn from *Fourth Generation Evaluation* (Guba & Lincoln, 1989) (see Chapter 5 for a fuller discussion of this approach). It enables a focus on key stakeholder groups such as users and staff in developing the evaluation agenda as well providing a forum in which to address different stakeholder priorities and concerns. Guba & Lincoln define stakeholders as 'persons or groups that are put at some risk by the evaluation, that is, persons or groups that hold a stake' (King & Appleton, 1999: 705). Three different groups of stakeholders are defined; agents, beneficiaries and victims:

- 'Agents' are defined as those 'who devise, operate, manage, fund, oversee, or otherwise contribute to the developments, establishment and operation of the evaluand'
- 'Beneficiaries' are defined those who 'profit, or are expected to profit, from the evaluand, and secondary beneficiaries related to them'
- 'Victims' are defined as 'persons who directly or indirectly are injured or deprived of some good by the implementation of the evaluand, including foregone opportunities'

(Guba & Lincoln, quoted in King & Appleton, 1999: 704)

Within this project the 'agents' may be viewed as the members of the strategy steering group, the nursing policy board and the trust board. The 'beneficiaries' for the evaluation strategy are viewed as the patients and service users, along with the practice developers and other practitioners. 'Victims' here were considered to be those excluded and/or not engaged with the strategy. For example, potentially this could include patient groups excluded because of age, language or mental health needs, or staff groups who fear the consequences of the evaluation, and those with a vested interest in 'keeping business as usual' and so are resistant to change! Guba & Lincoln argue that, in evaluating a project, there is no single reality 'but only multiple realities constructed by human beings' (Guba & Lincoln, quoted in King & Appleton, 1999: 704). They advocate that taking this view, stakeholders' potentially diverse perspectives are of paramount importance, and their approach attempts to elicit these differing views. The method by which this can be achieved is to capture the claims, concerns and issues of all stakeholder groups. Claims are defined as 'favourable assertions' about the subject of the evaluation, for example, 'discussing the strategy is helping me contribute to our shared vision'. By contrast concerns are described as 'unfavourable assertions', for example, 'I am concerned about my ability to prioritise this work against other Trust targets'. Issues are seen as questions which reflect what any reasonable person might be asking about the subject of an evaluation. In this case such questions might include, 'What strategies can I use to gain commitment for this work, from others who are not here today?' The benefits of using this method within the practice development workshops has been shared with the steering group. As the steering group was also comprised of many of the stakeholder groups it was used at the start of these meetings too.

The practice development strategy (see Box 11.3) was presented to the Trust board and approved. The workshops were dynamic, creative, hard work, enjoyable, challenging, inspiring and exhausting! The first cultural change became apparent at this time. This was

Box 11.3 The strategic objectives

1. To improve the patients' experience
2. To improve patient outcomes
3. To provide more opportunities for patient/user involvement
4. To increase evidence-based care
5. To promote access to all forms of evidence and enable practitioners to develop, critique, and use all forms of evidence
6. To develop corporate and local mechanisms for providing feedback on unit and departmental effectiveness
7. To develop a workplace culture that is person- and patient-centred
8. To develop everyone's leadership (interdisciplinary) potential across the trust
9. To develop a learning culture
10. To implement systems of clinical supervision/action learning in all areas
11. To introduce 360° feedback across the Trust

the improved teamwork which had been generated amongst the practice development team through working together in a strategic direction while all the time maintaining the local initiatives that were established prior to the project. The action learning sets provided the balance of high challenge and high support necessary to help the participants to explore and develop their practice development work. The sets were co-facilitated by set members initially with facilitation provided by the senior nurse for practice development and a facilitator from the practice development function at the Royal College of Nursing Institute (RCNI). The action learning sets are now co-facilitated by the set members. Many of the practice development facilitators are now facilitating sets in their local areas with groups of nurses, mainly targeting junior nursing staff.

The evaluation framework

The evaluation strategy was developed with the practice development nurses by identifying priority evaluation questions related to the vision. These questions in turn informed the selection of possible evidence-based tools that would:

- Enable a baseline of the current situation to be identified against which later changes may be compared
- Provide ongoing feedback on the journey towards achieving the vision
- Identify mechanisms which practice development nurses may use with colleagues to engage them in developing ownership of the vision through active participation

The framework focuses on four evaluation questions under which more detailed questions are posed, and possible tools identified (see Table 11.1). The remainder of the chapter addresses initial steps in addressing the strategic and evaluative goals of our work.

Putting the strategy into action: first steps

The key to the success of the strategy will be the development of ownership and engagement by all healthcare practitioners in the Trust. This is demonstrated in two of the objectives to improve patients' experience, and to develop the leadership potential of staff. The *Essence of Care* (DoH, 2001) benchmarks provide the opportunity to demonstrate best practice with the intention that the patient's experience should be enhanced. The clinical leaders need to be supported in developing their skills to work effectively with their teams, to deliver best practice, and to develop ownership and engagement

254

Table 11.1 The evaluation strategy: questions and sources of evidence.

Evaluation questions	Subsidiary questions	Sources of evidence

How do we demonstrate cultural change?	It is important to be able, first, to identify the culture (defined as 'the way things are done around here' (Drennan, 1992)) as it is now and to pose the following questions:
	
	• How are things done now?
	• Are interventions patient-centred/focused?
	• Do patients feel valued all the time by nurses?
	• Do patients feel confident and trusting with the care they are receiving?
	• Is change a norm in the culture?
	• Can staff articulate the vision in their own language?
	
	   • Ownership
	   • Common language
	   • Involvement/participation
	
	• What is the Trust/directorate/ward culture?
	• Does more than one culture exist?
	• What are the strategies for developing and working with cultures?
		• Aiken Tool (Aiken *et al.*, 1998) provides quantitative data for both organisational and directorate/unit factors influencing effectiveness
		• Cultural indicators of a transformational culture (Manley, 2001) – provide a framework for compiling a directorate/ward/unit profile (qualitative and quantitative data) in relation to what constitutes a transformational culture as well as enabling areas that need to be addressed to be identified
		• Observation of patient care
		• Staff stories

What impact is the strategy having on patient care?	• What structures are in place to enable measurement of clinical outcomes? • How is patient feedback collected, evaluated and acted upon? • What effect has the RCNI project had on the Practice Development nurses?	• Patient stories/narratives • Adverse events • Nursing database • Essence of care benchmarks/audit

Table 11.1 *Continued*

Evaluation questions	Subsidiary questions	Sources of evidence
To what extent is practice evidence-based?	• How is leadership developed within the clinical area? • How are staff supported to bring about change?	• Action Learning Set (ALS) analysis of processes and outcomes from documentary analysis of process notes and reflective diaries and reviews • Qualitative '360° feedback' (RCN, 2003) using semi-structured questions developed by each Practice Development practitioner to obtain feedback from their role set (i.e. the staff they interface with in everyday practice in their work) through either interview/ e-mail/telephone
What impact are the practice development nurses having in operationalising the strategy?		• Development of unit portfolios from Trust data, which provides information on patient outcomes and workplace culture e.g. staff turnover, incidents, MRSA rates etc. • Exploration of the quality of evidence used to inform practice decisions through use of audit tools yet to be developed • Essence of Care benchmarks (DoH, 2001)

with the strategy. The remainder of the chapter will outline the journey towards achieving elements of these two objectives.

Working with clinical leaders

The clinical leaders within the organisation were identified as key stakeholders in the success of the strategy. For the purposes of the strategy during this phase clinical leaders were identified as 'G' Grade Sisters/Charge Nurses or Midwives. The Trust negotiated with the RCN to 'buy-in' the RCN Clinical Leadership Programme (Cunningham, 2000). Initially 24 clinical leaders were supported to take part in the programme in the first year. It is envisaged that in the years that follow, further cohorts of healthcare practitioners will be supported through the programme, aiming to recruit potential leaders from across the interdisciplinary team. The clinical leaders are essential to the strategy and are a highly valued resource within the trust. As co-ordinators of patient care they are in a key position to engage with patients and the interdisciplinary team. The clinical leaders will take a key role in collecting patient stories and carrying out observation of care during the programme, and providing feedback on the outcomes of these two methods to the interdisciplinary ward or department team. The trust established a new post, that of Clinical Leadership Facilitator (CLF) to support the clinical leaders in the programme, their role is supported by the practice development team alongside the 'insider' and 'outsider' facilitators.

Participation in the programme has been voluntary. Participants have been recruited to the programme on the basis that they were supported by their manager and they could demonstrate the capacity to both give and receive feedback (the idea of 'emotional intelligence' (Goleman, 1999) informed our thinking here). Participants are supported throughout the programme by action learning sets and one-to-one clinical supervision.

Working with patients: using the Essence of Care benchmarks

The key stakeholder group that has been largely absent throughout the story of this journey is that of the patients. Participation, involvement and engagement of patients remains high on the priority list of all healthcare providers. The driver for this is coming from all directions, from local level through to government directives. There are many excellent examples of patient participation in areas of healthcare provision and healthcare providers value the sharing of experiences of effective engagement of patients/service users in healthcare planning and evaluation of service provision. The question is of how best to fully engage our patients in the process in a way that reflects the rich and diverse communities.

Nationally we have feedback from patients following the National NHS Patient Survey, we have data provided by our PALS (Patient Advice and Liaison Service), we have feedback and reporting mechanisms in place provided by other user and advocacy groups. We also have feedback through our complaints procedures and many wards and departments have a wealth of verbal and written feedback from patients who have used their service. Engagement of patients and their active involvement in the service planning, provision and evaluation of the service provided was the next challenge on our journey.

As part of our commitment to ensuring that users' views are at the forefront of delivering the strategy, we have used the English Department of Health's (DoH) *Essence of Care – Patient-focused Benchmarking for Healthcare Practitioners* pack (DoH, 2001). During 2000 across England and Wales over 2,000 patients, carers, health-care professionals and patient-representative groups were asked to identify the important aspects of care that they valued. Out of this exercise eight fundamental aspects of care were recognised as high priority for improvement (see Box 11.4). Using the benchmarking approach provides the opportunity for local interdisciplinary teams to celebrate and share their evidence of best practice. The priorities have been established as a quality initiative across England and Wales, the practice development strategy moved ahead in this area of establishing what patients value about the care they receive, and providing suggestions for improvement.

The benchmarking process fits into the quality framework along with the National Service Frameworks (NSF), the guidance from the National Institute of Clinical Excellence (NICE) and will be moni-tored through the Commission for Health Improvement (CHI). The benchmarks set standards for aspects of patient care and clearly articulate what patients want from the health service. It was agreed that undertaking the benchmarking process would enhance our patients' experience of receiving care. The work has contributed to the vision to create a culture of effectiveness across the Trust that has involved the commitment, contribution and valuing of all staff

Box 11.4 The Essence of Care priority areas (DoH, 2001).

1. Personal and oral hygiene
2. Privacy and dignity
3. Pressure ulcers
4. Continence and bladder and bowel care
5. Food and nutrition
6. Safety of patients/clients with mental health needs in general settings
7. Record keeping
8. Principles of self-care

involved in the delivery of direct patient care. The clinical bench-marking has been a nurse-led initiative. It involves nurses, as the co-ordinators of patient care, working in partnership with their patients and other members of the interdisciplinary team in the development of best practice. For many it has proved to be an opportunity to explore new ways of working and to celebrate the impact practitioners have on the patient's experience.

For each of the fundamental aspects of care the *Essence of Care* benchmarking toolkit contains:

- An overall statement, which expresses what patients/clients/consumers want from care (patient-focused outcome)
- Suggested indicators or information that is currently gathered which may indicate action is required to improve poor practice or that good practice exists which should be shared with others
- Elements of practice that support the attainment of the patient-focused outcome (factors)
- Key sources: policy documents, references, the evidence base used in compilation
- Patient-focused best practice in each of the factors; the benchmark
- A scoring continuum for each factor. These statements guide practitioners in awarding their own practice a score, and provide stepping stones for practitioners to consider taking, in order to achieve best practice
- Finally, there is a space for the identification of evidence that comparison group members agree would justify an A score in their particular area of practice
- Statements around best practice were identified by patients/clients, consumers and professionals and are included to help stimulate comparison group discussions

(DoH, 2001: 9)

The Nursing Policy Board agreed that the Trust would commence work on all eight of the fundemental aspects of care. This afforded the opportunity for individual wards and departments to be able to choose one or possibly two benchmarks that reflected an area of best practice that they wanted to celebrate and share with other teams. This supported the sharing of best practice across the Trust. It also enabled others to network with those clinical areas that wanted to learn from others' experience of the benchmarking process. It has resulted in a diversity of activity throughout the Trust that reflecting a commitment to establish priorities, based on local needs assessment. Clinical leaders and their teams, supported by their practice development facilitators have been identifying patient-focused aspects of care to benchmark. Having established a consensus the team then access the 'expert' members of that identified benchmark resource group. The creation of an innovative and dynamic intranet site has provided an excellent communication channel for supporting the wards and departments in getting started, and more importantly, the opportunity to surf 'across and into the waves of activity' throughout the Trust. Wards and departments become 'live' on the site as soon as they identify their area of best practice and commence the process of benchmarking.

Roadshows, open to all, were held on all hospital sites presenting the *Essence of Care* and providing an opportunity for discussion of the process of implementation. The roadshows now take place every six months and provide an opportunity for ward and department teams to celebrate the progress they are making to improve patient experience on their healthcare journeys, and to share best practice with their colleagues from across the Trust. The four nursing teams received a presentation at their meetings. Practice development nurses from all directorates have been exploring the benchmarking process during their workshops. They continue to act as a local resource for raising awareness of the fundemental aspects of care within their directorates.

Trust-wide groups have been established, providing a valuable resource to support wards and departments to introduce their chosen benchmark. Each group represents one of the fundamental aspects of care and becomes the 'expert' resource. There are existing and established multidisciplinary groups within the Trust that directly relate to the themes of two of the fundamental aspects of care: nutrition and tissue viability. Both groups agreed to facilitate the 'resource group' activity. They have provided a model for the remaining six groups.

Practice development facilitators are pivotal to the success of the project. They have the opportunity of setting the agenda for the corporate vision for practice development as well as supporting the identification of areas of best practice within their directorates. They are ideally placed to work in partnership with clinical leaders and their teams at a local level. Each practice development nurse has an 'Essence of Care toolkit' and facilitates local education and training on the benchmarking process.

Where are we now with Essence of Care?

At the time of writing (early 2003) all the resource groups had been established with an interdisciplinary membership. Many of the clinical areas had 'gone live' (i.e. completed the benchmarking process, and agreed a plan of action), addressing at least one fundamental aspect of care. The practice development intranet site had been established as an interactive means of communication, and was being used as the principle means of keeping stakeholders informed of progress. Consequently the core work of the project, the sharing of best practice, was underway across the Trust. The criteria for benchmarking communication as a fundamental aspect of care has been developed.

The biggest impact of Essence of Care is potentially on the patient journey. The complexity of the trust (nine directorates across three sites) presents a formidable challenge for identifying and celebrating progress. Take the example of a patient brought into the hospital via the helicopter following trauma received from involvement in a road traffic accident. They are admitted via the accident and emergency department, and transferred straight to the operating theatre. From there they are cared for in the intensive care unit before being stabilised and transferred onto a neurosurgical ward. Following their stay they are admitted to a rehabilitation unit and discharge plans are implemented for follow-up in the community under the care of the local primary care trust. During their hospital journey they have been cared for within five different directorates. If the teams, in those five areas, chose to 'benchmark' and share best practice in *one* of the fundamental aspects of care, for example the safety of people with mental health needs in general settings, the impact is likely to be considerable.

Conclusion

In conclusion, I would like to reflect on all the all issues and strategies explored and described throughout this chapter. What I would like to end with is an example on which I hope that readers will be able to reflect, as a patient or as a potential patient of our healthcare service . . .

Close your eyes (after reading this!) and think of all the things that you do when you arrive home at the end of a shift. Include everything that you do right up until the time you leave home the next day for work. What are the things you do to which you look forward, what are the routines, what are the chores, what are the pleasures, what are the things that you take for granted? What do you do with friends, with partners, in private, in the company of others? Now, I would like to think about doing all of those things, as usual, but make one small imaginary change . . . leave your front door open. What would you do differently? What would change?

How would you feel? You now may have a greater insight into how the patients that you have cared for all day or night feel – they are 'at home' during their stay with you in hospital, with the same difference, but for them it is the reality – the door is left open.

We are now two years along our practice development journey as a Trust. The 'recipe' has been written, discussed, critiqued and agreed by the 'cooks'. The ingredients have been identified and are in the process of being combined together. The temperature is right at this time, and despite some of the ingredients changing over time, the timer is set for an optimum outcome. The toolkit is expanding and being used by many members of the healthcare team now identifying themselves as 'practice developers'. The recipe is under review by the 'consumers' in partnership with the 'cooks' throughout the process. Our motto for this work is to 'trust the process' – we have a recipe for success! Success is achieving our vision 'to create a culture of effectiveness which is patient-centred and evidence-based'.

References

Aiken, L.H., Sloane, D.M. & Sochalski, J. (1998) Hospital organisation and outcomes. *Quality in Healthcare*, **7**, 222–6.

Cunningham, G. (2000). Follow your leader. *Nursing Standard*, **15**(12), 18–19.

Department of Health (DoH) (1998) *A First Class Service: Quality in the New NHS*. Stationery Office, London.

Department of Health (DoH) (1999) *Making a Difference: Strengthening the Nursing, Midwifery and Health Visiting Contribution to Health and Healthcare*. The Stationery Office, London.

Department of Health (DoH) (2000) *The NHS Plan*. The Stationery Office, London.

Department of Health (DoH) (2001) *Essence of Care: Patient-focused Benchmarking for Healthcare Practitioners*. HMSO, London.

Drennan, D. (1992) *Transforming Company Culture*. McGraw-Hill, London.

Garbett, R. & McCormack, B. (2002) A concept analysis of practice development. *Nursing Times Research*, **7**(2), 87–100.

Goleman, D. (1999) *Working With Emotional Intelligence*. Bloomsbury Press, London.

Guba, E.G. & Lincoln, Y.S. (1989) *Fourth Generation Evaluation*. Sage, Thousand Oaks, CA.

Johns, C. (1994) *The Burford NDU Model: Caring in Practice*. Blackwell, Oxford.

King, L. & Appleton, J. (1999) Pearls, pith and provocation: fourth generation evaluation of health services: exploring a methodology that offers equal voice to consumer and professional stakeholders. *Qualitative Health Research*, **9**(5), 698–710.

Kouzes, J.M. & Posner, B.Z. (1987) *The Leadership Challenge.* Jossey-Bass, San Francisco, CA.

McGill, I. & Beaty, L. (1997) *Action Learning.* Kogan Page, London.

Manley, K. (1992). Quality assurance: the pathway to excellence in nursing. In: *Nursing Care: The Challenge to Change* (eds. G. Brykczinska & M. Jolley). Edward Arnold, London.

Manley, K. (2000a) Organisational culture and consultant nurse outcomes. Part 1: organisational culture. *Nursing Standard*, **14**(36), 34–8.

Manley, K. (2000b) Organisational culture and consultant nurse outcomes. Part 2: consultant nurse outcomes. *Nursing Standard*, **14**(37), 34–9.

Manley, K. (2001) *Consultant nurse: concept, processes, outcomes.* Unpublished PhD thesis, University of Manchester/RCN Institute, London.

Royal College of Nursing Institute (RCNI) (2002) Definitions of practice development http://www.rcn.org.uk/practice_development/

Royal College of Nursing Institute (RCNI) (2004) *Expertise in practice project report.* RCN Practice Development Team, London.

Titchen, A. (2000) *Professional Craft Knowledge in Patient-centred Nursing and the Facilitation of its Development.* University of Oxford Dphil thesis. Ashdale Press, Oxford.

Commentary

Paddie Blaney

This chapter seeks to inform the organisational aspects of the corporate adoption of practice development as an approach to assuring and improving patient/client care. The context is a large acute training Trust but the corporate themes are not, I would suggest, context specific and would have validity in any setting in which health and social care is delivered. The writer here identifies a strategic and corporate journey and proposes a Practice Development recipe identifying the essential ingredients.

Health organisations are renowned for being large and complex and it is a significant challenge to have an enabling, creative and supportive culture. Viewing organisations as 'organic' (Burns & Stalker, 1961) provides the opportunity to consider the psychology of the organisation by which to change the organisational culture and inculcate a sense of patient/client/family/community centeredness which is care that is concentrated on the users' needs, which is implicitly expected to result in the best care.

Practice development approaches require an appreciation of the psychology of change processes and how these act upon individual members of the health and social care team to help develop team cultures that free up potential and facilitate real and sustainable change. In the same way, organisations should corporately engage in similar activities in order to effect a more positive corporate culture. The author identifies key concepts and theories and a practice development 'toolkit'. Most effective at the corporate level may be activities such as values clarification, establishing a shared governance approach, evaluation of the context of care, releasing and enhancing leadership potential, growing ownership and planning systematic improvements.

The policy context within which health and social care organisations exist must also value approaches that aim to create patient/client/family/community centeredness. The emerging modernisation policy context for all parts of the United Kingdom is a central driver in this regard. The levying of a statutory duty of quality on

Chief Executives, the governance agenda and establishment of structures such as the Commission for Health Improvement, the National Institute for Clinical Excellence and the Social Care Institute for Excellence as well as National Service Frameworks, all provide the regional or national context for organisations to commit to new approaches aimed at providing better care. Many of these developments are to be mirrored within Northern Ireland in the form of Health and Social Services Regulation and Improvement Authority and the Health and Personal Social Services (HPSS equivalent of the NHS) Standards and Guidelines Unit and Service Development Frameworks (see dhsspsni.gov.uk).

Whilst the policy context is vital it is also important that professional colleges, bodies and groups have a policy direction that promotes patient/client/family/community centeredness and can embrace practice development activities. A new organisation, the Northern Ireland Practice and Education Council for nursing and midwifery (NIPEC) embraces in its functions the development of practice approaches as a legitimate activity alongside educational developments in the professional development of all nurses and midwives providing healthcare in Northern Ireland. Mirroring such commitment at the regional and national level is to be encouraged. In England the DOH's initiative *Essence of Care* (DoH, 2001), referred to in this chapter, clearly provides a context within which teams of staff charged with providing such care might employ a practice development approach. An added challenge is to ensure that individuals properly engaged in practice development activities, have their contribution and involvement respected and given tangible value as part of their portfolio. NIPEC aims to ensure this happens as they lead the design of a Development Framework for all the nursing and midwifery professions in Northern Ireland.

Coherence between the various national, regional, professional and organisational contexts will do much to create corporate environments within which patient/client/family/community centeredness can exist and practice development approaches can be employed. Many positive outcomes should be evident including: improved care that is sustained and dynamic; improved communications; teams of staff emancipated; leadership potential maximised; and workforce benefits such as greater job satisfaction, reduced turnover, and improved retention.

Corporately these benefits should both be valued and expected. However, other realities of practice development approaches are challenging but they must be acknowledged and planned for. The investment in terms of time and in the individual roles such as that of facilitators is critical and must not suffer from short-term imperatives. Expectations of practice development must be viewed over the more medium term and plans must be made to handle the unease that will be experienced organisationally during the initial processes of developing a practice development approach.

The author identifies the 'cooking' time of the recipe from three years for notable changes and up to 15 years for sustained cultural change. Thus whilst the pay-off as outlined above is significant, investors must recognise the growth period of practice development activities. Stokes rightly identifies the importance psychologically of recognising and handling the concerns of staff groups engaged in practice development activity. Much of the time and effort involved in practice development is in view of this very aspect. The challenge is to ensure that this is understood at the corporate level particularly as it is probably the main reason for the time investment identified. What must be appreciated is that there are no short cuts if cultural change is to happen. Short-cutting this aspect of practice development will only result in short-term unsustainable advances at best and at worst can disillusion members of the workforce involved, neither of which are in the best interests of patients, clients, families or communities.

Organisationally, Chief Executives may be minded to consider the value of practice development initiatives, which contribute to them achieving their duty of quality responsibilities. They should be as confident in the infrastructure to meet a duty of quality as they are for the financial duty. Confidence in practice development approaches must be supported by evidence of the returns of the approach at the corporate and organisational level. The author identifies and discusses an evaluation framework to progress alongside practice development activities, and this must be seen as a critical aspect at the organisational/corporate level. This is also the challenge to all those involved in and promoting practice development as an approach to improving care.

Jane Stokes is to be applauded for stating that it is time to put the value back on the delivery of the fundamental aspects of direct patient care. Employing a corporate practice development approach can help achieve this.

References

Burns, T. & Stalker, G. (1961) *The Management of Innovation*. Tavistock, London.
Department of Health (DoH) (2001) *Essence of Care: Patient-focused Benchmarking for Healthcare Practitioners*. HMSO, London.

12. 'From Conception to Delivery'

A Journey Towards a Trust-wide Strategy to Develop a Culture of Patient-centredness

Jill Down

Introduction

Providing patient-centred and evidence-based care as well as developing a culture that fosters interdisciplinary teamwork and effectiveness, is central to NHS modernisation (Department of Health, 1999a, 2000, 2001; Bristol Royal Infirmary Inquiry, 2001). The skills necessary to make this a reality are the focus and expertise of practice development (Manley, 2001; Garbett & McCormack, 2002a, b). This chapter describes how a group of practice development facilitators (PDFs) at Addenbrooke's NHS Trust re-focused their work agendas and developed a Trust-wide practice development strategy to lead and facilitate initiatives that would deliver and evaluate the impact of improving and involving patients in their care. The achievement of the strategy has become a corporate objective.

Addenbrooke's NHS Trust is a 1,200 bedded teaching hospital in Cambridge that employs 6,000 people, 2,500 of whom are nurses. It acts as a District General Hospital to a local community of 600,000 people and provides tertiary or specialist services, such as organ transplantation, to a regional and national community. Similar to other Trusts, Addenbrooke's had sought a number of avenues to continually improve practice for the benefit of patients. A number of nurses were employed across the service directorates, whose job titles and roles had evolved and become known as practice development. In their own service areas they were perceived as having a dual role in that they would organise training and study days for nurses and provide clinical supervision and support for newly qualified nurses. This pattern of work continued until the group took on the challenge of refocusing its work to better reflect the needs of the Trust and its patients. At this time the practice development group had a membership of 15 nurses. The group identified the need to re-focus and re-define the role of practice development facilitators and their contribution to the Trust's Nursing and Midwifery Strategy and objectives and the impact on patient care. At this stage the group had:

- uni-professional membership;
- no shared or common understanding of what practice development was;
- a fragmented work agenda based in clinical areas resulting in duplication of work and focused on traditional training and learning based in clinical areas;
- not aligned their work to the Trust business plan or Nursing and Midwifery Strategy;
- focused on outcomes;
- few mechanisms for evaluating the effectiveness of its work.

There were a number of driving forces behind the desire to change and refocus the work of the group and individuals but the primary reason was a desire to make a real contribution to improve the patient experience using effective practice development processes. It was recognised that there was a need to work more effectively and strategically by sharing resources and skills across the hospital.

The journey of this group of practitioners is ongoing and evolving but the aim of this chapter is to:

- illustrate why this particular organisational approach to practice development was adopted;
- describe some of the approaches used;
- identify some of the challenges and lessons learnt in undertaking the initiative;
- highlight some of the successes achieved so far.

In order to make the work applicable, based in reality and meaningful to all healthcare workers, it was realised that the work needed to have a coordinated corporate approach but be delivered and evaluated in clinical areas. The route taken has sometimes been convoluted and we have been forced to re-evaluate our plan based on our learning and our eagerness to focus on outcomes rather than establish the processes needed. However, the process of refining and readjusting our plan has produced a much greater understanding of the processes involved with practice development, together with a recognition that the real life arena of clinical practice and practice development is messy, reflecting Schon's (1987) 'swampy lowlands'. The work is presented as an honest account of our experiences with the intention of sharing the learning, including the highs and lows of the processes, to stimulate discussion and critical debate, rather than as a model to be adopted by others.

Approaches to modernising practice development

First steps

Practice development facilitators (PDFs) are potentially a key resource for improving the patient experience. They play an important strategic and operational role in leading and facilitating patient focused changes in practice. Essentially PDFs continually seek to underpin practice with appropriate evidence, develop skilled and competent practitioners and teams, and enable the transformation of the context of care to one that is conducive to putting patients' needs first and where the culture is one of effectiveness (McCormack *et al.*, 1999). Nevertheless practice development is a concept that is widely referred to by all staff groups and managers and is often perceived as a solution to a number of challenges in the health care environment – this was also true of Addenbrooke's. Practice developers were delegated the management of nurse rotation schemes, education contract monitoring and training package development by local directorate managers, as these were thought to be practice development initiatives. Such a focus was driven by a desire to deliver a particular initiative in practice, with little co-ordination across the Trust. Whilst the work was valuable and of benefit to the organisation, in this 'technical approach' to practice development the focus was on delivery of specific initiatives rather than on the processes that enable practitioner ownership and sustained change (Manley & McCormack, 2003). The delivery of the work at that time lacked ownership by practitioners in clinical areas because of an approach that did not consider the different contexts and cultures of individual areas in which the change was being implemented. This was supported by learning from our previous practice development work when trying to implement evidence into practice. Namely, that the presentation of good evidence on its own does not guarantee effective implementation. Use of evidence in practice does not just rely on the quality of the evidence but also, more significantly, is influenced by two other factors: skilled facilitation, and the nature of the context and culture of care (Kitson *et al.*, 1998). This led to some frustration with a number of practice development nurses who did not fully understand how best to utilise their skills and knowledge to assist the service to meet its objectives and enable sustained change.

Skills for practice development

Making changes within the NHS and a large organisation requires an understanding and appreciation of several factors. These are: the changing pressures within the organisation; that there are many stakeholders to be considered; recognition of the interdependence of individuals and teams; and of the need to develop shared values within the organisation (Iles & Sutherland, 2001). The group thought they had the skills to undertake a change in work focus. Namely, those skills of problem solving and facilitation, an ability to identify the way forward (vision), an understanding of the organisational culture, expertise in clinical practice, research and change management (Kitson *et al.*, 1996). Work by Garbett & McCormack (2002a) with practice developers has also defined this as a skills set core to practice development, with the exception of research skills (although they argue that practice development is systematic and rigorous). The work of the Trust practice development group would support the need for research expertise and be identified as integral to the approach used. The group aspired to using transformational leadership processes in their work by valuing individuals as people and enabling them, by challenging and stimulating, by developing trust, by inspiring and communicating and by developing a shared vision (Kouzes & Posner, 1995).

Securing organisational support

Work continued on developing a shared view of the purpose of practice development based on available literature and personal beliefs and it was agreed that the primary purpose was to increase the effectiveness of patient-centred care (Garbett & McCormack, 2002b). The group was clear about the need to link their activities to those of the Trust Nursing and Midwifery objectives and to be able to facilitate initiatives in their own local areas in response to the needs of their particular client group, whilst working with the culture of that area. In essence, it was felt that there was a need for the practice development agenda to be linked to organisational policies within a Trust-wide strategy for practice development, that was delivered and evaluated in clinical areas and would, in turn then inform the organisational agenda in a cyclical process (McCormack *et al.*, 1999). Essentially we were targeting our development work at three levels, the organisation, teams and individuals.

The group was effective in developing and delivering key Trust practice development objectives that focused on the patient and linked with national and local policies:

- Improving patient care as linked to the Essence of Care standards (Department of Health, 2001)
- Exploring and developing the competencies required to be an effective ward manager linked to *Agenda for Change* (Department of Health, 1999b)
- Developing work-based learning and leadership development linked to *Making a Difference* (Department of Health, 1999a)
- Dissemination of practice development activities at a local and national level

Organisational sponsorship and support was secured resulting in the formation of a Steering Group with key stakeholders including representatives from patients, clinical governance team, Primary Care Trust, Medical Director, Non-executive Director, Chief Nurse, Community Health Council, Allied Health Professionals, Ward Manager, Education provider, project leader for Leadership Development and the Chair and Vice Chair of the Practice Development Group. This ensured a robust reporting system and a direct link with a number of key departments and stakeholders who could inform and challenge our work whilst integrating a number of agendas and promote practice development processes with a number of staff groups. Integration of leadership and *Essence of Care* initiatives with practice development was important if we were to work towards a co-ordinated patient centred approach rather than specific projects working in isolation. Practice development is an interdisciplinary concept and the quality of care provided to patients and users does not rest with just one discipline but requires effective team working, a characteristic of a learning organisation (Senge, 1990). We had engaged allied health professionals, a patient and the Clinical Audit and Effectiveness manager in the Trust Practice Development Group. There were now approximately 22 staff working in practice development or clinical practice supervisor roles engaged in the practice development work. Although there was a shared implicit view of what practice development was, the group had not at that point developed a vision statement that encapsulated their values and beliefs. We did not realise what a vital step we had missed.

Challenges

The nature of the journey had been convoluted and evolving with PDFs becoming more skilled in effective communication, providing each other with challenge and support, and becoming more politically astute, whilst remaining focused on achieving the objectives.

Empowerment and action learning

It was a difficult time for PDFs as several of them were comfortable performing a training and development role and they required support from the group and additional challenge and support from action learning to address local issues and facilitate change with staff more senior to them. Communication and active involvement of staff was and remains a constant challenge. PDFs worked with their directorate managers to ensure that the Trust practice development objectives were adapted and delivered locally to reflect particular local needs. Membership of an action learning set or professional supervision was a crucial mechanism to support and develop practice developers on their journey. It provides an opportunity to highlight some of the discrepancies of our own work, between what we say and the actions we actually take in practice, those actions that we often just take for granted (Manley, 2000). Fay (1987) describes this as 'enlightenment', the personal discovery of how we as individuals act in certain situations and is a precursor of 'empowerment'. If we do not understand and become aware of our own actions and those we take for granted in our everyday working we will not be motivated to act and make changes. 'Empowerment' is the motivating force resulting from 'enlightenment'. Having become aware of personal actions and the consequences of them in our everyday work we can be motivated and empowered to change things. The final step is 'emancipation' and is a powerful driver to actually take action on things we had previously taken for granted in our practice. Practice developers can enable themselves and other staff to see their work through a different lens that allows them to work with the patient, and gives staff support enabling them to reflect and challenge as an integral part of their work (Johns, 1998).

There was an agreement that action learning was a key practice development process and part of developing a learning organisation (Senge, 1990). The group made a commitment to facilitate action learning sets for other staff groups, with a particular focus on those who had undertaken the Leading an Empowered Organisation course.

There was a general acknowledgement of the positive change in the focus of work and of the energy and tenacity of the group to support real and lasting changes within the Trust. The literature available about practice development supported the approach to practice development called 'emancipatory practice development' (see Chapter 3). This approach is synonymous with sustainable improvement where, through skilled facilitation, the provision of quality patient care becomes the focus of all staff. This approach focuses on:

- enabling individuals and teams to develop;
- developing the culture and context within the workplace;
- practitioners generating ideas for action but encompassing strategy;
- processes and outcomes;
- an evaluation encompassing interventions, staff empowerment and cultural change.

(Manley & McCormack, 2003)

The group realised the enormity of the work agenda it had embarked upon and that to have a significant and lasting effect on the culture would take a number of years. It celebrated the successes so far whilst realising that it could be even more effective, particularly in the evaluation of the work and in the demonstration of the impact of practice development work on improving the patient experience. For example, the description in practical terms, of the effect of action learning at the patient interface; the impact of developing a learning culture in the clinical areas; and how developing an interdisciplinary team approach had impacted on quality issues affecting patient care such as privacy and dignity (Department of Health, 2001). In addition there was a need to refine objectives so that they were generated from clinical areas to inform strategy development rather than the other way round. It was at this point that we negotiated expert facilitation from the Royal College of Nursing Institute (RCNI) to work with us and focus on the evaluation of practice development. Our work therefore was to experience a further transition.

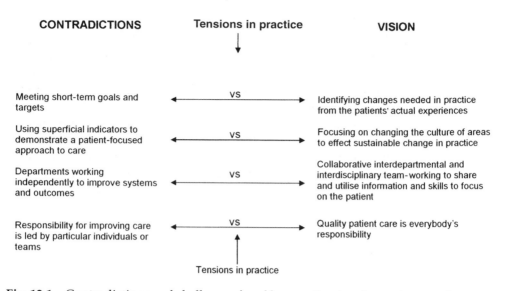

Fig. 12.1 Contradictions and challenges faced by practice developers in everyday practice when working towards the Practice Development vision: 'To work in partnership with patients ensuring they are the focus of effective care.' (Adapted from Manley, 2002)

Keeping the focus on the patient

Several issues facing the group have been indicated above but there are constant challenges to work with to overcome the barriers and contradictions in everyday work at all levels of the organisation. These are barriers to achieving a truly patient-focused approach (Fig. 12.1). Staff want to deliver good patient care but are often struggling with other pressures. The challenge for the practice developer is to work with all staff to develop change that is sustainable and reflecting the emancipatory rather than the technical approach to practice development (Manley & McCormack, 2003). The group had succeeded in gaining organisational support and continues to invest energies in working with staff to ensure integration and involvement of departments across the disciplines using skilled facilitation and high challenge and high support.

Developing a shared vision and objectives

One of the first discussions with the RCNI focused around being challenged to articulate our vision for practice development. We had made significant progress towards meeting objectives, widening membership, co-ordinating work across the Trust and securing support for the work, but had not developed a vision statement. The group knew what it wanted to achieve tacitly but was unable to articulate this in a succinct way that embraced the values and beliefs of practice developers and other key stakeholders. Being clear about our vision and subsequent purpose, as well as being able to articulate this became a priority and was achieved through using a values clarification exercise (Manley, 2000). Twelve practice developers, a patient, a manager, a midwife and the Assistant Chief Nurse undertook this process to begin to develop an explicit shared vision for ourselves that could be shared and contributed to by others.

A number of themes developed from the values clarification exercise reflecting the purpose of practice development as concerned with:

- Continuous evaluation
- Patient impact
- Enabling workforce
- Culture
- Evidence base

It is interesting to note that the themes generated from the values clarification exercise are also reflected in this definition of practice development proposed by Garbett & McCormack (2002b).

> Practice development is a continuous process of improvement towards increased patient effectiveness in patient centred care. This is brought about by helping healthcare teams to develop their skills and to transform the culture and context of care. It is enabled and supported by facilitators committed to systematic, rigorous continuous processes of emancipatory change that reflect the perspectives of service users.
>
> (p. 88)

This definition arising from a concept analysis does indeed cover all aspects of practice development as we perceived it. However, feedback from our presentations, written reports and users, identified that we needed to keep our language simple if we wanted to get our messages across effectively and make it important for all staff and patients. The final vision statement has endeavoured to use a language that is understandable to patients and staff alike and feedback on the language used has been obtained from patient and staff groups.

The vision for practice development at Addenbrooke's NHS Trust was therefore articulated as to work in partnership with patients ensuring they are the focus of effective care.

The means through which we believed this vision could be achieved were:

- Increasing patient involvement in care/service decisions
- Individuals and interdisciplinary teams taking responsibility for quality
- Continuous evaluation of care/services
- Providing evidence based care
- Developing a learning culture

Consultation with staff, the steering group and patient groups resulted in an agreement that the vision and the means for achieving it reflected our values and beliefs for practice development and the next stage was to refine our current objectives to progress the journey towards this vision. The resulting Trust-wide strategic objectives (see Table 12.1) were identified under four headings:

1. Patients
2. Culture
3. Practice development roles and processes
4. Evidence base

Developing an evaluation strategy

Having clarified our vision our attentions were turned to identifying methods to evaluate progress towards the vision and delivery of the objectives. Notes from the practice development workshop at this time identify that the purpose of an evaluation strategy is to:

> Identify evaluation questions within an overall evaluation framework which will help us to gain feedback on whether we are moving towards the vision. These questions, in turn will help us to identify the methods we will need to use and the data we need to collect and analyse in our everyday practice development activity. Such data is not used to just demonstrate pre and post differences but is the impetus for helping staff to begin to develop their practice into practice development locally.
>
> (Addenbrooke's NHS Trust Practice Development workshop notes, 2002, unpublished)

In order to evaluate the effectiveness of the practice development strategy across the Trust we realised we would need skills in research and evaluation. To date practice development studies have focused mainly on unit practice development activity rather than Trust-wide activity (Manley, 2000; Titchen, 2000); however, the group was keen to co-ordinate a Trust-wide evaluation. It wanted to integrate and enable clinical areas to receive feedback in relation to the provision of effective and evidence-based patient care whilst informing a corporate action plan. All ward areas would need to

276

Table 12.1 Summary of Addenbrooke's NHS Trust practice development strategy.

Title: An Action Research Study Implementing and Evaluating a Trust-wide Practice
Development Strategy.
Purpose: To gain information about the patient experience, culture, practice
development roles and evidence-based practice in each clinical area.
This information will *enable teams to work in partnership with patients ensuring they are
the focus of effective care* by developing robust action plans to improve care and share
good practices.

Objectives	Methods	Tools
1. *Patient focus* • To improve the patient experience • To meet the Essence of Care standards • To develop opportunities for patients/carers to be more involved in their care	• Interviewing service users (patients/families/carers) • Utilise Essence of Care standards Trust-wide • Robust systems utilising patient feedback	• Patient stories • Essence of Care standards • Collating Trust data on complaints, risk management and audit
2. *Culture* • To facilitate the development of work-based learning • To facilitate the development of a culture where quality is everyone's concern and staff are adaptable in responding to changing healthcare context • To promote inter-disciplinary working	• Assessing practice in clinical area • Interviewing clinical staff • Evaluating impact of audit on clinical practice	• Observations of practice • Staff stories and patient stories • Leadership development feedback • Essence of care audits • Indicators of effectiveness, e.g. turnover, absenteeism; length of stay, readmission rate etc.
3. *Practice development* (PD) *roles & processes* • To provide support and facilitation to help staff develop their practice • To ensure all practice development activity is evaluated • To engage staff and patients in achieving the PD vision and strategy	• Practice development staff appraisal • Analysis of previously collated Trust data • Analysis of action learning and clinical supervision	• 360° review • Set review sheets • Monitor performance against targets

Table 12.1 *Continued*

4. *Evidence-based practice*		
• To improve the quality of patient care by developing, implementing and evaluating evidence-based practice	• Appraisal of practice guidelines • Assess evidence base in clinical areas • Interviewing clinical staff • Evaluating impact of audit on clinical practice	• Guideline appraisal tool • Evidence base benchmark • Staff questionnaire • Evaluation of audits

become engaged in this work, receive feedback from the evaluation to reinforce elements of good practice and to identify areas where action plans needed to be implemented to improve practice. The focus for the activity was to be on the essential aspects of patient care, the evidence used to support practice and the development of a learning culture with leadership potential developed at all levels. The group identified useful data that was already collected across the Trust in relation to these areas such as, staff surveys, exit interviews, uptake of clinical supervision, and highlighted some key areas where additional information was required to give a complete picture from which to develop local and Trust action plans. The group particularly wanted to interview patients, carers and staff about their experience of being a patient and staff member at Addenbrooke's and to undertake observations of practice in clinical areas for the purpose of capturing the culture currently experienced.

Work was already underway to link results of patient satisfaction surveys, audit, clinical incidents and complaints at directorate level to enable work to commence on local action planning, but if we were to be true to our values and beliefs we needed to adopt an action research approach. This was the chosen methodology because of the consistency with the aims and values of practice development (Manley & McCormack, 2003), namely that it is empowering, collaborative, focuses on everyday actions and improving practice in the 'real world'. The purpose of action research is: to develop practice; to enable practitioners to develop; and to contribute to the refinement and development of theory (Greenwood, 1994). Fourth Generation Evaluation (Guba & Lincoln, 1989) would also be used to enable key stakeholder groups such as users and staff to develop the evaluation agenda as well as mutually educating each other about different stakeholder priorities and concerns. It was anticipated that any work undertaken would add to an understanding about the practice development processes necessary to achieve a culture of effectiveness, one that is patient-centred and evidence-based and importantly, how such outcomes can be demonstrated in day-to-day work. A successful ethics application was submitted and a time-frame of three years agreed. A summary of the objectives, proposed methods and tools is summarised in Table 12.1. At this point there was excitement that we were actually demonstrating congruency with our beliefs and our actions by using this approach to the work. There was also some apprehension about both the enormity of the task ahead and a sense of uncertainty associated with where this research would actually end. We had again to learn to trust the processes involved rather than focus on outcomes.

Successes – developing a shared governance structure for maintaining development

There have been many successes including: a 360° review being undertaken by all practice developers, resulting in individual action plans that will be co-ordinated into a corporate action plan; working with clinical leaders to understand the patient experience in their areas by developing a shared approach to undertaking patient stories and developing action plans in response to this feedback; the involvement of clinical areas who were initially reluctant to work in a collaborative way and many others. Space dictates a focus on key areas of success, namely the organisation of practice development activity, developing skills and guidelines for practice, and user involvement.

Organisation of practice development activity

The development and co-ordination of practice development activity across the Trust has required that we were clear about the structure, membership and purpose of each forum. This is now established as shown in Fig. 12.2. A project plan with key milestones has been developed that enables PDFs to focus on key steps without being too overwhelmed with the total project. Four practice developers have been identified as the lead for each of the four evaluation areas and afforded additional support for co-ordinating and facilitating progress in the form of mentoring and action planning time, whilst maintaining their practice development roles in a clinical area.

Practice Development Forum

The Forum monitors progress towards the Trust practice development objectives in local areas. Each directorate has developed an action plan with clinical leaders and key personnel, based on the Trust practice development objectives and adapted to meet particular needs of their areas. Information on successes and useful strate-

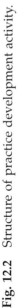

Communication strategy

Involvement of all stakeholders

Workshops

Co-ordinate evaluation
- Monthly
- Open membership
- Project plan refinement
- Develop skills and guidelines for evaluation
- Develop action plans in response to feedback

Steering group

for practice development, leadership and Essence of Care
- 3-monthly
- Key stakeholders
- Report progress against project plan
- Gain support
- Identify implications of the work
- Utilise expertise

Practice development vision

To work in partnership with patients ensuring they are the focus of effective care

Local activity in clinical areas
- Develop local action plans
- Evaluation activities
- Facilitate interdisciplinary team working
- Action learning sets

Dissemination of work

Action learning

Practice development forums

Monitor progress against corporate and local objectives
- Monthly
- Rotating practice development chairperson
- Practice development representative from each area
- Share learning and resources
- Identify additional learning needs

Fig. 12.2 Structure of practice development activity.

gies are shared and the production of simple monthly 'performance against targets' reports by each area has focused the group on the need to identify progress in a structured way. 'Performance against targets' also enables the co-ordination of Trust-wide information on progress towards, for example, Essence of Care standards (Department of Health, 2001). Presentation of information in this way has the added advantage of providing evidence to demonstrate activities across the organisation that are patient-centred and evidence-based, for example, for Commission for Health Improvement (CHI) reviews and also to support performance indicators. It remains a constant challenge for all practice developers to manage their time to meet timescales. However, such is the impetus of the work that there is now much sharing of resources and skills such as coaching and co-facilitation to support each other across different directorates. The group has become empowered to continually develop themselves and is self-energising and self-organising.

Workshops

This forum develops the skills and processes for undertaking the evaluation using a variety of approaches ranging from dramatisation, role-play and utilisation of evidence from clinical areas. Each practice development workshop now has 20 to 25 participants including staff from areas initially reluctant to get involved. As some of the more tangible effects of the work are becoming visible, other staff not in dedicated practice development roles have become interested, endorsing the fact that all practitioners can be practice developers. The group has established an open and honest approach in their workshops that always identifies concerns, claims and issues for each participant and others with whom they were working (Guba & Lincoln, 1989 (see Chapters 3 and 5)). Initial reviews of the themes arising from the concerns and issues have focused on how to make practice development work real to others and how to capture what is important to stakeholders in any presentations about the work.

Developing skills and guidelines for practice

The real success of the workshops has been the ongoing development of guidelines and skills for different aspects of the work that have been generated by practice developers themselves. Particularly in the areas of:

- undertaking stories from patients and staff
- giving feedback to clinical areas
- thematic analysis of stories
- developing action plans from results of personal 360° reviews

Rather than the traditional approach to learning, the group has striven to continually develop their own practice and self-knowledge using a practical approach. An example of how this works in practice can be illustrated by the description of a particular piece of work.

When preparing to undertake patient stories in clinical areas it was identified that, as a group we were novices (Benner, 1984). The workshop therefore focused on work based learning, integrating theoretical principles and critical debate by:

1. Preparation
   * Familiarisation with the ethics proposal to be clear about processes and inclusion and exclusion criteria prior to the workshop
   * To have read the patient information sheets and consent forms
2. Perform
   * Perform a dramatisation of the whole process of taking a patient story with PDFs playing nurses, a patient, a carer and the rest of the group watching and taking notes
3. Communicate, critical analysis and questioning
   * 'Freeze framing' at intervals when individuals were struggling and also at intervals along the way to identify, discuss and make notes to form guidelines for the process including:
     * what approaches were working well?
     * how could it have been more effective?
     * identify strategies for dealing with specific issues, documentation, crises and ethical issues
     * identify the responsibilities of the researcher
4. Formulation of learning into practical guidelines
   The result of this work has been the development of guidelines for undertaking patient stories that have been refined to enable production of similar guidelines for staff stories and integrating some approaches and questions to support practitioners in this work. These are refined and updated as information from practical experiences of undertaking stories in clinical areas is generated.

A portfolio of practical guidelines for staff in the particular areas of undertaking staff and patient interviews, giving feedback, undertaking a 360° review and for thematic analysis of information generated from interviews has been generated through this process. This approach encapsulates the purposes of action research by developing practice; enabling practitioners to develop and to contribute to the refinement and development of theory (Greenwood, 1994). The knowledge and skills developed both as a team and as individuals in this approach has been tremendous and beyond our hopes and expectations when embarking upon this work. It is important to recognise that this has also generated the skills to be more effective practice developers in everyday work, as they are the same skills utilised in different settings and with different staff groups.

User involvement

A patient representative sits on the steering group, as an active and regular workshop member, a proof-reader of written work and latterly, a co-presenter of the work at a conference. She is an advocate for practice development who has been part of the journey we have undertaken, is considered a colleague by the group and makes a significant contribution to the work. She provides a user perspective on all aspects of our work by promoting, sharing and receiving feedback from user groups affiliated to the Trust and provides us with a different perspective in the workshops. The group particularly values her comments and questions about our use of language and jargon, whilst recognising the risk that she may perhaps absorb it as she is now so involved in the work. She will be supporting the work in undertaking staff interviews, and undertaking observations of care in clinical areas. Identifying changes needed in practice from the patient's actual experience is a key element of the evaluation strategy. It has been a privilege to hear these experiences and a powerful form of evidence to share with clinical teams in order for them to develop action plans and share good practices. The approach demonstrates a real desire of practitioners, teams and the organisation to learn from patients, rather than the use of superficial indicators to demonstrate a patient focused approach to care where the emphasis is on ticking boxes (Manley, 2000).

Lessons learnt

Many lessons have been learnt in developing this work. They are underpinned by practice development processes and have been described within the text. When the group began its work it had:

- uni-professional membership. It now has interdisciplinary membership and established good working partnerships with departments such as Clinical Audit and Effectiveness, Patient Advisory and Liaison Service, Communication department and Allied Health Professionals;
- no shared or common understanding of what practice development was. It now has a vision for practice development on which to focus the work;

- a fragmented work agenda based in clinical areas and resulting in duplication of work and focused on traditional training and learning based in clinical areas. It now has a systematic approach to practice development that is developing the culture of each area and working with clinical teams to be more effective;
- not aligned their work to the Trust business plan or Nursing and Midwifery strategy. It now has a strategy and objectives that reflect the needs of the organisation and its stakeholders;
- focused on outcomes. It now understands and invests time in setting up the processes to support sustained change and understands that these processes are fundamental to effective practice development;
- few mechanisms for evaluating the effectiveness of its work. It now has a robust action research approach to evaluation of the work at clinical and corporate levels and mechanisms to action plan in response to this evidence.

The journey towards the practice development vision, 'to work in partnership with patients ensuring they are the focus of effective care', is well established and ongoing. The development of a vision involving users and stakeholders has provided a real focus and impetus for the work. We were absolutely wrong to have thought we could have developed our work without one – it underpins all our work and serves as a signpost for us whenever we are feeling momentarily overwhelmed by the work. The nature of action learning with ongoing spirals (Coghlan & Casey, 2001) is being experienced in practice and our plans are adapted to meet the needs of issues identified and skills to address them are developed. As a group we have developed a way of working that really does value everyone's contribution and embraces all staff. There is a sense of excitement and passion because we can visualise the purpose, direction and outcomes of the work. This sometimes becomes private irritation when others cannot see the benefits of collaborative and interdepartmental working to focus all work on the patient. However, this, too, provides us with an opportunity to learn and develop. We have learnt to adapt our language to suit the audience and to highlight particular aspects of the work that will engage them and make them interested (RCN, 2002/www.rcn.org.uk/pd).

Impact on the organisation

The organisation has supported the development of this work, particularly in terms of resourcing the RCNI involvement. It has required some courage on the part of the organisation to invest in

284

a programme of work that does not seek 'quick fix' answers, but is prepared to invest in the processes to develop a culture that nurtures real and lasting change.

The organisation now has work that is focused on the patient, is systematic and evaluated and focuses on sustainable change by working to develop a learning culture (Manley & McCormack, 2003). We have developed a system that monitors 'performance against targets' in clinical areas and supports the need of the organisation to provide evidence for external monitoring purposes. This evidence must be embedded in the culture rather than allowing the system simply to undertake superficial monitoring (Manley, 2002). This will support the business planning process in the Trust. The Trust now has a widening group of interdisciplinary practitioners who are actually undertaking research, not having it done to them (Greenwood, 1994).

The impact on teams and individuals

There is a sense of excitement from clinical teams, that this work will provide them with information to support changes in their practice based on a range of evidence. It makes sense to them; they understand it; it feels as though they are able to make changes in their own areas; that it will influence the care they give and that it meets the needs of their patient group (verbal communication with a ward manager). This ward manager was feeling emancipated (Fay, 1987) and was describing a sense of renewed purpose where she felt able to work with the team towards the vision. Clearly not all teams view the work in this way, some are currently working to a different agenda but others are at different stages of enlightenment (raising awareness), and empowerment (becoming motivated to act) and this, too, is healthy. It means that we can learn from those teams undertaking the processes now and can utilise that learning for those following, whilst demonstrating an understanding of the different cultures within each area with which we need to work.

The group actively promotes practice development as an interdisciplinary concept with the quality of care provided to patients and users a result of effective team working. However, much of the facilitative and enabling, non-technical work, is invisible to others and it remains a constant challenge for the group to demonstrate promotion of this aspect across the Trust. It has highlighted that even with a strategy to communicate activities across the Trust, there is always a need to do more and we continue to try and model transformational leadership behaviours (Kouzes & Posner, 1995). The work has developed practical skills to support practitioners in their everyday work within a shared direction and purpose. Individuals and teams are now able to take responsibility for their own practice and introduce innovations whilst being supported and challenged by colleagues.

It is a challenge to ensure that all the care is centred on the needs of the patient and it requires energy, tenacity and a real desire to involve everyone in the process in a way that will have a positive and practical impact on care. The work of this group demonstrates some of the processes we have used and highlights areas where we could have been more effective. It is based in the real world of practice and we continue to learn and implement our learning into practice, adjust our plans in response to the challenges and based on feedback from stakeholders, whilst continuing our journey towards patient-centred care.

References

Benner, P. (1984) *From Novice to Expert.* Addison Wesley, Menlo Park.

Bristol Royal Infirmary Inquiry (2001) Kennedy, I. (Chairman) *Learning from Bristol: The report of the public inquiry into children's heart surgery at the Bristol Royal Infirmary 1984–1999.* Bristol Royal Inquiry, Bristol.

Coghlan, D. & Casey, M. (2001) Action research from the inside: issues and challenges in doing action research in your own hospital. *Journal of Advanced Nursing,* **35**(5), 674–82.

Department of Health (DoH) (1999a) *Making a difference: Strengthening the nursing, Midwifery and Health Visiting Contribution to Health and Healthcare.* The Stationery Office, London.

Department of Health (DoH) (1999b) *Agenda for Change: Modernising the NHS Pay System.* The Stationery Office, London.

Department of Health (DoH) (2000) *The NHS Plan. A Plan for Investment. A Plan for Reform.* The Stationery Office, London.

Department of Health (DoH) (2001) *Essence of Care: Patient-focused Benchmarking for Healthcare Practitioners.* Department of Health, London.

Fay, B. (1987) *Critical Social Science: Liberation and its Limits.* Polity Press, Oxford.

Garbett, R. & McCormack, B. (2002a) The qualities and skills of practice developers. *Nursing Standard,* **16**(50), 33–6.

Garbett, R. & McCormack, B. (2002b) A concept analysis of practice development. *Nursing Times Research,* **7**(2), 87–100.

Greenwood, J. (1994) Action research: a few details, a caution and something new. *Journal of Advanced Nursing,* **20**:13–18.

Guba, E.G. & Lincoln, Y.S. (1989) *Fourth Generation Evaluation.* Sage, Thousand Oaks, CA.

Iles, V. & Sutherland, K. (2001) *Organisational Change: A Review for Healthcare Managers, Professionals and Researchers.* National Co-ordinating Centre for NHS Service Delivery and Organisation R&D. London.

References

Johns, C. (1998) Opening the doors of perception. In: *Transforming Nursing Through Reflective Practice* (eds. C. Johns & D. Freshwater). Blackwell Science, Oxford.

Kitson, A.I. & Ahmed, L.D., Harvey, G., Thompson, D. & Seers, K. (1996) From research to practice: one organisational model for promoting research based practice. *Journal of Advanced Nursing*, **23**(3), 430–40.

Kitson, A., Harvey, G. & McCormack, B. (1998) Enabling the implementation of evidence-based practice: a conceptual framework. *Quality in Healthcare*, **7**, 149–58.

Kouzes, J.M. & Posner, B.Z. (1995) *The Leadership Challenge.* Jossey Bass, San Francisco, CA.

McCormack, B., Manley, K., Kitson, A., Titchen, A. & Harvey, G. (1999) Towards practice development – a vision in reality or reality without a vision? *Journal of Nursing Management*, **7**, 255–64.

Manley, K. (2000) Organisational culture and consultant nurse outcomes. Part 2: consultant nurse outcomes. *Nursing Standard*, **14**(37), 34–9.

Manley, K. (2001) The Bristol Royal Infirmary inquiry: the agenda for practice development? Editorial. *Nursing in Critical Care*, **6**(5), 213–15.

Manley, K. (2002) Keeping focused on patient and user experiences. Editorial. *Nursing in Critical Care*, **7**(6), 1–2.

Manley, K. & McCormack, B. (2003) Practice development: its purpose and methodology. *Nursing in Critical Care*, **8**(1), 22–9.

Royal College of Nursing (RCN) (2002) Definitions of practice development for different purposes. RCN Practice Development website/www.rcn.org.uk/pd

Schon, D. (1987) *Educating the Reflective Practitioner.* Jossey Bass, San Francisco, CA.

Senge, P. (1990) *The Fifth Discipline: The Art and Practice of the Learning Organisation.* Doubleday Currency, New York.

Titchen, A. (2000) *Professional Craft Knowledge in Patient-Centred Nursing and the Facilitation of its Development.* Ashdale Press, Oxford.

Commentary

Rob Garbett

An adage within the environmental movement for many years has been, 'Think globally, act locally'. Reading Jill Down's chapter demonstrates how relevant this idea is in modern health services (or indeed in any complex modern organisation). The power of this simple phrase is that it stresses how important it is for us to be able to relate our day-to-day actions to broader ideas and principles in order to achieve progress.

Jill describes a journey that started with a group of people with conviction, energy and enthusiasm but whose skills and commitment had not been entirely harnessed. Their work, while valuable, did not move them or their organisation in a particular direction. Instead they reacted and responded to the challenges that came their way. Their work was not necessarily shared, supported or valued because it was not part of a larger picture. By the end of the journey they have demonstrated the potential of the repertoire of perspectives and activities gathered together under the banner of practice development to unite the efforts of their own team and to engage with their organisation, with patients and with directions in NHS policy: actions may be local but they relate to more global ideas about health service delivery. Crucially they have done this in a way that involves practitioners. What is more they have done so in a way that has moved practice development in their organisation from being the concern of nurses to being the concern of people drawn from all parts of the organisation.

Part of the journey therefore has been to take emerging concepts and ideas from the practice development literature and try them out. These ideas, which form the content of this book, have emerged through inductive work over many years across a range of organisations and settings. However, the work described here (as well as the work described in Chapter 11 by Jane Stokes) represents a particularly ambitious use of the ideas because of the sheer scale of the undertaking. Although similar in some respects the work described by Stokes in Chapter 11 and that described by Jill Down above had quite distinct starting points as well as occurring in different contexts. For Jill and her colleagues the challenge has been to pull together a range of disciplines in order to develop a more strategic approach to enhance the effect of existing work. While in Jane Stokes' chapter the challenge of pulling a policy framework (*Essence of Care*) and existing practice development activity together is the focus. The chapters both demonstrate the importance within practice development of balancing where an organisation 'is at' with the demands of national agendas but to do so in a way that reflects the particular needs of an organisation. In other words, one size does not fit all!

Anyone who has attempted to bring about change in the smallest of settings will know how complex it is. To attempt it on an organisational scale and to be able to demonstrate success requires courage, commitment and (I suspect) sheer bloody-mindedness. However, it also requires principles and approaches that make sense to those involved. This chapter shows how ideas drawn from a body of practice development work have been taken, used, tested and refined.

Working in the health service all too often feels like jumping on board a train that is hurtling away into the distance. It feels like there is no time to collect your thoughts and plan your journey, all you can do is cling on and hope for the best. However, by creating the opportunities to talk and listen, Jill Down and her colleagues found a way for colleagues and patients to talk about how things were and how they wanted them to be. Through making sure that there was a broad involvement they were able to create links between the concerns of patients and staff as well as being able to relate those concerns to the broader agenda for the Trust as a whole. As a result the potential has been created to replace episodic and ad hoc activity on isolated projects with activity that has both strategic (so helping the Trust meet its objectives) and local (so responding to the concerns and issues of clinicians and patients) relevance.

The chapter is a dialogue about existing ideas, tools and approaches and their robustness and utility in a new setting. Having material like this is crucial to our understanding of the possibilities of practice development. Having identified critical social science as an underpinning framework for practice development work we need to expose the ideas to critique and examination so that they can be refined in readiness to be used again (and again). And it would be in the spirit of critique that I would suggest that Jill's account would benefit from the kind of detail that would bring the experience of those involved in the work alive, for example, first-hand accounts and the richness of qualitative data. However, any such critique must be balanced against the enormity of the task of accounting for a far-reaching and complex body of work that does justice to the range of activity undertaken.

For the reader the chapter reiterates a profound challenge that has been present in other practice development work, the challenge is that these approaches take time if they are to reach their full potential. This account is about changing a culture. Changing culture is very much part of contemporary health service discourse. Policy initiatives call for cultures which are more responsive to service users' needs (DoH, 1998) and which learn from mistakes rather than burying them and blaming scapegoats (BRI Inquiry, 2001). There can be no argument with the desirability of such cultural shifts. But the danger lies in the ways in which they are brought about.

Jill's chapter demonstrates just how much preparation is required, how much energy is needed to provide the opportunities for everyone with a stake in healthcare to have their say and identify how they can contribute. The time and resources involved in this process are considerable, but without them good ideas can become empty rhetoric. The work of Binnie & Titchen (1999) and Manley (2000) amongst many others reinforces the work described in this chapter in demonstrating that the pace of this work is dictated by its depth and the fact that it takes place against an unpredictable and frequently hostile backdrop of service provision, and as such may take years to reach fruition (and indeed should become a continuous process). Investment in skilled facilitation and in the development of work contexts that foster growth and learning requires long-term vision. In a health service all too often attracted by quick fixes, chief executives need to be investing in practice developers to work alongside practitioners over years, not months, to develop work cultures that will truly foster clinical effectiveness.

References

Binnie, A. & Titchen, A. (1999) *Freedom to Practice: The Development of Patient-centred Nursing*. Butterworth-Heinemann, Oxford.

Bristol Royal Infirmary Inquiry (2001) Kennedy, I. (Chairman) *Learning from Bristol: The report of the public inquiry into children's heart surgery at the Bristol Royal Infirmary 1984–1999*. Bristol Royal Inquiry, Bristol.

Department of Health (1998) *A First Class Service: Quality in the NHS*. Department of Health, London.

Manley, K. (2000) Organisational culture and consultant nurse outcomes. Part 2: consultant nurse outcomes. *Nursing Standard*, **14**(37), 34–9.

13. *Developing and Implementing a Family Health Assessment*
From Project Worker to Practice Developer

Kate Sanders

Many healthcare practitioners engage in activities that aim to develop practice and improve care. Sometimes these activities are undertaken with limited experience of the process of facilitating change and perhaps with little insight into the knowledge, skills and support that may be required to achieve a successful outcome. This chapter focuses on my own experience of taking on the role of project worker to introduce a family health assessment into health visiting practice in just this situation.

The first part of the chapter is largely descriptive, providing background information about the origins of the project and an account of how the Family Health Assessment (FHA) was developed and implemented into practice. It could be suggested that this section corresponds to the first phase of the reflective process as defined by Kim (1999). However, I am also aware that it could represent the way in which I was practising at the time – focusing more on 'what' needed to be achieved rather than the 'how' and 'why'. A critical reflection of the process I adopted when developing practice follows in the second part of the chapter with the key lessons that have been identified discussed in light of future work to be undertaken.

Background

Health visitors work with families to promote health. Many health visitors spend a lot of time working with families who have the greatest health needs, supporting and working with parents to help them cope with the stresses of parenting and other life events (Appleton, 1996; Department of Health, 2001). Searching out health needs and stimulating clients' awareness of health needs are two key principles of health visiting practice (Chalmers, 1993). Such practice is supportive of the health visitors' role as defined by the government in the following publications, *Saving Lives: Our Healthier Nation* (Department of Health, 1999a) and *Making a Difference* (Department of Health, 1999b).

Currently there is no standardised approach by which health visitors identify those families who are at greatest risk of developing poor physical, psychological and/or social health. This chapter is based on a project that aimed to develop and implement a family health assessment to identify those families with the greatest health needs. In the main, it is a personal reflection on the process I adopted when developing practice which was triggered by my realisation that the health visitors who had been involved in the development of the FHA were reluctant to use it.

Getting started

The project developed from an incident in the mid 1990s when a social worker contacted the health visiting manager late one Friday afternoon to make inquiries about a family about whom someone had expressed concerns. The manager said she would check the health visiting notes and report any relevant information back to the social worker. On finding the notes, it was identified that a previous health visitor had expressed some concerns about the family, but at that time the family were attached to a caseload which was currently vacant and therefore had not had any contact with the health visiting service for over six months. As a consequence, the health visiting manager proposed that a system needed to be in place that enabled health visitors to identify those families with the greatest health needs, often described as 'vulnerable families', thereby ensuring that services could be offered to these families even in situations when caseloads were vacant.

A small group of health visitors began to explore ways in which this need could be met and created a checklist tool to identify those families with the greatest health needs, based on a small literature search and discussion around the use of professional judgement. The tool was piloted by several health visitors and then implemented into practice across the Trust. After the tool had been in use for approximately a year, the group who had developed it asked the clinical audit department for support with an audit of its use. It was at this stage, however, that it was realised that the validity and reliability of the tool had not been tested during the development phase. Following this realisation, discussions started about how the tool was being used in practice. It began to emerge that health visitors were questioning the validity of the tool. They were able to identify many situations where a family had a high score when assessed using the checklist tool and therefore should be considered 'vulnerable', yet the health visitor did not have any particular concerns about the family situation. Similarly, there were families who did not score highly when assessed using the tool but about whom the health visitor might be very concerned.

In response to this situation, the primary care nursing and health visiting managers, supported by the Trust's research and development committee developed a project proposal. The project aims were to:

- develop a standardised assessment that health visitors could use to identify those families with the greatest health needs;
- test the assessment for validity and reliability;
- implement the assessment across the Trust.

A successful application for funding was made to the Foundation of Nursing Studies to support the project and I was appointed as project worker in February 1999.

Approach to developing practice

In this section, I outline the process that was adopted when developing practice. As suggested in the introduction, it is largely descriptive, with the focus being mainly on the task assigned to me as project worker, i.e. to develop and implement a family health assessment. I now recognise that the approach was strongly influenced by my belief at the outset of the project that practice should be based on evidence. This belief is reflected in the structure of this section as it illustrates how evidence was collected, shared with others and used, to develop the Family Health Assessment.

Collecting the evidence

I started the project by searching the literature to explore how 'vulnerable' families were defined and to gain ideas about how they might be assessed. Whilst there was not a great deal of literature that related specifically to health visiting, a few key papers were identified which began to stimulate ideas about possible ways of developing an assessment (Aday, 1994; Appleton, 1994a, b, 1996, 1997; Rogers, 1997; Williams, 1997; Flaskerud and Winslow, 1998). Further evidence was gained by meeting with researchers and 'experts' in the field. At this time, I had a very strong feeling that I needed to share the information from the literature and my ideas about the development of the assessment with other health visitors. I wanted to confirm if the ideas that I had, which were stimulated by the literature and my own personal experiences of health visiting, reflected the thoughts and views of others. Ultimately I wanted to engage a group of health visitors in the development of the assessment. I was conscious, even at this early stage, that if I was developing an assessment for health visitors to use in practice it seemed logical that they should be involved in the developmental process. I believed that it was important to ensure that the assessment would be seen as user-friendly and of value to health visitors and clients. I anticipated that by actively involving some health visitors in the development of the assessment, they would act as change agents when it was ready to be used in practice.

Establishing the project group

Following discussion with the health visiting manager, a group of health visitors were approached and invited to become involved in the project. Health visitors were approached to ensure that:

- a variety of health visiting experiences from both within, and outside the Trust, could be brought to the group;
- all areas of the Trust were represented;
- group members had been practising for varying lengths of time.

In addition, an open invitation was extended to any other health visitors within the Trust. Initially, the group explored the concept of vulnerability and what this meant, as this term is commonly used in health visiting practice to describe those families that health visitors consider to have the greatest health needs (Appleton, 1996). Discussions centred on the health visitors' understanding of the term 'vulnerability' and their experiences of identifying those families with the greatest health needs. Evidence from the literature was used to trigger and inform these discussions.

The group members wanted to confirm that their experiences and opinions reflected those of the rest of the health visitors within the Trust. With the help of group members and the clinical audit department, a questionnaire was developed. This was sent to all health visitors within the Trust to explore their experiences of using the current checklist tool and to gain ideas about the factors which influenced whether a family was vulnerable or not. The responses to the questionnaire reflected those of group members. A consensus of opinion was evident with regard to the concept of vulnerability, both across the literature, and from among group members and other health visitors working within the Trust. General agreement was reached about the factors that contribute to a family becoming vulnerable, and those factors which are protective. It was also agreed that 'vulnerability' is often due to a combination of factors.

It was recognised at this stage that the term 'vulnerability' would not be appropriate to use on the new assessment as the group members felt that this may appear stigmatising to clients. There was agreement amongst the group members that what we were trying to develop was an assessment of family health and it was therefore agreed that 'family health assessment' would be a more suitable phrase to use when discussing the project with clients. Similarly, the use of the term 'tool' seemed inappropriate as it could imply that something was 'being done' to the clients, rather than focusing on an 'assessment' which the health visitor and client could discuss together.

Developing the Family Health Assessment (FHA)

Using all the available evidence, a list of factors that contribute to the health of a family in either a positive or negative way was identified and these were clustered into categories. Discussions were then held involving group members, academics, researchers and clients to determine how these categories could be turned into questions relating to family health that could be worded in a sensitive and non-threatening way. These questions developed into what became known as 'trigger questions' and collectively as the Family Health Assessment (FHA).

The FHA was designed with the intention that the health visitor and client should discuss it together, each question providing an opportunity for the client to consider a different aspect of their lives which may affect the health of themselves or their family members. It was anticipated that health visitors would follow up the responses to the questions, where appropriate. It was recognised that the health visitor's knowledge of the factors that contribute to family health needs and the issues around responding to cues and gaining entry as identified in the work of Luker & Chalmers (1990) and Chalmers (1993) may influence this process.

In addition to the questions, a Family Health Assessment Summary was developed to summarise the family situation in light of the issues raised using the trigger questions. Underlying the development of this summary was the desire to:

- focus on the positive aspects of a family's situation as well as those which may be detrimental to health;
- recognise the role of social support in promoting health;
- provide a method for summarising the family situation which could easily be reviewed with the client and be used to develop packages of care appropriate to the needs identified by the client.

The summary was based on the concept of 'zones' stimulated by Rogers' (1997) model of vulnerability, and Anthony's (1974) matrix which illustrates the relationship between vulnerability, risk and psychiatric disorders, cited and discussed by Rose & Killien (1983). The client is asked to rate themselves on a scale of 0–10 for 'stress' and 'support' and these measures are recorded on two axes at right angles to each other. These terms reflect the concept of vulnerability that suggest that it depends on an individual's/family's ability to cope with stress and the support that is available to them (Appleton, 1994b). The result is four zones/quadrants with varying combinations of high/low 'stress' and 'support'. The resulting quadrant is used to discuss the family situation overall and then to develop an appropriate plan of care/intervention and a date for reassessment. Where the family place themselves in the quadrants can be used to assess their situation over a period of time and in response to input from health visiting and/or other services.

Piloting the Family Health Assessment

The FHA was piloted between June and August 2000 with 20 families with pre-school children who lived in the area covered by the Trust for which ethical approval had been gained. The aims of the pilot study were:

- To determine whether using the FHA was a valid and reliable way for health visitors to identify those families who have the greatest health needs;
- To gain feedback from clients on their views about the value of the FHA as a way of identifying aspects of their everyday life which may affect health and thereby ensuring user involvement in the future development of the FHA.

Whilst only a small scale pilot, a variety of methods were employed to test the validity of the FHA. A theoretical sampling approach was used whereby families from the caseloads of the health visitors involved in the designing of the FHA were approached. The health visitors used their current knowledge of the families and their professional judgement to allocate the family to one of the four quadrants within the FHA Summary. In this way, it could be ensured that the sample would include families with a variety of 'stresses' and levels of 'support'. Although statistical testing would not be appropriate due to the small sample size, the pilot study found that there was a high level of agreement between the responses given to the trigger questions, the scores on the FHA Summary, and the comments and scores from two other validated assessments used. There was a high degree of acceptability for the FHA and the assessment process amongst the sample client group. No negative comments were recorded. A few adjustments were made to the FHA in response to comments from clients.

It was not possible formally to test the reliability of the FHA as part of the project as many of the methods that could be used, such as split-half technique, require larger sample sizes, or depend on testing large batteries of questions. Internal consistency, however, could be considered by comparing the responses to trigger questions with the responses to the FHA Summary and a structured assessment format was created to reduce user-bias. It was anticipated that the reliability of the assessment would be further enhanced by the development of a training package and by recommending that health visitors who use the assessment have the opportunity to reflect on their experiences with peers on a regular basis.

Using the Family Health Assessment in practice

In the very early days of the project, it had been anticipated that once the FHA had been piloted, all the health visitors in the Trust would be trained and begin to use the assessment in their everyday practice. However, having completed the pilot study, the limitations of the purposive sampling and small sample size were recognised. These were discussed with the working group and as a result, they agreed to use the FHA in practice over a period of several weeks to find out how a larger number of clients who had not been specifically selected responded to this new approach. A date was arranged when I would meet with the group to obtain feedback about their experiences, comments from clients, and their ideas about the further development of the assessment.

It was during this meeting that it became apparent that the health visitors had been reluctant to use the FHA in practice. Much of their feedback related to situations when the client and health visitor appeared to have different views about the health needs of the family. They reported that on occasions they felt 'uncomfortable' and also that they felt that their professional judgement was being threatened. The focus of their feelings seemed to be directed at the FHA and questions were asked about how useful it was. This reluctance to use the FHA obviously came as a great disappointment to me and I had to consider deeply why the health visitors had responded in this way.

Initially I questioned whether there may be a fundamental problem with the FHA but realised that this could only be answered if I gained more information about how it was used in practice. To address this issue, I shared information about the project with health visitors and their managers in neighbouring localities. Those who expressed an interest were invited to use the FHA in practice for a period of a few weeks. Meetings were arranged with groups of the health visitors involved so as to gain feedback about their experiences. Whilst there were health visitors in these groups who had not used the FHA on many occasions, there were others who had used it many times and were positive about their experiences. These health visitors were able to offer case scenarios that illustrated how it had enabled them to work with clients to:

- identify health needs
- prioritise health needs
- develop appropriate packages of care
- measure the outcome of interventions
- identify public health issues
- provide evidence to support the development of services

I was therefore faced with the reality that the working group members' reluctance to use the assessment in practice may be a consequence of the way in which the FHA had been developed and implemented. Support for this possibility was reinforced by a text I was reading at that time. Unsworth (2001) cites the work of Lancaster (1999) when he discusses the potential reasons for reluctance to change practice and summarises some assessment criteria that can be used to identify resistance in the following questions:

- How great is the change?
- How reasonable is the change?
- How much are participants emotionally invested in the old way of working?
- How threatening to the participants is the new way of working?

- Will it alter their role and power?
- Will it alter the content of their job?
- Will it alter the person's freedom to perform their job?
- How do participants feel about the change agent?
- How clear are people about what is expected of them?

(Unsworth, 2001: 88)

When considering these questions, I realised that little if any thought had been given to these issues during the project. I could also see that by asking health visitors to use the FHA, they may have had to alter the way in which they were working, which in turn could have had an impact on their role, their power and the content of their job. Recognising this stimulated me to reflect critically on the processes I had used to develop practice.

Reflection on the approach I adopted to developing practice

Before I could reflect critically on the process I had adopted to develop practice, I recognised that I first needed to identify the nature of the process involved. This may seem somewhat surprising, but I realised that up until this point, I had not given this issue a great deal of consideration. In this section, I consider the literature on evidence-based practice and practice development in relation to my own experiences. Through this process, I was able to explore the different approaches to developing practice and reflect on the ways in which these may influence how change is achieved and sustained.

Task or process?

When starting the project I was very aware of the increasing emphasis being placed upon evidence-based practice and the need to demonstrate the value of health visiting. This emphasis is reflected by Kendall (1999) who argues that clinical effectiveness in health visiting 'relies on the best possible care being provided, based on the best available evidence' (Kendall, 1999: 31). I was, however, unaware of literature that explored how this could be achieved. To a large extent, my approach to developing and implementing the FHA was guided by a perceived need to base practice on evidence and my assumption that to do this, one collected and critiqued 'the evidence', presented it in a format that would be acceptable to practitioners, and then as a consequence, practice would change.

With hindsight, I now recognise that my approach to developing practice was naïve, a view that is supported by Rycroft-Malone *et al.* (2002) who also suggest that it is 'linear and logical' (Rycroft-Malone *et al.*, 2002: 174). It was only when I started to reflect on the project that I became aware of the increasing amount of literature focusing on the complexities of implementing evidence into practice. Kitson *et al.* (1998) offer a conceptual framework to show how research findings can be successfully implemented into practice. They suggest that successful implementation is dependent upon 'equal recognition being given to the level of evidence, the context into which the evidence is being implemented, and the method of facilitating the change' (Kitson *et al.*, 1998: 158). Reflecting on the key elements of this framework has made me recognise that successfully implementing evidence and changing practice is a far more 'complex and messy task' (Rycroft-Malone *et al.*, 2002: 174) than I first realised. At times during the project, I would have believed that:

- due attention had been given to the evidence, as research, experience from practice, and client feedback had all been considered;
- the health visitors in the working group were clear about their role and involvement in the project, and my role as project worker, thereby clarifying the context;
- in my role as facilitator of the group, I was there to make things easier for the group and achieved this by taking on the greatest share of the work.

However, I now realise that these views were largely based on assumptions that were never explored and in turn reflected an approach which was focused on the task rather than the 'means' by which the task could be achieved or one that considered the stakeholders involved.

Consequently, I began to recognise that the process that is adopted when developing practice is far more important than the task or outcome alone. This led me to consider the literature on 'practice development', a term that is being increasingly used when referring to activities that aim to change practice and improve patient care (Unsworth, 2000; Garbett & McCormack, 2002). Two papers were of particular benefit when exploring the purpose and processes involved in practice development and how this might enhance my understanding of my own experiences. Unsworth (2000) and Garbett & McCormack (2002) use different approaches to analysing the concept of practice development in an attempt to clarify this widely used but poorly defined term (Clarke & Proctor, 1999).

Unsworth (2000) used a framework developed for the study of nursing concepts by Walker & Avant (1995). This approach starts with exploring the body of knowledge, and how the concept is used to develop and clarify critical attributes, antecedents and consequences of the concept. Following a review of definitions of practice development and the use of the term in the literature, Unsworth (2000) is able to identify a number of attributes. Through the development of cases these attributes are tested so as to identify those that should be present in all examples of practice development. Four critical attributes of practice development are identified from this process, each of which can be identified within the project to develop and implement the FHA and are outlined in Box 13.1.

Having reflected on these findings it could be argued that the nature of the project I had been involved in was practice develop-

Box 13.1 Unsworth's critical attributes of practice development applied to the FHA development and implementation.

Unsworth's (2000) critical attributes of practice development	Developing and implementing the FHA
New ways of working which lead to a direct measurable improvement in care or service to the client	We were developing a new assessment process to identify those families with the greatest health needs in order that appropriate services could be offered.
Changes which occur as a response to a specific client need or problem	The need to develop a system that enabled health visitors to identify those families with the greatest health needs had been identified.
Changes which lead to the development of effective services	It was anticipated that this intervention would lead to the health visiting service being used more effectively by those families with the greatest health needs.
The maintenance or expansion of business/work	It could be regarded as maintaining the business of the health visiting service i.e. identifying health needs and offering appropriate interventions to meet these needs.

ment when judged against Unsworth's (2000) attributes; however, this realisation alone did little to help me understand why the approach I had adopted had not been effective in achieving the changes in practice that were needed for the successful implementation of the FHA.

In comparison, the concept analysis by Garbett & McCormack (2002) focuses more on the processes of practice development and as a result provided greater insight into why I had not been successful in bringing about a change in practice. They adopt a dispositional view to understand the concept which involves trying to capture the meaning of the concept in the 'real world', i.e. as seen by those who use it. Qualitative methods are used to analyse primary and secondary sources of data as suggested by Morse (1995). This included data collected from a search of the UK literature, telephone interviews and focus groups with practitioners involved in practice development. Through the thematic analysis and cognitive mapping of a rich data source four main themes relating to practice development emerged:

1. It is a means of improving care.
2. It transforms the contexts and cultures in which nursing takes place.
3. It is important to employ a systematic approach to effect changes in practice.
4. Various types of facilitation are required for change to take place.
(Garbett & McCormack, 2002: 92)

Whilst, both the papers by Unsworth (2000) and Garbett & McCormack (2002) support the view that the purpose of practice development is to improve patient care, the essential difference between the two is that Garbett & McCormack (2002) emphasise the importance of the people involved. Recognition of this difference led me to realise that this was an aspect of the project to which I had given little consideration. Garbett & McCormack (2002) believe that practice development is concerned with the transformation of the context and culture of care and suggest that this is achieved through a process of facilitated change (see Chapter 2). Whilst I recognised the need to involve health visitors in the project, I now realise that I did not have the knowledge and skills to involve them in a way that would enable sustainable change.

Technical or emancipatory?
To a large extent, the two views of practice development emerging from these concept analyses are reflected by the two worldviews of

practice development as identified by Manley & McCormack (2003). These are 'technical' and 'emancipatory' practice development, informed by Habermas's (1972) different knowledge interests and Grundy's (1982) three modes of action research (see Chapter 2).

In technical practice development, the intention is to use research findings to improve patient care with the focus being on the outcome rather than the processes used to get there. Technical practice development is generally a top-down approach that is based on the assumption that once practitioners have the evidence their practice will change: 'Development of staff, if it occurs, is a *consequence* of practice development rather than a *deliberate* and *intentional* purpose' (Manley & McCormack, 2003: 24). In comparison, developing and empowering staff is a specific purpose of emancipatory practice development, as is the creation of a transformational culture (Manley, 2001) such that: 'quality becomes everyone's business; positive change becomes a way of life; everyone's leadership potential is developed; and, where there is a shared vision, there is an investment in and valuing of staff (Manley, 2000a, b) (see Chapter 4).

Reflecting on these two worldviews has enabled me to take a closer look at the approach to practice development that I had adopted. I now recognise that in the main I had adopted a 'technical' approach to practice development as defined by Manley & McCormack (2003). As suggested earlier, I believe that the adoption of this approach was not intentional, but largely driven by my beliefs at the start of the project about evidence-based practice. Having considered the literature, however, I now recognise that there are consequences of having adopted this approach and these have ultimately influenced the outcome of the project.

Manley & McCormack (2003) suggest that in technical practice development: 'the goal is known, and the focus is on achieving the outcome . . . rather than being concerned with the means of achieving it' (Manley & McCormack, 2003: 24). The first part of this statement rings very true as during the project I would have suggested that all those involved would perceive that the aim was to develop an assessment to identify families with health needs and to implement it into practice across the Trust. Becoming aware of this, however, has enabled me to recognise that the project was in fact based on the assumption that using a standardised assessment to identify family health needs would be better than what was currently happening in practice. As a consequence of the approach adopted, this assumption was never explored and other assumptions were made as a result. The key stakeholders, i.e. clients, health visitors and managers, were never consulted as to whether they thought a standardised approach to the assessment of health needs would be better.

As already outlined, impetus for the project initially came from management, a factor which again reflects the 'technical' nature of the project. There was a desire to have a system in place that would help health visitors to identify those families with the greatest health needs, thereby ensuring that even in times when there were shortages of health visiting staff, these families could be offered the support they required. It could be suggested that this represented a risk management agenda.

But did health visitors share the view that a standardised assessment would be better? I was aware that the checklist tool that we (health visitors) were currently using to identify health needs had many flaws. Personal experience and anecdotal evidence from other health visitors suggested that it was not valid and the way in which it was presented did not encourage health visitors to share it with clients as it may be perceived as threatening. As a result, clients may not have been aware that their health needs were being assessed and recorded. For these reasons, I saw the benefit of developing an assessment that:

- was evidence-based;
- was valid and reliable;
- health visitors could share with clients.

Whilst I did not assume that all health visitors would welcome this initiative, I must have assumed that those who agreed to join the working group believed that there was some value in developing a standardised assessment. Implicit in this is the assumption that as a group we must share some common beliefs about how health needs should be identified. I now recognise that this was a huge assumption to make and was challenged when to a large extent the health visitors in the working group showed a reluctance to use the FHA in practice.

And what about clients? Although clients were involved informally in the development of the FHA and those included in the pilot study were asked to give their views on the assessment, they were never actually asked how they thought health needs should be assessed.

By assuming that all those involved agreed that a standardised approach to assessing health needs was the way forward, the project followed a technical approach with the emphasis being on the development of the assessment and getting it into practice

(Manley & McCormack, 2003). I now realise that this influenced both the focus of the group and the way in which it was facilitated.

Project worker or practice developer?

Recognising that the process I had adopted influenced the way in which the group worked, I have had to look critically at my role as project worker. Manley & McCormack (2003) cite the work of Grundy (1982) when they suggest that in technical practice development:

> ... the practice developer is perceived as an expert authority figure in the sense they know what has to be done, to what standard, and the criteria for success pre-exists in their mind. . . . It is the facilitator's ideas, which direct a project, their focus is on an end point already in their mind. . . . Staff are the instrument through which the outcome is to be achieved and therefore through which practice is improved. The danger here is that staff may be 'pawns' who are unconsciously manipulated for the facilitator's or organisation's ends.
>
> (Grundy, 1982)

On reflection, I can relate many of the points made in this view to my involvement in the project and this has led me to consider the way in which I facilitated the working group. As already acknowledged, my focus was mainly upon the task. I do not believe that this was to the exclusion of all other considerations, as I did recognise the need to involve other health visitors in the change process. But I did not possess the knowledge and skills to 'enable others' and did not know where to source this support. This inexperience meant that I 'did for others', probably as this was a role with which I felt comfortable and familiar. I was also influenced by the fact that I was the only member of the group that had allocated time for the project and therefore felt that I needed to be doing something visible with this time. This role is recognised by Harvey *et al.* (2002) when they surmise that: 'the purpose of facilitation can vary from providing help and support to achieve a specific goal to enabling individuals and teams to analyse, reflect and change their own attitudes, behaviours and ways of working.' When represented on a continuum, the extreme points show a focus on the 'task' at one end, and a 'holistic' approach at the other.

I recognise the facilitation skills and attributes that I contributed to the project to a large extent as those identified by Harvey *et al.* (2002) in their summary of the 'Oxford Model' (Allsop, 1990 cited in Harvey *et al.*, 2002). This model of facilitation has been applied to health promotion where again the emphasis is more on the achievement of a goal. The skills/attributes include supplying technical or clinical advice, networking, offering suggestions, formulating solutions, helping shift attitudes, political skills, vision and energy. My role included: searching and appraising literature and then presenting it to the group in a format that was relevant to the project; gathering information from other sources including 'experts' in the field and feeding this back to the group in the form of suggestions and ideas; and working with the group to identify a vision of the assessment in order that we could work towards trying to develop it. I have to recognise, however, that the adoption of this approach may have resulted in the group members viewing me as the one who had the knowledge and expertise, and that I was driving the project towards achieving an outcome.

When considering the outcomes of the project, in terms of the 'task', it could be suggested that the group were successful in achieving the development of the FHA and in part this success may be attributed to the use of 'technical' facilitation skills. However, with regard to the implementation of the FHA, its use in practice within the trust was limited.

As a group, we had knowingly created an assessment that actively involved the client in the assessment of family health, but by adopting a technical approach to achieve this, we had not considered how using the FHA may affect the way in which we practiced as health visitors. I began to realise that to be successful in this, the skills and attributes of a 'holistic/enabling' approach to facilitation would have been more effective.

Towards an emancipatory approach to practice development

Ongoing development of the project has been encouraged by the large amount of interest that has been shown in the work to date from health visitors all around the UK. This interest is perhaps being driven by the need for health visitors to strengthen their family-centred public health role as outlined in the Department of Health's (2001) health visitor practice development resource pack. In many localities, health visitors are being charged with the task of developing family health assessments and are keen to learn from the experiences of those who have already been involved in this work. In light of my learning, this interest has raised two questions:

- What aspects of the work undertaken do I want to share?
- How can this best be achieved?

When considering these questions, it would be very easy to once again concentrate on the outcome and adopt a technical approach to sharing this work. In this way, the focus would be on informing health visitors about the FHA and offering guidelines for how it could be used in practice. However, such an approach was used during the later stages of the project when I met with the health visitors from neighbouring localities and whilst the assumption is made that once the health visitors have this information they will use the FHA in practice, I now recognise that in reality this often does not happen.

The health visitors who attended these introductory meetings appeared enthusiastic about the new approach, yet their plans to use the FHA in practice were not always realised when they got back to the workplace. Some reported feeling unhappy about introducing a new way of working at a time when they felt under pressure from the day-to-day burden of their caseloads. Others tried using the FHA and then gave reasons why it didn't work for them. As a consequence, the FHA was rejected and these health visitors continued with or returned to their usual ways of practising. Grundy (1982) (cited in Manley & McCormack, 2003) recognises the different responses shown by these health visitors to the implementation of the FHA as a consequence of a technical approach to developing practice.

Although some health visitors did incorporate the FHA into their work and have used it to inform and support their practice, on reflection, I would suggest that successful implementation in these cases was neither related to the technical approach or the facilitation of its introduction, rather it was due to the readiness and ability of these practitioners to challenge and reflect on existing practices.

Consequently, there seems little to be gained from continuing to share the FHA in this way. I now believe that by adopting a technical approach to this activity, there is a danger that attention will be given to the FHA alone. If health visitors see the FHA simply as a solution to the challenge of assessing family health, it is possible that attempts to implement the FHA into practice will occur at the expense of first developing a shared understanding about the purpose of using such an assessment. Also, there may result a lack of regard for the issues that introducing new ways of working may raise for practitioners.

By reflecting on the approach I adopted to developing practice, I became aware that as a group we had never clarified the ultimate purpose of assessing family health. Instead, the FHA was developed on the assumptions that it would be a means of:

- identifying those families with the greatest health needs;
- actively involving clients in the assessment process.

Because the development of the FHA was based on these assumptions, the values and beliefs that underpinned this work were never made explicit and as a result, we were unaware of whether we were currently practising in a way that was compatible with these values. Instead, we used our experiences from practice to confirm how we thought things should be, rather than as a means of challenging how they really were. This can be illustrated through the following example.

When developing the FHA all the group members agreed that clients should be actively involved in the assessment process. Because this espoused value was just accepted and never explored we must have assumed that clients were currently being involved in this way. By making this assumption, we failed to recognise that when using the FHA, some health visitors may in fact be required to work in a way that was incongruent with their current practice.

Having recognised the reality of this situation, the relevance of an emancipatory approach to developing practice became apparent. By adopting such a critical social science approach to practice development, Manley & McCormack (2003) state that the following will have occurred:

- critical reflection resulting in clarity about the values and beliefs being held about *health visiting* [my italics];
- recognition of any contradictions between the values and beliefs espoused and practised;
- increasing awareness of the barriers within the workplace that prevent values being practised;
- removing the barriers identified so as to practice in a way consistent with the values and beliefs espoused.

(Manley & McCormack, 2003: 25)

Considering these actions made me realise that successful implementation of the FHA could only have been achieved if the health visitors in the working group had been facilitated through a process that enabled them to:

- establish the purpose of assessing family health;
- identify the values and beliefs that underpin this purpose;
- critically reflect on their current practice to determine if it was consistent with their values and beliefs;
- be supported in developing new ways of working.

Through this process consideration is given to the development of the health visitors and recognition is given to the need to develop a culture that is supportive of change.

It now becomes evident that when sharing my experiences from this project, the FHA itself is secondary as it is unlikely that health visitors will use it in practice if its implementation is the main focus of any initiative. Instead the emphasis should be on clarifying the values and beliefs about the assessment of family health. Once these have been established, the FHA may be considered as one of many ways in which these values and beliefs can be realised in practice. In this way, implementation of the FHA would not be seen as an end point. Health visitors may start to use the FHA assessment as a means of assessing family health, but as a result of reflecting on their experiences and considering the views of clients and other key stakeholders, changes may be made to the FHA at a local level, as in action research or reflexive research (Rolfe, 1996).

Conclusion

This chapter presents a project that attempted to develop an assessment of family health and to implement it into health visiting practice. In the main it is based on my own personal journey from project worker to practice developer. By reflecting critically on the approach I adopted to developing practice I became aware of my own naïvety at the outset about the complexities of facilitating change. Whilst the last few years have seen an increase in the amount of literature focusing on the complexities of this process, the challenge remains to make this literature both accessible and relevant to all practitioners. By sharing my experiences and through considering the two worldviews of practice development in relation to the work undertaken, I hope I have been able to demonstrate how consideration of the process when developing practice may influence the effectiveness of an initiative in a way that is pertinent to readers from all areas of practice.

References

Aday, L.A. (1994) Health status of vulnerable populations. *Annual Review of Public Health*, **15**, 487–509.

Anthony, E.J. (1974) The syndrome of the psychologically invulnerable child. In: *The child in his family: children at psychiatric risk* (eds Anthony, E.J., Koupernik, C. & Chilland, C.). John Wiley and sons, New York.

Appleton, J.V. (1994a) The role of the health visitor in identifying and working with vulnerable families in relation to child protection: a review of the literature. *Journal of Advanced Nursing*, **20**, 167–75.

Appleton, J.V. (1994b) The concept of vulnerability in relation to child protection: health visitors' perceptions. *Journal of Advanced Nursing*, **20**, 1132–40.

Appleton, J.V. (1996) Working with vulnerable families: a health visiting perspective. *Journal of Advanced Nursing*, **23**, 912–18.

Appleton, J.V. (1997) Establishing the validity and reliability of clinical practice guidelines used to identify families requiring increased health visitor support. *Public Health*, **111**, 107–13.

Chalmers, K. (1993) Searching for health needs: the work of health visiting. *Journal of Advanced Nursing*, **18**, 900–11.

Clarke, C. & Proctor, S. (1999) Practice development: ambiguity in research and practice. *Journal of Advanced Nursing*, **30**(4), 975–82.

Department of Health (DoH) (1999a) *Saving Lives: Our Healthier Nation.* HMSO, London.

Department of Health (DoH) (1999b) *Making a Difference: Strengthening the Nursing, Midwifery and Health Visiting Contribution to Health and Healthcare.* HMSO, London.

Department of Health (DoH) (2001) *Health Visitor Practice Development Resource Pack.* HMSO, London.

Flaskerud, J.H. & Winslow, B.J. (1998) Conceptualizing vulnerable populations. Health related research. *Nursing Research*, **47**, 69–78.

Garbett, R. & McCormack, B. (2002) A concept analysis of practice development. *Nursing Times Research*, **7**(2), 87–100.

Grundy, S. (1982) Three modes of action research. *Curriculum Perspectives*, **2**(3), 23–34.

Habermas, J. (1972) *Knowledge and Human Interests*, trans J.J. Shapiro. Heinemann, London.

Harvey, G., Loftus-Hills, A., Rycroft-Malone, J., *et al.* (2002) Getting evidence into practice: the role and function of facilitation. *Journal of Advanced Nursing*, **37**(6), 577–88.

Kendall, S. (1999) Evidence-based health visiting – the utilisation of research for effective practice. In: *Research Issues in Community Nursing* (ed. J. McIntosh), pp. 29–52. Palgrave Macmillan, Basingstoke.

Kim, H.S. (1999) Critical reflection inquiry for knowledge development in nursing practice. *Journal of Advanced Nursing*, **29**(5), 1205–12.

Kitson, A., Harvey, G. & McCormack, B. (1998) Enabling the implementation of evidence-based practice: a conceptual framework. *Quality in Health Care*, **7**(3), 149–58.

Luker, K. & Chalmers, K. (1990) Gaining access to clients: the case of health visiting. *Journal of Advanced Nursing*, **15**(1), 74–82.

Manley, K. (2000a) Organisational culture and consultant nurse outcomes. Part 1: Organisational culture. *Nursing Standard*, **14**(36), 34–8.

Manley, K. (2000b) Organisational culture and consultant nurse outcomes. Part 2: Consultant nurse outcomes. *Nursing Standard*, **14**(37), 34–9.

References

Manley, K. (2001) *Consultant nurse: concept, process, outcome.* Unpublished PhD thesis, University of Manchester/RCN Institute, London.

Manley, K. & McCormack, B. (2003) Practice development: purpose, methodology, facilitation and evaluation. *Nursing in Critical Care*, **8**(1), 22–9.

Morse, J.M. (1995) Exploring the theoretical basis of nursing using advanced techniques of concept analysis. *Advances in Nursing Science*, **17**, 31–46.

Rogers, A.C. (1997) Vulnerability, health and healthcare. *Journal of Advanced Nursing*, **26**, 65–72.

Rolfe, G. (1996) *Closing the Theory–Practice Gap: A New Paradigm in Nursing.* Butterworth-Heinemann, London.

Rose, M.H. & Killien, M. (1983) Risk and vulnerability: a case for differentiation. *Advances in Nursing Science*, **5**(3), 60–73.

Rycroft-Malone, J., Kitson, A., Harvey, G., *et al.* (2002) Ingredients for change: revisiting a conceptual framework. *Quality and Safety in Health Care*, **11**, 174–80.

Unsworth, J. (2000) Practice development: a concept analysis. *Journal of Nursing Management*, **8**(6), 317–26.

Unsworth, J. (2001) Managing the development of practice. In: *Developing Community Nursing Practice* (eds S. Spencer, J. Unsworth & W. Burke). Open University Press, Buckingham.

Walker, L.O. & Avant, K.C. (1995) *Strategies for Theory Construction in Nursing*, 3rd edn. Appleton & Lange, New Jersey.

Williams, D.M. (1997) Vulnerable families: a study of health visitors' prioritization of their work. *Journal of Nursing Management*, **5**, 19–24.

Commentary

Kate Gerrish

Kate Sanders' honest and insightful account of her experiences of seeking to introduce a change in health visiting practice aptly illustrates the complexity of undertaking practice development in the real world. It also highlights a number of important principles that merit consideration when taking forward practice development initiatives.

First, it is made clear that technical models of practice development which adopt a linear approach to change are not well suited to the messiness and unpredictability of introducing change in the practice environment. Our attention is drawn, instead, to the need to adopt participatory and empowering approaches to practice development in which equal consideration is given to process and outcome. To this end, the account resonates with the need for those involved in practice development to understand the change process and be skilled in change management in order to facilitate the process. However, achieving a balance between process and outcome can be difficult for a project worker appointed with a particular task to achieve in order to meet the expectations of those commissioning the change, in this case the managers. The skills of project management are not the same as the skills of change management, yet as this chapter points out, the practice developer needs to be multi-skilled.

The issue of ownership, although not stated explicitly, is also highlighted. Change theory emphasises the need for change to be recognised and owned by those whose practice is the focus of the intended change. As this chapter illustrates, consultation and a degree of involvement in the development process is not sufficient to ensure a commitment to implementing change, particularly where personal interests are at stake. Whereas management initiated proposals for change can and do meet with success, ownership of the need for change at grass roots level needs to be secured for successful implementation (Gerrish, 1999). As Kate Sanders implies, ownership is problematic where the proposed change represents a direct challenge to an individual's underlying values and beliefs and his or her established, comfortable ways of working.

The author also reflects upon her role as a facilitator of practice development. Facilitation within the context of practice development can range from discrete task-focused activity to multi-faceted approaches to enabling individuals, teams or organisations to change (Harvey *et al.*, 2002). My own work on the implementation of integrated community nursing teams (Gerrish *et al.*, 1998) highlights the complexity of an external facilitator's role in supporting practice development in terms of balancing support from the side lines to enable individuals to develop at their own pace, providing leadership, giving direction, and providing practical assistance. In taking account of the changing practice context the facilitator, rather than adopt a particular approach, needs to employ a range of strategies at different times during the lifetime of a particular practice development initiative.

We also need to recognise that whereas practice development is often concerned with planning and introducing a change in practice, the impact extends beyond changing what practitioners do. As Kate Sanders points out, the attempts to introduce a new assessment tool challenged fundamental values underpinning the practice of individual health visitors which were reflected in the way health visitors interacted with the clients on their caseload. Professional ideologies, in this case involving clients in the assessment process, were not necessarily evident in the everyday work of health visitors.

This chapter also draws the readers' attention to other issues that are alluded to but not considered in depth. First, there is the issue of client involvement in practice development. Clients, we are told, were involved in discussions regarding the development of the assessment tool and in providing feedback as part of the pilot exercise. However, the opportunity to involve clients more actively throughout the whole process of practice development is considerable and appears to be largely missed.

Second, the timing of practice development initiatives merits consideration in that it may influence the success or otherwise of an initiative. Kate Saunders hints at this when she mentions that interest in the assessment tool has gained momentum following the recent introduction of the Department of Health's resource pack to develop the family-centred role of health visitors. A particular initiative may well be difficult to implement in isolation; however, when a number of related drivers are introduced which support the initiative, effective change may be easier to achieve. To this end, it is important to remember that the receptiveness of practitioners to changing practice is context bound and that the context is constantly changing.

Finally, the need to consider the evaluation of practice development from the outset is not highlighted. So often in service development, consideration is given to evaluation strategies once an innovation has been implemented, but this should form part of the development process. Whereas the original intention had been to develop a standardised assessment tool that health visitors could use to identify families with the greatest health needs in order to direct health visiting resources to areas of greatest need, other objectives are mentioned. These include involving clients in the assessment process, focusing on positive aspects of the family's situation, using the assessment to develop packages of care appropriate to the needs of family clients, etc. Each of these should be addressed as a part of the evaluation strategy and consideration given to how successful or otherwise the initiative has been in achieving these objectives. However, as the initial attempts to implement the assessment tool illustrate, evaluation should also consider the process of implementation and how the change is viewed by all those involved. Pluralistic approaches to evaluation which take account of various stakeholder perspectives and encompass subjective perspectives of process as well as objective measures of outcome lend themselves to evaluating practice development initiatives (Gerrish, 2001).

References

Gerrish, K. (1999) Teamwork in primary healthcare: an evaluation of the contribution of integrated community nursing teams. *Health and Social Care in the Community*, **7**(5), 367–75.

Gerrish, K. (2001) A pluralistic evaluation of Nursing/Practice Development Units. *Journal of Clinical Nursing*, **10**(1), 109–18.

Gerrish, K., Pollard, J. & Ross, B. (1998) Integrated nursing teams: the community nursing facilitator's role. *Primary Health Care*, **8**(8), 12–14.

Harvey, G., Loftus-Hills, A., Rycroft-Malone, J. *et al.* (2002) Getting evidence into practice: the role and function of facilitation. *Journal of Advanced Nursing*, **37**(6), 577–88.

14. *A Clearer Vision of Practice Development?*

Brendan McCormack, Rob Garbett & Kim Manley

In this chapter we explore the practice development journey undertaken in this book. Whilst there are multiple journeys set out in the various chapters, ultimately this has been a shared journey, exploring the many facets, dimensions and tensions embedded in the seemingly simple term, practice development. We will extrapolate some key issues and outcomes arising from the chapters and explore these in the context of the concepts underpinning practice development as set out in Part 1 of this book. The contributors to this book have identified a number of issues and potential outcomes that arguably require further investigation, clarification and discussion.

In Part 1, we explored a conceptual framework for practice development, drawing upon the research and practice development work of a number of colleagues. There is a perceived lack of clarity and uniformity in the way that the term practice development is employed and thus in Part 1 we have endeavoured to clarify the term. Achieving a greater sense of clarity, it is argued, may help practice developers, clinicians and managers apply the concept with greater awareness of its attributes and possibilities. This in turn may result in a more internally consistent body of work and the easier identification and evaluation of successful approaches and strategies to developing practice. The chapters contributed by practitioners in Part 2 of the book continue this iterative process, with each contributing new insights to our understanding of practice development. For example, Mary Golden & Steve Tee's (Chapter 10) work with service users challenges the whole idea of user involvement in practice development. There are now a wide variety of resources available to practice developers that can assist with involving users in development projects. For example in the UK the Department of Health's 'Modernisation Agency' provide detailed information about how to involve users in modernising services and practice (http://www.modern.nhs.uk/improvement guides/patients/home.html). However, in their honest account, Mary and Steve bring out the many challenges and pitfalls to be faced when involving users. They do not try to provide us with a sanitised account, but instead present it 'as it is' – complex, challenging and fraught with difficulty. However, despite this, it is clear that there are many benefits to be achieved from engaging in this work. Most significantly, the authors demonstrate how the image of acute mental health services at an organisational level can become more highly valued through the processes of user-focused practice development.

We have argued that the term practice development is not used consistently and it covers a broad and sometimes contradictory range of activity. Nonetheless, we would argue that greater clarity could be provided in key areas, by defining the purpose, attributes and activities that comprise practice development. We have defined practice development as:

> a continuous process of improvement towards increased effectiveness in patient centred care. This is brought about by enabling health care teams to develop their knowledge and skills and to transform the culture and context of care. It is enabled and supported by facilitators committed to systematic, rigorous continuous processes of emancipatory change that reflect the perspectives of both service users and service providers.
>
> (Garbett & McCormack, 2002: 88)

We have illustrated this definition graphically (Fig. 14.1), placing improvement at the centre couched in a need to address cultural

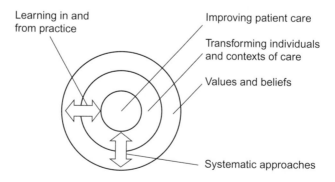

Fig. 14.1   A concept map of practice development.

aspects of care as well as the need to address the (evidence-based) knowledge and skills of those practitioners that deliver it. The whole is contained within a system of values and beliefs that emphasises the central importance of facilitating practitioners to learn from their everyday work experience. In Part 1 of the book we have illustrated the importance of clarifying values and beliefs concerning key components of practice development work (e.g. team working, the meaning of patient-centredness, clinical leadership or the purpose of the practice development work). The practice development process needs to be systematic and rigorous in order that lessons can be learnt and applied. This definition, we believe, states clearly and simply the key concerns of practice development. In so doing it reflects the way in which the concept is operationalised and provides the basis for promoting the concept of practice development. It is a deliberately global definition subsuming to some extent continuous quality improvement and clinical effectiveness activities. We would not claim that practice development can be entirely differentiated from such activities, although it could be argued that such activities are not always undertaken with emphasis on the processes by which the care delivered by practitioners is changed.

The definition incorporates six themes that are present to a greater extent throughout the chapters in this book:

- an emphasis on improving patient care
- an emphasis on transforming the context in which nursing care takes place
- the importance of employing a systematic approach to effect changes in practice
- the involvement of service users and service providers
- the nature of the facilitation required for change to take place
- the use and development of eclectic sources of evidence

We would also argue, however, that the emphasis placed specifically on the development of new skills and knowledge needs to be made more explicit. For practice developers professional development that accompanies practice development provides necessary new skills and knowledge to allow practice to change through raising awareness. It also provides motivation for those involved with development, especially in a health service culture in which accredited learning in particular is a form of currency. As Binnie & Titchen (1999) point out, professional development is important. It demonstrates an investment in practitioners as individuals, helping them to learn about their abilities and to acquire new knowledge and skills which allow them to progress and challenge issues arising in their working environments. Jill Down in Chapter 12 makes explicit the importance of integrating professional and practice development in an organisation-wide approach. The differentiation between professional and practice development is often nebulous and we have found that practitioners often make little or no differentiation between the two terms. However, the main differentiation is that practice development starts with the patient and user, whereas professional development starts with the practitioner. We would assert that the development of skills and knowledge is subordinate to and dictated by the needs of patient care but that it is an important component of practice development. Of course such conceptual hierarchies can only ever be tentative when the boundaries between concepts such as professional and practice development are blurred. This blurring is accentuated in Chris Caldwell's chapter (Chapter 9). Chris describes how a study module in a master's degree programme became a catalyst and a platform for significant changes in practice to occur. The chapter highlights the importance of flexible learning and the importance of course structures and processes being able to 'hold' practice innovation as a component of the overall learning endeavour.

But at the end of this journey (or perhaps the beginning of a new one!) are we any clearer about the purposes, attributes and consequences of practice development? The purposes of practice development are:

- Increased effectiveness in patient/person-centred care;
- Enabling individuals and healthcare teams to transform their care and the culture within which it takes place.

The attributes of practice development are:

- Being systematic (although, as will be discussed below, we would argue for a plural and broad notion of what constitutes a systematic approach to practice development)
- Being rigorous
- A continuous process
- A process founded on facilitation

As far as consequences are concerned we would acknowledge that accounts to date rarely give a complete or satisfactory picture. Nonetheless we would suggest that logically these would consist of:

- Outcomes for users in terms of improved experience and outcomes;

- Outcomes for practitioners such as increased flexibility and creativity, new knowledge and skills, raised awareness of their own abilities and contribution, raised awareness of the structures within which they work;
- Outcomes for team effectiveness as a building block of learning organisations;
- Outcomes for workplace culture towards developing a culture of effectiveness where quality is everyone's concern;
- Outcomes for organisational effectiveness in terms of cross-boundary working, corporate and strategic systems that support and optimise practice development at a local level.

Purpose

Increased effectiveness in patient-centred care

We would argue that practice development is unambiguously concerned with the improvement of patient care and services. Although in practice the term can be confused with the development of skills and knowledge that can lead to such improvements, such activity is clearly subordinate to the central aim of ensuring that the quality of care is addressed. Increasingly, policy developments within the NHS stress the importance of service developments reflecting the expressed needs of service users and the growing importance of incorporating the views of patients. The notion of improving patient care should therefore be understood to include the central importance of improvements reflecting the needs of those who receive a service, although as Clarke & Procter (1999) have observed, practice development and research are often seen as separate and optional activities within professional practice. On one level this concern can legitimately be located within the ethics, purpose and function of a professional group. Such a conviction is evident within the Nursing and Midwifery Council *Code of Professional Conduct* (NMC, 2002) and has been proposed as a compelling rationale underpinning the need for continuously appraising and improving standards of care (Draper, 1996; McMahon, 1998) – something that has been explicitly addressed by Jane Stokes in Chapter 11. Jane has described a strategic approach to practice development that focuses on the *Essence of Care* (Department of Health, 2001). In the project described, it is clear that the quality of individual care is the central focus of the practice development work. The outlined strategic approach to practice development uses this drive to create a wave of change throughout the organisation that ultimately focuses on sustaining quality patient-centred care. On another level, a commitment to services that reflect the needs of individuals and populations (as opposed to the needs of those that provide them) is a feature of a consumerist culture that has increasingly found expression in government policy in successive NHS reorganisations over the last 15 years (for example, Department of Health, 1991; Department of Health, 1998b). Assuming a patient-centred perspective can also be seen as a form of strategic lever. A concern with users' interests is congruent with policy discourses and so can be seen as a means of exercising power, an interpretation that can be applied to accounts by practice developers of using feedback from patients as a basis for reshaping services (as described by Mary Golden & Steve Tee in Chapter 10 and Jill Down in Chapter 12, for example). However, to progress beyond a token involvement of patients to ensure that all groups, no matter how frail or affected by ill health, can participate in both day-to-day care and the development of the services that they receive, requires considerable thought, tenacity and ingenuity. This is evident in Chapter 8 in which Jan Dewing & Emma Pritchard give an account of approaches that have been developed to involve older people with a dementia in the development of their care. Jan and Emma provide real examples from their own research and practice development activity to articulate methodological issues of user involvement. The outcomes from this work are clearly complex and not always amenable to linear approaches to outcome measurement. Instead they challenge us to go beyond the rational logical voice and to engage with the whole being of the person with dementia – perhaps a challenge that should underpin all work with service users!

Transforming workplace cultures

For the most part descriptions of practice development activity problematise change. Rather than assuming a linear and uncomplicated relationship between knowledge and practice they, in Schön's (1983) terms, juxtapose the 'swampy lowlands' of practice with the high hard ground of pure knowledge. For this reason practice development is not only concerned with securing change in behaviour in relation to a particular aspect of practice, rather it is concerned with developing cultures of work in which practitioners can learn from their work and be responsive to the needs of service users. As McCormack *et al.* (1999) have argued, such a culture may need to be in place at the level of the interface with service users, at an organisational level and at a strategic level. We would suggest, however, that while practice development is frequently seen as a unidisciplinary activity it may be more fruitful to see it as inclusive of any staff who have an impact on a service user's experience. Kim Manley makes such importance a reality in Chapter 4. The systematic approach adopted to changing workplace culture, did not just involve nursing staff (although nurses clearly led the initiative), but instead had as its primary focus the needs of patients. The systematic practice development work over many years resulted in sustained changes in workplace culture and the development of a service that was recognised as being person-centred.

The practical complexity of Manley's work is not to be underestimated, however. Cutcliffe & Bassett (1997) have argued that the complexity of healthcare organisations is such that attempting large scale change is futile and that local change is the most appropriate way forward. Practice developers contributing to this book point to the difficulties inherent in achieving strategic direction within large organisations. However, as Manley suggests, it is apparent that core values around the importance of users' experience and an organisational design that is enabling and supportive are highly valued. Whatever the approach used, however, it can be argued that addressing practice development is more usefully conceived of as an iterative activity that has a cumulative effect on individuals and organisations, improving the capacity to adapt to new demands and respond to problems. Such cultures, by their very nature, cannot be imposed but they can be changed through leadership. They are the product of an enabling approach that helps practitioners identify and resolve issues for themselves, and so build confidence and repertoires of new skills and knowledge.

Attributes

The situated, contingent and 'messy' nature of a transformational and enabling approach relates to the attributes of practice development. It could be argued that to advocate systematic and rigorous approaches to such a concept is paradoxical given the recognition of its situated and complex nature. However, we would argue that acknowledging the messiness and unpredictability of naturalistic settings actually demands careful, systematic and rigorous approaches precisely because of their complexity so that lessons can be learnt and inferences drawn with a degree of confidence about the relationships between activities and outcomes.

Being systematic and rigorous

It can be argued that the need to continuously improve care delivery is central to the professional duty of any healthcare practitioner because healthcare contexts are continuously changing. How then is practice development, as an activity, differentiated from this professional imperative? We would argue that the key difference lies in the strategic intent to address such issues across a whole service in an orchestrated way, represented by the importance placed on using a systematic approach to bringing about change and evaluating its impact. For us the idea of systematic practice development incorporates the importance of:

- Clarifying beliefs and values about the purposes of practice development work and the processes used
- Assessment of the needs and perspectives of key stakeholders as a precursor to change
- Planning
- Action
- Evaluation of the impact of practice development activity

The extent to which the beliefs and values underpinning practice development work have been made explicit is variable. Where such beliefs and values are made explicit they are rarely subject to critique. For the most part alignment with particular values and beliefs tends to be implicit more than explicit. However, the majority of chapters in this book do indicate to some extent that value is placed on the notion of clarifying values and beliefs as a precursor to practice development activity.

The notion that practice development should be seen as a systematic activity can arouse a degree of controversy with practice developers. Garbett & McCormack (2002) found that the majority of the literature sources advocated that practice development should be systematic, while, with exceptions, practice developers themselves had reservations about the necessity and desirability of systematic approaches to their work. This in part could be attributed to the notion of what constitutes the idea of being systematic being understood in different ways. For us the idea incorporates a broad range of possible methodological approaches in which the stimulus to develop practice could be deductively or inductively derived and the design of the work could incorporate a variety of data collection techniques, managerial approaches and so on (see for example Kitson *et al.*, 1996). The defining feature is therefore concerned with attention to rigour and transparency through identifying clear audit trails rather than a particular design.

We would contend, however, that a plural view of systematic approaches that seeks to reflect the complexity of a practice setting should be able to account for serendipitous and reflexive activities.

Indeed the 'emancipatory approach to practice development' (Chapter 3) has as a primary intention, increasing participation among practitioners through their engagement in reflexive activities that contribute to an overarching systematic practice development framework. Kate Sanders demonstrates this in Chapter 13, where the importance of participation in the development of ownership is central to an emancipatory approach. We would also contend that while systematic approaches do indeed reflect the interests of those stakeholders working in management and higher education, they also reflect the interests of practitioners inasmuch as they provide an audit trail of decision-making and give rise to practical and strategic information. As such we would argue that systematic approaches are uniquely able to integrate the interests of all those with an interest in developing practice. In addition, rigorously accounting for the decisions, approaches and activities while developing practice contributes to a deeper understanding on a theoretical level, and is more likely to have political and strategic impact. By contrast more ad hoc approaches to developing practice, while intrinsically valuable if they have an effect, are less likely to have a broader or cumulative impact. Returning to the notion of improving care, having an ethical and professional imperative it seems logical to argue that demonstrating effectiveness of practice development has a similar dimension.

In summary we would argue that practice development that is systematic and rigorous in nature is more likely to fulfil the requirements of a range of stakeholders as well as contributing to the body of knowledge about the processes of developing practice that could be transferred to other settings. Whilst we would acknowledge that such approaches may under some circumstances be constraining and alienating, we would also contend that locating such work methodologically within approaches that emphasise broad involvement and participation is more likely to be personally and professionally enriching for those who are involved as well achieve greater sustainability. Moreover, the idea of a systematic and rigorous approach to developing practice fits closely with the requirements of policy initiatives within the NHS. The cultural aspects of clinical governance (Department of Health, 1998a) fit closely with the purpose and attributes of practice development activity. For example, *Clinical Governance: Quality in the New NHS* (Department of Health, 1998a) describes the need to change organisational culture in a 'systematic and demonstrable way, moving from a culture of "blame" to one of learning' (p. 5). Similarly, the Modernisation Agency (2002) promotes an approach to practice change that involves the 'Plan, Do, Study, Act (PDSA) cycle'. This model has many similarities to action research, a key evaluative approach in practice development, as described by McCormack & Manley in Chapter 5.

Practice development is continuous

The notion that practice development is concerned with transforming culture and enabling individuals suggests also that it is characterised by being a feature of a work environment rather than an intermittent and external event. We would argue that practice development is concerned less with discrete projects and more with the development of a culture characterised by a willingness and ability to question practices and respond to feedback from users, practitioners and policy changes. Indeed this assertion is reflected in the majority of chapters in Part 2 of this book. Not describing discrete projects in these chapters could be seen as a weakness. However, we would contend that this orientation to practice cultures within which specific projects are located, more accurately reflects broad cultural change focusing on increased effectiveness in patient-centred care. Such a culture enables sustainable quality to be achieved independent of the original change agent.

Facilitation

Practice development takes place against a complex and dynamic background. The pace of change within the NHS is unprecedented and the subtext of developing practice is about equipping practitioners with the necessary flexibility to respond to such an environment. The emphasis is therefore not only on changing practice but also on increasing the repertoire of skills and knowledge that the practitioner can bring to bear on their practice in the future. The accent is therefore increasingly on developing learning organisations in which practitioners are helped to identify their own learning needs. The notion of facilitation has therefore assumed increasing importance (Harvey *et al.*, 2002). We have identified a range of features associated with facilitative approaches:

- It is a form of helping relationship in which the facilitator employs skills (such as the ability to think laterally) and strategies (such as supporting and encouraging refection on practice);
- Facilitation can take place at an individual group or organisational level;
- It can occur both formally and informally;
- It involves helping practitioners identify learning needs and means of meeting those needs (which can involve helping with

access to professional development in the form of materials and/or courses);
- It is necessary for helping practitioners optimise the use of evidence in and from practice.

Titchen's (2000; 2001) critical companionship model described in Chapter 7 was founded on work on a clinical unit to develop patient-centred nursing and is now being tested in other practice development projects and through the exploration of facilitation within educational programmes such as the practice development 'summer schools' run by the RCN in conjunction with university departments and organisations such as the Foundation of Nursing Studies across the UK and beyond. Practice developers themselves describe drawing on a range of adult education and professional supervision concepts. However, further work could usefully be done to investigate the range and utility of the facilitative approaches used.

We believe that the work presented in this book helps us to identify a range of attributes required of practice developers (Box 14.1). It could be argued that such attributes do not differentiate the notion of a practice developer from a senior clinical role, such as a ward leader. We would argue that while these characteristics are common to a number of roles, practice developers might reasonably be expected to demonstrate particular aptitude in certain of the areas. For example, practice developers interviewed in Garbett & McCormack's study (2002) talked at length about the need to develop a complex network within an organisation, learning the 'language' that different stakeholders used in order to negotiate with them. To this end establishing credibility with a range of colleagues seems to be important. For practitioners, credibility seems

Box 14.1 Characteristics of a practice developer.

- Clear values and beliefs
- Commitment to improving patient care
- Enabling not telling
- Facilitative skills
- Energy and tenacity
- Flexibility, sensitivity and reflexivity
- Knowledge
- Creativity
- Political awareness
- 'Being in the middle'
- Credibility

to be associated with the ability to demonstrate clinical know-how. The value and importance of practice developers demonstrating clinical credibility through role modelling is eloquently demonstrated by Binnie & Titchen (1999) who state that: 'Her (Alison Binnie's) presence as a role model was pivotal because, through her own behaviour in the ward and her work with patients, she was able to provide a living image of a style of nursing that the staff had not seen before' (1999: 219). Practice developers also place emphasis on achieving credibility through their abilities to help practitioners identify and resolve problems.

Practice development roles can give rise to some ambiguity. The clinical leadership role of some practice developers, for example, seems to overlap with that traditionally associated with clinical leaders such as ward managers. The vital importance of clinical leadership within nursing is enjoying a renewed emphasis at present with the government's recognition of the value of Clinical Leadership programmes. New roles such as consultant nurse posts also demonstrate this commitment (Manley, 2000a, b). However, there remains a need for a systematic evaluation of how various approaches to practice development function. In particular there is a need to examine various models of practice development posts in terms of their impact.

Consequences

The consequences associated with practice development are clearly congruent with the clinical governance agenda within the NHS at the present time. Clinical governance has been established to address the need to identify the activities involved in delivering high quality care to patients (Department of Health, 1998a). Within clinical governance the need to recognise the contextual and situated nature of such a project is acknowledged. Practice development approaches explicitly address these concerns as well as others arising from local and national policy.

The primary purpose of practice development is increased effectiveness in patient-centred care. Logically it can therefore be argued that a consequence of practice development should be to reflect that purpose. It is, however, difficult to always clearly demonstrate that impact. The complexity of organisations within which practice development takes place and the interdependence of so many factors means that relating processes to outcomes can be difficult. However, we would venture that a number of consequences can be extrapolated from the purposes and attributes identified. These can be seen as concerned as much with *process outcomes* as they are with more traditional forms of *clinical outcome*. Earlier chapters in this book (Chapters 2–7) have raised a number of methodological issues for framing practice development work so that process outcomes are made an explicit part of development frameworks. Largely, these chapters are concerned with the processes of development work in order to achieve a specific outcome, i.e. increased effectiveness in patient-centred care. We have not focused on outcomes to do with particular technical aspects of practice as we believe that these are secondary to the creation of an overall culture of effective patient-centredness. Thus, many of the chapters in Part 2 of the book privilege emancipatory development processes and thus the outcomes from their work are located in this approach. So what consequences (outcomes) can be seen in the chapters of the contributors? These can be stated as:

- Development of individuals, teams and organisations enables the delivery of evidence-based, person-centred care.
- Use of frameworks that are sensitive to the needs and abilities of service users and providers enable their voices to be heard.
- Use of emancipatory learning processes can result in changes in practice thus challenging the relationship between professional and practice development.
- Effective leadership (individual, organisational and strategic) is crucial to effective practice development.
- Systematic approaches to practice development can be defined as those that are flexible to the changing landscapes of healthcare whilst remaining focused on the collective vision for practice and the provision of evidence that demonstrates those changes that have occurred.

As has been discussed, the pace and scope of change within the health service implies the need to help practitioners become more flexible and responsive in order to be able to adapt to and assimilate change. These are the intended outcomes of the approaches talked about in the practice development literature, by practice developers themselves and attested to by practitioners themselves. The outcomes arising from the contributors' chapters in this book reinforce the need for flexibility in undertaking practice development work in order to realise the potential breadth of outcomes that are possible. Adopting a facilitative approach also implies helping practitioners identify organisational factors that impede progress and helping them find ways around such barriers. Another consequence of practice development can therefore be construed as being concerned with promoting awareness of the impact of organisations on practice.

Concluding comments

In this book we have explored the concept of practice development. However, the writing of the book and the contributions of others to our understanding of practice development raise even more questions. The organisation of practice development roles (for example, at what organisational level should practice developers be positioned?) is one such issue. Little work has been undertaken to systematically evaluate the role of practice developers, their authority to affect change in practice and their sphere of accountability. Given that these are issues of primary concern to practice developers then it seems ironic that little progress has been made in clarifying these issues for practice developers themselves. The advantages and disadvantages of different approaches to practice development (for example should practice development constitute a separate role or should practice development be a component of senior clinical roles?) and their impact on services and practitioners is a further dimension of role complexity and one that requires further attention. In addition, whilst there are increasing systematic accounts of practice development activities in the literature, few studies, as yet, explore (or make explicit) the theories, values, beliefs, strategies, skills and knowledge that practice developers draw upon in this work. We would argue that, armed with a clearer idea of practice development, evaluative case studies of different models of practice development around the United Kingdom and beyond could usefully be undertaken as a means of producing clearer and more complete accounts of good practice. This in turn would lead to more consistent application of effective approaches to practice development. That journey is only just beginning.

References

Binnie, A. & Titchen, A. (1999) *Freedom to Practice: The Development of Patient-centred Nursing*. Butterworth-Heinemann, Oxford.

Clarke, C. & Procter, S. (1999) Practice development: ambiguity in research and practice. *Journal of Advanced Nursing*, **30**(4), 975–82.

Cunningham, G. & Kitson, A. (2000) An evaluation of the RCN Clinical Leadership Development programme: part 2. *Nursing Standard*, **15**(13), 34–40.

References

Cutcliffe, J.R. & Bassett, C. (1997) Introducing change in nursing: the case of research. *Journal of Nursing Management*, **5**(4), 241–7.

Department of Health (DoH) (1991) *The Patient's Charter*. HMSO, London.

Department of Health (DoH) (1998a) *Clinical Governance: Quality in the New NHS*. Department of Health, London.

Department of Health (DoH) (1998b) *The New NHS. Modern. Dependable.* HMSO, London.

Department of Health (DoH) (2001) *Essence of Care: Patient-focused Benchmarking for Healthcare Practitioners*. HMSO, London.

Draper, J. (1996) Nursing development units: an opportunity for evaluation. *Journal of Advanced Nursing*, **23**(2), 267–71.

Garbett, R. & McCormack, B. (2002) A concept analysis of practice development. *Nursing Times Research*, **7**(2), 87–100.

Harvey, G., Loftus-Hills, A., Rycroft-Malone, J., *et al.* (2002) Getting evidence into practice: the role and function of facilitation. *Journal of Advanced Nursing*, **37**(6), 577–88.

Kitson, A., Ahmed, L.B., Harvey, G., Seers, K. & Thompson, D.R. (1996) From research to practice: one organisational model for promoting research-based practice. *Journal of Advanced Nursing*, **23**(3), 430 40.

Kitson, A., Harvey, G. & McCormack, B. (1998) Enabling the implementation of evidence-based practice: a conceptual framework. *Quality in Healthcare*, **7**, 149–58.

McCormack, B., Manley, K., Kitson. A., Titchen, A. & Harvey, G. (1999) Towards practice development – a vision in reality or a reality without vision? *Journal of Nursing Management*, **7**(2), 255–64.

McMahon, A. (1998) Developing practice through research. In: *Research and Development in Clinical Nursing* (eds B. Roe & C. Webb). Whurr, London.

Manley, K. (2000a) Organisational culture and consultant outcomes. Part 1: Organisational culture. *Nursing Standard*, **14**(36), 34–8.

Manley, K. (2000b) Organisational culture and consultant nurse outcomes. Part 2: Consultant nurse outcomes. *Nursing Standard*, **14**(37), 34–9.

Modernisation Agency (2002) Managing the human dimensions of change: working with individuals. In: *Improvement Leaders' Guides, Series 2*. Modernisation Agency, NHS, Ancient House Printing Group.

Nursing and Midwifery Council (NMC) (2002) *Code of Professional Conduct*. Nursing and Midwifery Council, London.

Schön, D.A. (1983) *The Reflective Practitioner*. Temple Smith, London.

Titchen, A. (2000) *Professional Craft Knowledge in Patient-centred Nursing*. University of Oxford, DPhil thesis. Ashdale Press, Oxford.

Titchen, A. (2001) Skilled companionship in professional practice. In: *Practice Knowledge and Expertise in Health Professions* (eds J. Higgs & A. Titchen), pp. 69–79. Butterworth-Heinemann, Oxford.

Index

methods used, 230–33
outcomes/achievements, 233–9
reflections/evaluation, 237–40
staff/provider concerns, 232
user concerns, 230–31
communication issues, 189–92
culture and status, 232
see also dementia care
mentoring, 19–20
methodology
for conceptual analysis of practice
development, 34–48
identification of value systems, 34–6
for evaluation of practice development, 87–114
see also evaluation; values, beliefs and
assumptions
Modernisation Agency, 217
and 'Plan, Do, Study, Act' (PDSA) cycle, 323–4
and user involvement, 315–16
Morrell, C. *et al.*, *140*
Morris, K., 222
Morse, J.M., 11–13
motivation, 27
Muir Gray, J.A., 119
multidisciplinary initiatives, 17–18
mutuality, 157–8

National Institute for Clinical Excellence (NICE),
119
National Service Frameworks
acute mental health services, 226, 242
child health services, 217–18
for dementia care, 181
networking, 216, 224, 325–6
The NHS Plan, 51
NHS restructuring, impact on services, 210–11,
227–8, 239–40
Northern Ireland policy context, 265
Noyes, J., 222
nursing development units (NDUs), 7, 18
and action research, 24
Graham's report, 16
research on workplace culture, 55–61
see also transformational culture
nursing profession, 208–211
clinical leaders as practice development
facilitators, 62–3, 110–12
staff recruitment/retention, 60–61, 211, 226, 242

observation exercises, in dementia care, 187–9
organisational culture, 52–4, 260, 264–6, 284–5,
321
background studies and interpretations, 51–4
barriers to change, 210–11, 320–21
and decision-making, 57–9
espoused v. culture-in-practice, 55–9, 61
and evidence-based healthcare, *123*, 131–3
in specific services, 320–21
acute care mental health services, 226
child healthcare nursing, 210–11

dementia care, 177–82
family health visiting, 307–308
and technical practice development, 42, 302–305
values, beliefs and assumptions, 36–9, 54–9,
64–6, 75–6, 264–6, 308
see also transformational culture
Ouch! Sort it Out: Children's Experiences of Pain, 129
outcome indicators, 108, 237–8, 326–7
evaluation of consequences/impacts, 25–6,
29–30, 59–61, 318–19
process measures as evaluation tool, 62–3, 326–7
traditional measures, 41–2, 61, 327
Owen, J.M. & Rogers, P.J., 84–6
ownership, 233, 307–309, 312–13
of research findings, 118
Oxford Model (health promotion), 138, 305–306

PACE *see* Promoting Action on Clinical
Effectiveness programme
Page, S., 215–16
PARIHS *see* Promoting Action on Research
Implementation in Health Services
participation, 59–61, 69, 89–91, *94*
staff attendance, 214, 238, 257, 259–60, 285–6,
307–308
therapeutic v. harmonious working, 58
whole systems approach, 61, 69, 72–3
see also ownership; stakeholders; user
involvement
particularity, 159
patient involvement *see* user involvement
patient journey, and benchmarking, 261
patient stories, 206, 281–3
see also role-modelling
patient-centred care
barriers and challenges, 232–3, 274
and cultural change, 17, 57
in dementia care settings, 192–3
The Essence of Care benchmark targets, *258*
Government policy, 320
multidisciplinary v. unidisciplinary
approaches, 18
personalised approaches, 38–9
role of practice development, 16–18, 34–5, *277*,
319–20
patient-staff disassociation, 182, 192
The Patients Charter, 21
Pawson, R. & Tilley, N., 96–101
PDFs *see* practice development facilitators
peer supervision, 111, *165*, 216, 224
'Plan, Do, Study, Act' (PDSA) cycle, 323–4
political awareness, 21, 28, 325
political/policy context, 4, 17–18, 119–20, 264–5
Northern Ireland, 265
see also Government policy
portfolios, 111–12
positivism v. constructivism, 96–7
power dynamics, 73–4, 210–11, 226
children v. adult, 208
in dementia care, 182–5, 198